AF841701

THE CHRONIC PSYCHIATRIC PATIENT IN THE COMMUNITY

THE CHRONIC PSYCHIATRIC PATIENT IN THE COMMUNITY:

Principles of Treatment

Edited by

Ivan Barofsky, Ph.D.
Health Services Research
and Development Center
The Johns Hopkins Medical
Institutions

Richard D. Budson, M.D.
Director, Community Residential
Services, McLean Hospital
Department of Psychiatry
Harvard Medical School

SP

SP MEDICAL & SCIENTIFIC BOOKS
a division of Spectrum Publications, Inc.
New York

Dedicated to

Anna-Lisa
and
Jeremy

Sandy,
Andrew,
and
Vickie

Copyright © 1983 by Spectrum Publications, Inc.

All rights reserved. No part of this book may be reproduced in any form, by photostat, microform, retrieval system, or any other means without prior written permission of the copyright holder or his licensee.

SPECTRUM PUBLICATIONS, INC.
175-20 Wexford Terrace
Jamaica, NY 11432

Library of Congress Cataloging in Publication Data
Main entry under title:

The Chronic psychiatric patient in the community.

Includes index.
1. Mentally ill–Care and treatment. 2. Community mental health services. I. Barofsky, Ivan. II. Budson, Richard D. [DNLM: 1. Mental disorders–Therapy. 2. Community psychiatry. WM 30.6 C557]
RC480.53.C48 1982 362.2 82-7338
ISBN 0-89335-164-4

Printed in the United States of America

PREFACE

The purpose of this book is to present an integrated approach to the treatment of the chronic psychiatric patient living in the community. This requires that topics as diverse as pharmacokinetics, psychotherapy and community organization be appropriately coordinated. Such an approach is partly complicated by the wide range of differences among patients, in terms of social skills, intellectual capacity and psychiatric diagnosis. In addition, unclear, insular or overlapping roles of various mental health disciplines further confound integrated treatment efforts.

Given such complexity, any single clinician's point of view is subject to the distortion inherent in specialization. Too often a volume in the field of mental health focuses either on only one aspect or presents only one clinician's unique perspective of a task that is, in fact, multifaceted. We have tried to avoid this pitfall by having representatives from many of the concerned professions present a variety of treatment approaches and associated issues in one text. Further, the editors have attempted to illuminate the relevant clinical and/or administrative interrelationship between the subjects of each section through a succinct introductory commentary.

The book is divided into five sections. The first section represents an attempt to address some of the interactive sociological, psychological and pharmacological background issues common to all attempts at treatment of this population.

A detailed presentation of each of the psychosocial modalities follows, including individual and group approaches to the patient and his family as well as to his social, vocational and residential needs. The management of medication selection, side effects and drug refusal is presented next. These basic principles of treatment thus elucidated, their application is explored in selected urban and rural settings. Recognizing that comprehensive clinical care does not exist in a cultural void, but rather is intrinsically tied to current sociological realities, the volume continues with a section addressing advocacy, cost analysis and judicial issues. Finally, the editors conclude with two summarizing chapters focused on clinical principles and research tasks regarding this population.

The rationale of this volume is based upon the conviction that the patient and his particular needs must be sustained as the primary raison d'être of the entire care delivery system. It is thus incumbent upon the network of clinicians within that system to so operate as to deliver treatment which is understandable, thoughtful and comprehensive. The unacceptable alternative is fragmented services, which are likely not only to bewilder, frustrate and demean the patient, but also, in such circumstances, to be rendered ineffective. We strongly believe that each clinician within the treatment system must therefore develop effective collaboration which is predicated upon a developing knowledge of how all of the parts work together to help the individual patient. The editors hope that this volume will make some contribution to this end by providing assistance to the entire interdisciplinary array of developing and practicing mental health professionals—including psychiatrists, nurses, psychologists, social workers, vocational rehabilitation counselors and all of the allied paraprofessionals.

To what extent we have attained our ideal is unclear. We are aware that the individual authors may not have related their own specialties to the rest of the care system as much as we had hoped would be possible. The organization of the book as well as our sectional commentaries represent our effort to coordinate the overall text and thus to prevent the subject matter from being experienced by the reader as a compendium of isolated topics. The extent of the editors' effort required to unify the text is testimony to the integrative challenge to the clinician in the field.

Perhaps the most instructive lesson to be learned from the experience is the extent to which we must respect the patient's position, in his own need to understand the full nature of his condition and its treatment in his quest to be a full partner in its management.

The idea for the book can properly be said to have grown out of a meeting held in Boston, Massachusetts, entitled "The New England Conference on the Chronic Psychiatric Patient in the Community." The success of the meeting prompted the editors to invite some of the participants to prepare manuscripts on the basis of their contributions. Additional authors were solicited to ensure the comprehensiveness of the material included.

The conceptualization, format, composition and overall content of the book represent the combined but equal efforts of two health care professionals: one of them (Dr. Budson) is primarily a clinician, and the other (Dr. Barofsky) is primarily a researcher. The background of each editor insured that the contributions to the book reflected information which is clinically relevant, as well as clinical statements that can be supported by available data. The authors are listed in alphabetical order without indication of priority.

ACKNOWLEDGMENTS

The authors are grateful to their respective institutions for providing the academic environment conducive to the pursuit of a comprehensive work in this field. Additional acknowledgment is given for all of the support services provided which facilitated the completion of this volume. Specifically, Dr. Barofsky is grateful to Mr. Sam Shapiro, Director, Health Services Research and Development Center, Johns Hopkins Medical Institutions, for his support, as well as to Pearl German, Sc.D., for her thoughtful comments. Dr. Budson acknowledges Shervert H. Frazier, M.D., Psychiatrist in Chief, as well as Francis de Marneffe, M.D., General Director, McLean Hospital, for their encouragement and support of the development of community mental health programs at McLean.

Mrs. Dorothy Schwartz for Dr. Barofsky, and Ms. Pamela Healey and Mrs. Mary Lou Silverman for Dr. Budson are thanked for their secretarial assistance throughout the preparation of the manuscript.

We gratefully acknowledge the efforts of Mr. John Staffier, Senior Associate of Sandoz Pharmaceuticals, who was instrumental in expediting financial support for the meeting from which this book evolved.

The authors thank their families for their support and understanding during the months of preparation of this manuscript.

CONTENTS

III. PHARMACOLOGIC TREATMENT PRINCIPLES

IV. SELECTED APPLICATIONS OF TREATMENT PRINCIPLES

V. ADMINISTRATIVE ISSUES IN THE APPLICATION OF TREATMENT PRINCIPLES

VI. OVERVIEW

CONTRIBUTORS

Donna Conant Aguilera
University of California
at Los Angeles
Los Angeles, California

William A. Anthony
Sargent School of Allied
Health Sciences
Boston University
Boston, Massachusetts

Janet Archer
The Johns Hopkins University
School of Hygiene & Public
Health
Baltimore, Maryland

Leona L. Bachrach
University of Maryland
Baltimore County
Baltimore, Maryland

Ross J. Baldessarini
McLean Hospital
Harvard Medical School
Belmont, Massachusetts

Ivan Barofsky
The Johns Hopkins Medical
Institutions
Baltimore, Maryland

Richard D. Budson
McLean Hospital
Harvard Medical School
Belmont, Massachusetts

Jonathan O. Cole
McLean Hospital
Harvard Medical School
Belmont, Massachusetts

Catherine E. Connelly
George Mason University
Fairfax, Virginia

Marien E. Evans
Boston, Massachusetts

Samuel Grob
Dept. of Psychiatry
Tufts University School
of Medicine
Boston, Massachusetts

Ernest M. Gruenberg
The Johns Hopkins University
School of Hygiene & Public
Health
Baltimore, Maryland

Muriel Hammer
New York State Psychiatric
Institute
New York, New York

Hans R. Huessy
University of Vermont Medical
School
Burlington, Vermont

Norman C. Hursh
Sargent School of Allied
Health Sciences
Boston University
Boston, Massachusetts

Louis E. Kopolow
National Institute of Mental Health
Washington, D.C.

H. Richard Lamb
University of Southern California School of Medicine
Los Angeles, California

Julian P. Leff
Institute of Psychiatry
London, England

Jeffrey Rubin
Rutgers State University of New Jersey
New Brunswick, New Jersey

Alfred H. Stanton
McLean Hospital
Harvard Medical School
Belmont, Massachusetts

Leonard I. Stein
University of Wisconsin School of Medicine
Madison, Wisconsin

Mary Ann Test
University of Wisconsin School of Medicine
Madison, Wisconsin

Theodore Van Putten
Brentwood VA Hospital
University of California at Los Angeles
Los Angeles, California

Stephen L. Washburn
McLean Hospital
Harvard Medical School
Belmont, Massachusetts

PART I

BACKGROUND

EDITOR'S COMMENTARY: PART I

The care of the chronic psychiatric patient can truly be said to be in the midst of a revolution. Radical changes are occurring in the primary place of care, which have dictated essential changes in the nature of this care. The clinical experience and research evidence required for a consensus on the essential elements of care are now only slowly emerging. There is also increasing recognition that no one therapeutic option is without its cost and benefit, nor without its limits in effectiveness. Efforts to minimize the cost and maximize the effectiveness of therapy for the chronic psychiatric patient call for the integration of the multiple elements of a treatment program. In this way psychiatric care can take advantage of the synergic effects that result from the combination of separate elements of care. This first section of the book addresses some of the core issues in this ongoing revolution.

Bachrach discusses the meaning and definition of the term deinstitutionalization. She points out that reassignment of the site of care of the chronically disabled psychiatric patient from an institution to the community is something which is ongoing, that it is a process which itself requires programmatic efforts, but that it is also a philosophy governing the organization of care. She suggests that a systems approach is needed to insure both the optimum placement of the patient in the community and development of program objectives. Bachrach would also see the integration of the elements of therapy (e.g., pharmacotherapy, psychotherapy and social therapy) as evolving from the system providing care. This system or operations research approach is an example of an organizational approach to the integration of treatment.

Gruenberg and Archer argue that the system of care provided the patient should be organized around the nature of the dysfunction of the patient—the breakdown in the social functioning of the patient. The treatment of episodes of the social breakdown syndrome (SBS) will vary as a function of their origin (e.g., in the community, in the institution, etc.) but will be more successful if they are preventative in nature. Thus, Gruenberg and Archer would not argue for the integration of all elements of currently available treatment, as if each were equally efficacious, but instead would select and weigh the components of treatment in terms of their potential for dealing with the SBS.

The Hammer article follows naturally from the Gruenberg and Archer paper and deals with a major aspect of the SBS—the social network that makes up the structure of the patient's social relationships. Hammer argues that attending to and enhancing the social network of the patient could improve the patient's "micro-level social skills" and in this way contribute to the patient's adjustment. This article is particularly relevant to the issue of how to design the optimal social environment of the chronic psychiatric patient. As has been pointed out by Wing (1978), the chronic psychiatric patient may need a very special type of environment which neither over- nor underexposes the patient to social stimuli. A social network approach provides a model for the development and assessment of the design of such an optimal social environment.

The Barofsky and Connelly chapter represents an exploration of the complexity involved when a clinician prescribes medication to a patient. Through an in-depth analysis of the problem of medication compliance, the intricate nature of the use of psychoactive drugs is examined. Thus, the seemingly unidimensional clinical event actually embrances psychological issues such as clinician–patient alliance, systems issues such as social supports, and pharmacological issues such as chemical side effects and the attainment of desired efficacy.

The four chapters set the stage for a direct discussion of treatment options. They have sketched some of the issues that a reader must consider when dealing with the integration of treatments. The papers indicate that successful integration will require the selection and weighing of individual components of treatment for patients as organized in a system of care. The nature of some of these individual components of care is discussed in the subsequent two sections of the book.

REFERENCE

Wing, J. K. *Schizophrenia: Towards a New Synthesis.* London: Academic Press, 1978.

CHAPTER 1

CONCEPTS AND ISSUES IN DEINSTITUTIONALIZATION

LEONA L. BACHRACH, Ph.D.

INTRODUCTION

Deinstitutionalization of services for persons with chronic mental disorders is but one manifestation of a social reform momentum that for a number of postwar years prevailed in the United States. Closely related to such notions as "normalization" (Wolfensberger 1970) and "mainstreaming" (Anonymous 1977; Omang 1979; Silverman 1979), deinstitutionalization for the chronically mentally ill has counterparts in an increased emphasis on community-based services for the developmentally disabled, the physically disabled and juvenile and adult criminal offenders.

There are currently some 2,000,000 persons suffering from chronic mental disorders in the nation (Goldman, Gattozzi and Taube 1981). These individuals, who reside in a multitude of settings, require a wide variety of services related to their mental health care. And although the deinstitutionalization movement has achieved some notable successes in providing such services in various kinds of nontraditional and noninstitutional environments, it is widely acknowledged that the target population in its entirety is today less than adequately and humanely served by existing programs. When it comes to caring for chronic mental patients, service systems are typically reported to be fragmented and unresponsive, and the most seriously ill are more often than not described as "falling through the cracks" (Bachrach 1980b).

Accordingly, after a quarter of a century's experience in designing, implementing and attempting to perfect plans for community-based care of these patients, many care-givers and service planners are now questioning both the assumptions and procedures of past deinstitutionalization efforts (Bassuk and Gerson 1978; Halpern et al. 1978; Langsley 1980; Scherl and Macht 1979). The deinstitutionalization movement has, in fact, been accused of overlooking the needs of the very people it was originally intended to serve, those whose mental illnesses are most persistent and most disabling (Zusman and Lamb 1977). There is a fair degree of consensus that community mental health services tend de facto to be geared toward patients who can, for the most part and most of the time, look after themselves; and the most seriously ill are alleged to have been shortchanged in the deinstitutionalization movement.

Certain basic circumstances are today understood to strain the provision of services targeted toward this particular patient population. First, individuals suffering from chronic mental disorders are characterized by a wide range of disabilities and service needs that often endure as lifelong conditions (Bachrach and Lamb 1982). In sharp contrast to the breadth and variety of these needs, service delivery tends to be planned with a view toward pragmatic simplicity. Hansell (1978) suggests that in general community-based programs for the chronically mentally ill irrelevantly place "unwarranted emphasis on the single-episode user of services" and thus exhibit a "deficiency of interest in people with lifelong disorders."

Second, many efforts ostensibly designed as deinstitutionalization programs resist the treatment of the most severely impaired chronic mental patients and are not realistically directed toward their needs (Link and Milcarek 1980; Stern and Minkoff 1979; Task Panel 1978). Miller (1977) writes of an "inverse system of care" in which "the most trained and skilled clinicians deal with the most articulate, interesting and likely to succeed clientele," while the existence of those patients most in need is largely ignored. Halpern and associates (1978) draw the parallel that "expecting the chronically mentally ill patient to use the current mental health system is like expecting a paraplegic to use stairs. . . . The chronic long-term mentally ill person can't use the current mental health system because it's oriented toward people who have motivation, who have the capacity to develop insights, to change behaviors, to accommodate through socially acceptable behaviors" (p. 19)—characteristics not generally descriptive of persons with chronic mental impairments.

Third, the delivery of community-based services to the chronically mentally ill takes place against a backdrop of stigma that is exceedingly difficult to penetrate (Budson 1979; Johnson 1980; President's Commission 1978; Talbott 1980).

Fourth, fragmentation of services and authority in addressing the needs of the chronically mentally ill is a serious and difficult problem that reduces the quality of the care available to them (Bachrach 1976, 1979; President's Commission 1978; U.S.G.A.O. 1977). In past years most persons with chronic mental disorders were admitted to state mental hospitals where many remained—often for the rest of their lives. They comprised an essentially static population pool that changed primarily as the result of new admissions and deaths. Providing care was relatively simple: virtually all services could be delivered within a single physical setting. Today, by contrast, authority for providing for the needs of chronic mental patients is divided among numerous mental health and human service agencies in the public and private sectors. Successful deinstitutionalization programs require the fine tuning of initiatives that originate with separate, sometimes competing, authorities—a process far more complicated than what was suggested in John F. Kennedy's utopian "bold new approach" to mental health service provision (1963).

Fifth, deinstitutionalization programs are designed and implemented within a context of semantic confusion that both reflects and sustains service delivery problems (Bachrach 1980a, 1981; Carpenter 1978; Moos and Igra 1980; Peele and Keisling 1980). A potent barrier to effective care, conceptual vagueness results from, and underscores, a general failure to assess adequately the complexities that attend deinstitutionalization. The semantic context of deinstitutionalization is discussed in greater detail below.

If increased sensitivity to the problems associated with deinstitutionalization has not altogether generated definitive solutions, it has at least increased our ability to ask some appropriate questions—a necessary step in program planning (Bachrach and Lamb 1982). Indeed, a number of mental health program and statewide mental health system authorities have recently begun to review policies that were initiated when the deinstitutionalization movement was young and that have apparently, over the years, generated unanticipated problems complicating the delivery of services to the target population of chronic mental patients (Cannon and Kotkin 1979; Christensen 1980; Cramer 1978; Salzman 1975; Scherl and Macht 1979).

This chapter reviews the meaning and the background of deinstitutionalization, examines some of the problems that are associated with the movement and discusses effective confrontation of these problems.

THE SEMANTICS OF CARE FOR CHRONIC MENTAL PATIENTS

As a sociologist, I usually make the assumption that most culture traits exist for a purpose: that they do not occur by chance. This holds for words, as well as for other items of culture. The use of language has social functions that extend beyond mere denotation and description. The words that we use, and the ways in which we use them, reflect our ideology, our beliefs and our social status. Words determine what questions we ask—and, coincidentally, what questions we fail to ask. Even imprecision in language, though not necessarily intended, may itself have certain functions. Imprecision can be used in an effort to protect vested interests. Or it can cover up inaction. Or it can perpetuate the status quo.

Concepts like "least restrictive setting" and "continuity of care," which are central to the notion of deinstitutionalization, are generally inadequately defined in the mental health literature (Bachrach 1980a, 1981). These concepts, which are intended to serve as aids in deinstitutionalization planning, are too vague and too unrefined to fulfill that function. In order for a concept to be useful as a planning device, it must be precisely defined, and its empirical referents must be clearly designated; but these conditions are not met with the concepts of continuity of care and restrictiveness.

Nor are these terms unique in their vagueness in the area of deinstitutionalization planning. The word "community," which is implicitly or explicitly inherent in every definition of deinstitutionalization, provides another example. Panzetta (1971) writes that this term "can be applied in a variety of situations and so is versatile as a one-word concept." But at the same time, Panzetta cautions, this term is "prone to multiple connotative meanings and so can be easily misunderstood."

In fact, the word "community" has come to be used so loosely in deinstitutionalization planning that it has lost its original meaning and become synonymous with "noninstitution." The semanticist Hayakawa (1972) reminds us that "fine-sounding speeches, long words, and the general *air* of saying something are effective in result, regardless of what is being said" (p. 103). Because the word "community" *sounds* right, many persons have, by some faulty logic, confused the word with the quality of *gemeinschaft*, which refers to community of spirit. But merely calling something a "community-based" facility does not automatically invest it with *gemeinschaft*. In reality, chronic mental patients in the "community" are to be found in a wide variety of environments, including independent residences, family homes, halfway houses, apartment hotels, foster homes and board and care facilities. Each of these residential categories is highly variable in degree of restrictiveness, and there may be as much (or more) variation *within* these categories as *among* them (Bachrach 1980a). Indiscriminate use of the term "community" to refer to any place that is not a state hospital has greatly reduced the utility of that concept.

Another example of semantic confusion is provided by the concept of chronicity. Peele and Palmer (1980) identify six different criteria that have been used to judge mental patients' chronicity: deficit in function and/or responsiveness to treatment, dependent life style, diagnosis, time spent in institutions, legal eligibility for entitlements and indefinite need for supportive services. Yet discussions of "chronic mental patients" in the literature have only very recently, after several decades of deinstitutionalization experience, begun to identify which of these, or possibly which other dimensions (Minkoff 1978; Robins 1978; Task Panel 1978), are being used to establish chronicity in a specific instance. One recent outstanding effort to identify and quantify chronic mental illness in the United States is provided by Goldman, Gattozzi and Taube (1981).

Finally, the very word "deinstitutionalization" is itself surrounded by uncertainty and a basic absence of consensus. At times, persons associated with the care of chronic mental patients have become quite impatient with that word and have expressed a wish to do away with it—as if getting rid of the word will somehow also eliminate the problems that it implies. It must be remembered, however, that this word, while perhaps cumbersome, is really neutral. Although it suggests the breakdown of traditional (or "institutional," in the sociological sense) ways of dealing with the problems of the mentally ill, it carries no value judgments as to whether these techniques are good, bad, adequate or indifferent; it merely indicates social *change*. It is up to planners, service providers and researchers to evaluate that change.

The concept of deinstitutionalization, in fact, tends to be perceived disparately by the various persons concerned with it. It may, for example, have quite different connotations for the hospital-based psychiatrist, the community-based nurse making a home visit and the program evaluator attempting to make sense of difficult-to-trace patient movements. It is doubtless variously understood by the many patients it affects—those who have been hospitalized for several decades and whose future continues to be linked to institutional care;

those who are about to be released to the "community" after varying periods of residence within the state hospital; and those whose admission or readmission to a state hospital is effectively barred by admission diversion policies (Sullivan 1979a, 1979b).

TOWARD AN UNDERSTANDING OF DEINSTITUTIONALIZATION

I should like to suggest a working definition of deinstitutionalization that allows for these discrepant points of view. Deinstitutionalization may be defined as *a process involving two elements: the eschewal, shunning or avoidance of traditional institutional settings, particularly state hospitals, for the care of the chronically mentally ill; and the concurrent expansion of noninstitutional facilities for the care of this population.* For purposes of this chapter, chronicity is defined loosely to include all persons who are, have been, or might have been but for the deinstitutionalization movement, on the rolls of long-term mental institutions, especially state hospitals. This conceptualization of chronicity, while lacking operational precision, nevertheless captures the dynamics of population reassignment that characterize the deinstitutionalization movement.

The important point in the definition of deinstitutionalization proposed here is that it is a mistake to view deinstitutionalization unidimensionally, as if it refers exclusively to patients leaving state hospitals. We shall presently see that it is a much broader event, which affects even people who have never been hospitalized.

The sense of this definition of deinstitutionalization is conveyed in a statement by the medical director of a children's hospice in New York City: "'A hospice is not a place, but rather a concept'" (Teltsch 1980). It is also captured by North Carolina's Governor James Hunt who defines deinstitutionalization as "'the most appropriate care for the mentally ill in the most appropriate setting'" (Anonymous 1980). Governor Hunt is, incidentally, a pioneer in the effort to establish a statewide mental health plan that specifically assigns high priority to the needs of the chronically mentally ill in service planning (Governor's Task Force 1980).

Implicit in this conceptualization of deinstitutionalization is the notion that sociological as well as physical phenomena are involved. Physically, deinstitutionalization refers to the creation of new environments for the chronically mentally ill. It is a geographical event that is reflected in the rapid and continuing depopulation of large state hospital facilities and the equally rapid expansion of community-based services and facilities. Sociologically, the concept of deinstitutionalization implies widespread and basic adjustments in traditional patterns of care for this basically dependent and persistently disabled population.

ASPECTS OF DEINSTITUTIONALIZATION

There are at least three separate but closely interrelated aspects of deinstitutionalization. Deinstitutionalization is a process. It is also a philosophy. And it is also a fact.

Deinstitutionalization Is a Process

More than the simple depopulation of large public facilities, deinstitutionalization may be understood as *a dynamic and continuing series of adjustments involving constant accommodation of all the components of the mental health service system*. Because of the dynamic nature of deinstitutionalization, the chronically mentally ill are today found in a wide variety of demographic settings, and at least five separate population subgroups can be identified—two in the hospital and three in the community.

A first subgroup within the target population consists of *hospital dischargees*, and it is very difficult to deliver adequate services to two somewhat diametrically opposed subsets of this subgroup—those patients who are highly visible as they go again and again through the revolving doors of the service delivery system, and those who become virtually invisible (i.e., "fall through the cracks") as they exit from the doors of institutions and become, for all intents and purposes, lost to the service delivery system.

Although patients discharged from mental hospitals are most often associated with the term "deinstitutionalization," they in fact make up only a portion of the target population and are by no means the only chronically ill persons affected by the movement. A second subgroup within the target population consists of *never hospitalized individuals* who probably would have been institutionalized several decades ago, and who, as the direct result of deinstitutionalization policies and practices, represent an ever increasing percentage of the target population. A 1977 study of chronically mentally ill persons living in San Mateo County, California, for example, establishes that two in five (39%) have never been hospitalized (Lamb and Goertzel 1977). Pepper and associates (1980) report that 79% of patients served in Rockland County, New York, outpatient mental health clinics have never been hospitalized, and a large, though unspecified, portion of these patients suffer from chronic mental disorders. The medical, psychiatric and social service needs of these individuals are very different from those of the ever-hospitalized.

Deinstitutionalization has also affected patterns of care for a variety of patients who, despite deinstitutionalization efforts, continue to utilize state hospitals (Shore and Shapiro 1979). Thus, a third subgroup of the chronically mentally ill consists of *old long-stay patients*—veteran residents of state hospitals who were admitted long ago and have remained in the hospital despite deinstitutionalization efforts. Estimates from the National Institute of Mental Health (NIMH) indicate that in recent years 59% of all state hospital residents have lived in those institutions for five years or longer (Division of Biometry unpublished data).

The hospital also contains a fourth subgroup of the chronically mentally ill, *short-stay patients* who will soon be released to the community. According to NIMH estimates, nearly one quarter of all admissions to state mental hospitals are released within a week of admission, and nearly 40% are released within 14 days of entering the hospital (Division of Biometry unpublished data).

Finally, the hospital also contains a fifth subgroup of the chronically mentally ill—*new long-stay patients*, who represent a buildup of long-term residents from among recent admissions that are unlikely to be considered good risks for community care and probably will not be discharged. Smith and Hart (1975) estimate that 2% to 5% of new admissions to state hospitals in Illinois will "remain too disturbed ever to be discharged from the hospital."

A study conducted by Dorwart (1980) at a state hospital in Massachusetts confirms that the residue of patients treated in state hospitals today tend to have distinctive clinical and management needs that have been "accentuated by deinstitutionalization." These patients tend to exhibit acute psychotic symptoms, to be dangerous to themselves or others, to require intensive care and to lack social skills. It is certainly likely that the continuing diversion of resources toward the expansion and improvement of community-based services may work to the detriment of those patients whose special needs require the financing of well-organized, well-staffed in-hospital programs (Ashbaugh and Bradley 1979).

The boundaries of these five subgroups of the chronically mentally ill population are fluid in varying degrees, and the revolving door phenomenon may be understood conceptually as their ongoing realignment.

We see, then, that deinstitutionalization is a complex, multifaceted process that continues to alter patterns of patient care. Although current planning initiatives frequently tend to stress "aftercare," programming for deinstitutionalization should ideally accommodate all five of these patient subgroups, not only discharged hospital patients. Because each subgroup represents, in its own way, fallout from the deinstitutionalization movement, individuals in all of them must be regarded as legitimate beneficiaries of planning efforts that are intended to improve patient care in this era of deinstitutionalization. At a time when financial constraints make it necessary to be as parsimonious as possible, we are thus faced with the task of arranging a multitude of services for a variety of patient groupings in numerous settings. And in reality, our planning efforts have been spread so thin that on a nationwide basis none of these subgroups appears to be receiving adequate coverage in planning efforts.

Deinstitutionalization Is a Philosophy

When we view deinstitutionalization as a process, we can begin to understand something of its intellectual foundation, or the philosophy that underlies it. The philosophy of deinstitutionalization proceeds from at least three fundamental—and largely untested—assumptions concerning community mental health care. First, there is an assumption that community mental health is a good thing—*that community-based care is preferable to institutional care for most, if not all, mental patients.* A second underlying assumption is *that communities not only can, but also are willing to, assume responsibility and leadership in the care of the most seriously ill.* And a third assumption regarding deinstitutionalization is *that the functions performed by mental hospitals can be equally well, if not better, performed by community-based facilities.* It is believed, in other words, that the community is capable of providing the same range of services that is available inside the hospital.

These three assumptions, taken together, lead to an understanding of the *goal* of deinstitutionalization. Deinstitutionalization has assumed no less a task than that of "humanizing" mental health care—

of reversing the dehumanizing influences that are widely understood as accompaniments of institutional residence. In this sense, deinstitutionalization shares a great deal with other social efforts to enhance the lives of individuals. The deinstitutionalization movement was, and continues to be, the product of many forces. The development of antipsychotic drugs provided a technological base that was necessary for the active pursuit of deinstitutionalization. But the availability of these drugs provides only a partial explanation.

Deinstitutionalization was, in fact, all tied up with a social reform ideology that characterized postwar human services planning and reached a peak in the 1960s. At that time, a generalized philosophy of social reform stressing society's responsibility to help the individual and placing strong emphasis on civil rights prevailed. In other times in our history, we have pursued social progress by trying to change the individual, not society. But in that era of social reform, modification of the environment was emphasized as the primary avenue to social betterment (Hersch 1972).

In its broadest sense, then, deinstitutionalization may be understood as a protest movement. Like other civil rights protests, it is ideologically committed to improving the lot of persons who are seen as helpless in gaining access to life's entitlements. It is a movement dedicated to the dignity of the individual, and as such it emphasizes the rights of dependent individuals and their legitimate claims on society.

But it is important to note that ironically deinstitutionalization also owes much of its popularity to its appeal to more conservative forces. Acceptance of the progressive philosophy of deinstitutionalization has been facilitated by its attractiveness to persons who are more interested in fiscal reform than social reform—a situation making for strange bedfellows among the movement's proponents. When the movement began, deinstitutionalization was, and continues to be, widely believed to be cheaper than institutional care. At least in the early phases of a movement the accuracy of this kind of belief is much less important than its prevalence, even though disillusionment may eventually settle in. The fact that people *do* believe in the money-saving powers of deinstitutionalization is one of the factors that has made the movement acceptable to many who might otherwise have opposed it.

In addition to the presumption of cost-savings in community-based care, there has also been a desire on the part of state legislatures to reduce their own budgets by shifting the cost and responsibility of of the formerly institutionalized to a different level of government (Cramer 1978). With the closing of large institutions, many disabled persons have relied on federal public assistance funds for support. It is not difficult for states to justify reduced fiscal responsibility in the light of what is regarded so widely within the helping professions as a more humane system of care.

In short, the fact that the philosophy of deinstitutionalization has been allied with a coalition of opposing or contradictory political streams has accounted in large part for the rapid spread of the movement. Progressive reformers and fiscal conservatives alike have found something to support in the deinstitutionalization movement. Recent developments on the American economic scene have, however, generated suspicion that the wedding of these different views is coming to an end and that the ideological commitment to deinstitutionalization is being diluted. Although support is still widespread, the philosophical basis for deinstitutionalization is fragile because it is subject to the fickleness of political winds, particularly in times of inflationary stress. Thus, for example, an article in the Washington *Post* states that, "The explosive growth of government social welfare programs that has dominated domestic politics for the past quarter-century has come to an end," and it quotes the Dean of Columbia University's School of Social Work as predicting that this represents the " 'end of an era' " in social programming (Rich 1979).

Some of this ideological shift has to do with the fact that the fiscal superiority of deinstitutionalization has never been firmly established (Cramer 1978; Talbott 1980). It is now generally agreed that providing high-quality care for the chronically mentally ill is not cheap, no matter how the locus of care is shifted. Deinstitutionalization has not proved to be the overall money-saving solution that had been anticipated. Not only is the cost of community-based care high, but beyond a certain point in resident population reduction the per capita costs of running an institution must, obviously, increase. The savings that were supposed to accompany the depopulation of institutions simply have not materialized on a nationwide basis. To illustrate this point, suit was recently filed by two patients and the Mental Health Association of California against Governor Edmund Brown. The plaintiffs pointed out the high economic costs of community care and claimed that the state's increase of $25 million over the previous year's budget for this purpose was " 'woefully inadequate' " and " 'barely keeps up with inflation' " (Kotkin 1979).

Deinstitutionalization Is a Fact

In addition to its being a process and a philosophy, deinstitutionalization is also a fact with measurable dimensions. That it really is occurring is reflected in nationwide statistics concerning the depopulation of large institutions. For the mentally ill there has been a marked decrease in the resident population of the nation's state hospitals. That population peaked in 1955 at 558,992. Ten years later it stood at 475,202, and 20 years later at 193,436. Thus, the resident population of these facilities showed a decrease of 15% over one decade and a striking decrease of 65% over two decades (Division of Biometry 1979). The most recent NIMH statistic for the resident population of state mental hospitals indicates that at the beginning of 1977, 170,619 individuals lived in these facilities (Witkin 1979).

Other data provide additional reinforcement for the fact of deinstitutionalization. In 1955 about half of all psychiatric patient-care episodes occurred in state mental hospitals; in 1977 the corresponding figure was only about 9%. By contrast, in 1955 outpatient services accounted for only 23% of all patient-care episodes, but in 1977, more than seven out of ten patient-care episodes took place in outpatient settings. In 1977 federally funded community mental health centers, which did not even exist prior to the passage of the Community Mental Health Centers Act of 1963, provided the locus for 27% of all patient-care episodes (Witkin 1980).

UNDERSTANDING THE PROBLEMS OF DEINSTITUTIONALIZATION

The perspective that deinstitutionalization is a process and a philosophy as well as a fact permits a better understanding of the problems that are associated with the movement. Were deinstitutionalization merely concerned with the exchange of settings for patient care, many of the problems known to exist would not have arisen. The community would simply have replaced the hospital as the locus of care, and resultant problems would have been of a logistical nature, easily negotiated and resolved.

The fact is, however, that deinstitutionalization has, since its inception, encountered obstacles every step of the way. Fiscal disappointments are only one reality. There are many other issues associated with deinstitutionalization, and experience of the past two decades reveals that these problems are sometimes very difficult to resolve. A taxonomy of the issues associated with deinstitutionalization, which have been addressed extensively in the literature (Bachrach 1976), is presented in Table 1.

Table 1. A Taxonomy of Issues in Deinstitutionalization*

I. Issues related to the selection of patients for community care.
   A. Chronically ill patients
   B. Patients inadequately prepared for life in the community
   C. Disadvantaged and minority groups
II. Issues related to the treatment course of patients in the community
   A. Inadequate range of treatment services
   B. Fragmentation and lack of coordination in treatment services
   C. Inaccessibility of treatment services
   D. Questionable quality of care in community services
III. Issues related to the quality of life of patients in the community
   A. Inadequate community support systems
   B. Residential facilities and living arrangements
IV. Issues related to the greater community
   A. Community resistance and opposition to mentally ill individuals
   B. Effects on communities to which patients are released
   C. Ecological impact on hospital staff
   D. Ecological impact on hospital community
   E. Effects on patient's family
V. Issues related to manpower
   A. Training and retraining of staff for community work
   B. Maldistribution of personnel
   C. Role-blurring
   D. Attitudes of staff toward working with chronically mentally ill
VI. Financial and fiscal issues
VII. Legal and quasilegal issues
VIII. Informational issues and accountability
   A. Necessity for evaluation studies
   B. Difficulties in locating and following patients in the community
   C. Inadequacy of existing followup studies
IX. Additional issues resulting directly from process of deinstitutionalization
   A. Timing: precipitate implementation of new programs
   B. Inadequate attention to patients' desires
   C. Problems related to providing adequate services in hospitals during phase-out
   D. Failure to establish liaison between hospitals and community-based facilities
   E. Disenchantment with the deinstitutionalization movement: resistance to further change

*Adapted from Leona L. Bachrach, *Deinstitutionalization: An Analytical Review and Sociological Perspective*. Rockville, Md.: National Institute of Mental Health, 1976.

Clearly, it is time to reassess the deinstitutionalization movement, and one approach to doing so is through a sociological analysis of these issues. As noted above, one of the philosophical assumptions underlying the deinstitutionalization movement is the premise that the functions performed by traditional institutions can be performed equally well, if not better, by community-based facilities. What, exactly, are these functions? A review of the literature suggests that the array of functions performed by institutions for the mentally ill is surprisingly complex and is far more extensive than might at first glance be supposed (Bachrach 1976). An attempt to isolate the functions of mental hospitals as identified in the literature yields a list of 21 separate items as shown in Table 2. This listing includes only those functions explicitly stated in the literature. Were it to be expanded by including additional functions that are implicit, it would doubtless be even longer.

Some of the functions listed in Table 2 apply exclusively to patients and some to other elements of society. It is safe to say that some of these functions were not originally intended but have evolved as the system of institutional care in the nation has grown. The listing includes the widely acknowledged functions of providing long-term treatment for chronically disturbed individuals. It also includes the functions of asylum and custody that are frequently understood as important aspects of institutional care. But the listing goes further than this by also including a series of additional functions that are less readily perceived or acknowledged—such as rendering relief to the patient's family, or providing a kind of hiding place outside the community for some of its less attractive members, or providing an economic base for the hospital community.

An important observation emerges when the listing of functions in Table 2 is compared with the issues in deinstitutionalization presented in Table 1. The issues fall into two major groups vis-à-vis mental hospital functions. Either: (a) the issue has at least one referent among the functions listed, or (b) the issue has come into being as an unanticipated consequence of the deinstitutionalization movement itself. Thus, for example, Issue IV-E in Table 1, "effects on patient's family," has the functional referent of "relieving the patient's family from disruptive social interaction." And Issue III-B, "residential facilities and living arrangements," has the functional referent of "providing a residential environment for the mentally ill."

It is clear that efforts to reduce the stature of mental hospitals, or to eliminate them, have too often overlooked or neglected to stress the necessity for alternatives to the full range of functions listed. Not

Table 2. Functions of Mental Hospitals*

Providing long-term treatment for chronically disturbed individuals
Providing crisis intervention for patients undergoing acute stress
Providing respite for the patient from mounting pressures
Removing the patient from his usual environment and from whatever pathological influences that environment may have
Protecting the patient from exploitation by others
Providing a residential environment for the mentally ill
Providing constant and continuous monitoring and review of the patient's course of illness
Providing a social structure within which the role of the mentally disturbed individual is clearly defined
Providing the mentally ill individual with an alternative to due process of law
Providing the patient with a place to which he may escape from the greater society
Providing a means by which society can segregate some of its deviants
Relieving the patient's family and community from disruptive social interaction
Protecting society from the acts of dangerous individuals
Supplying an ostensibly relatively inexpensive form of patient care
Providing an economic base and employment for a community or a portion of a community
Providing job security and other job perquisites for numbers of employed persons
Providing a tax base for local communities
Providing for mental health professionals a funnel for the removal of unattractive and often poor patients
Diverting attention from the need for local planning and expenditures by creating an illusion that the mentally ill are being adequately treated elsewhere
Providing a place for research on mental illness
Providing a place for the training of mental health professionals

*Adapted from Leona L. Bachrach, *Deinstitutionalization: An Analytical Review and Sociological Perspective*. Rockville, Md.: National Institute of Mental Health, 1976.

even the central functions of treatment and asylum have been assured for deinstitutionalized individuals, not to mention the various other functions that have an impact on other elements of society. It is inevitable that any movement that so ignores the institutional makeup of society will encounter severe opposition. And it has.

It is also apparent that the zeal and dedication that have motivated deinstitutionalization have left in their wake a series of dysfunctional elements resulting directly from rapid, sometimes heedless implementation of incomplete program plans. A variety of serious problems have arisen as the result of efforts to implement the deinstitutionalization philosophy. In their zeal to move quickly on behalf of the chronically mentally ill, service planners have frequently confused geography with program substance. Although a number of successful community-based efforts on behalf of the chronically mentally ill have indeed been developed, these tend to be small and quite localized and do not meet the global needs of widespread deinstitutionalization.

Generally speaking, deinstitutionalization planning has not been conducive to clients' continuity of care (Bachrach 1981). It has too often taken place precipitately, without the prior development of necessary community-based facilities, particularly for those patients who are most severely handicapped. Planning has thus too often occurred in a functional vacuum. It has certainly failed to address adequately the needs of all five patient subgroups described above. In short, the philosophy, the process and the fact of deinstitutionalization have tended to be disjunctive.

CONFRONTING THE PROBLEMS OF DEINSTITUTIONALIZATION

Recent literature indicates an increasing awareness of the complexities of deinstitutionalization planning. Recognition of the full range of functions associated with institutions is becoming more prevalent, and this recognition is often accompanied by pleas for more realistic and more sensitive planning so that whole groups of people are not automatically excluded from program initiatives.

In the early years of social policy formulation in deinstitutionalization, the needs for developing "model programs" for the care of chronic mental patients was stressed. Mental health planners sought to develop such programs so that their essentials might be reproduced in other settings. It is being increasingly recognized today, however, that although model programs have valuable research potential, their diffusibility is quite limited for a variety of sociological and economic reasons. There are serious problems connected with transporting model programs to other settings. Moreover, because these programs tend to be limited in concept and highly selective in their target populations, they cannot provide solutions to the complex problems that affect mental health service delivery systems (Bachrach 1980b).

Although some planners and planning agencies continue to stress the development of model programs as solutions to the problems of deinstitutionalization, the discrepancies between successful isolated model endeavors and mental health service system "failures" are becoming more apparent. As a consequence, the need for new planning strategies is being increasingly recognized. To this end a number of analysts are calling for the application of systems theory in the development of mental health services (Bachrach 1982; Bradley 1978; Holder 1977; Johnson 1980; Marmor 1975; Moran 1980; Stratas and Boyd 1981). According to Miser (1980), systems theory asks questions that involve the critical examination of the social purposes of an intervention, that explore alternative ways of achieving goals and that estimate the "impacts of various courses of action."

The literature is now just beginning to explore some systems issues that must be resolved if deinstitutionalization efforts are to meet with success and chronic mental patients are to be cared for humanely in noninstitutional settings. One recent conceptualization by Johnson (1980) defines the systems context of mental health facilities in terms of four environments: (1) the *core-level environment* of the facility itself, with its distinctive charter and mandates; (2) the *specific environment*, including the agencies, associations and individuals interacting with the core-level facility—such as patients' families, hospitals and other health and human service delivery agencies; (3) the *supportive environment*, including government agencies, educational institutions and professional associations that provide finances, staffing and legitimation to the facility; and (4) the *general environment*—i.e., the "broad context" or sociological framework within which the facility operates. Aspects of the general environment include demographic and economic circumstances, political conditions, legal mandates and constraints, specific technologies for treatment intervention and such attitudinal considerations as the extent to which the community is "committed to caring for its impaired or impoverished members, or the extent of toleration of deviant behavior" (p. 74). Since the problems accompanying deinstitutionalization may be generated in any of these environments, solutions must take all of them into consideration.

Application of systems theory in deinstitutionalization planning permits the analysis and confrontation of problems that are essentially overlooked by more molecular planning approaches. One such problem concerns the setting of priorities in mental health systems. In order for chronic mental patients to be provided with adequate care, they must be assigned top priority in the service system (Bachrach 1980b). There is evidence that in the history of the deinstitutionalization movement, the requirements of the most seriously ill have been subordinated to those of patients who are essentially "healthy but unhappy" (Zusman and Lamb 1977). When the most seriously impaired patients, with their peculiar combination of service requirements, chronicity and impotence, have had to compete for scarce resources with others who are less severely impaired and more socially acceptable, the chronically ill have not fared well. A systems approach to deinstitutionalization has the potential for recognizing, and hence correcting, service inequities.

A systems approach also is necessary for addressing the placement needs of patients with chronic mental illnesses, particularly those for whom there appears to be no ready niche in a community-oriented system of care. This is an issue that has recently begun to surface in the literature, and it concerns patients whose needs are somehow anachronistic in, or at least out of tune with, current service delivery modes.

There are probably several varieties of these patients who "do not fit." Frequently they are people whom Neill (1979) describes as "black-listed 'difficult' patients . . . whose presence engenders strong negative feelings" among treatment staff. Bean and associates (1979) refer to them more generally as "system misfits." An article in the Washington *Post* describes increasing numbers of "deinstitutionalized people" living in suburban motels (Mansfield 1980). Bassuk and Gerson (1980), who have encountered patients who appear not to fit into the system in the psychiatric emergency ward of an urban general hospital, describe them as individuals "who, despite persisttent efforts to engage in an ongoing treatment process, keep returning to the emergency ward" where they constitute a familiar revolving-door population. Lamb (1980) refers to those emergency ward regulars as "psychiatric hoboes."

Closely related to, or part of, the problem of patients who do not fit in the service system are two other placement problems. One concerns patients whose preference and/or need for either long- or short-term hospitalization is not accommodated (Colen 1977; Rosenblatt and Mayer 1974; Simon 1965; Smith and Smith 1978; Spiegel and Keith-Spiegel 1969). Subtle clues to the dimensions of this particular problem are provided in two studies of the reasons that former patients visit those wards in general hospitals where they were once hospitalized. Kramer and Rubinson (1978) write that visits by former patients frequently reflect either "meaningful relationships with staff members and other patients" or "continuing treatment needs of various kinds." Similarly, Gruber, Brown and Mazarol (1978) write that visits by these patients represent a "response to real but unarticulated needs that are not being met by the mental health system" and that "while hospital readmission is commonly thought to indicate failure, it may be better to look on the brief hospital admission as an episode of temporarily increased dependency in the course of a long-continuing disability."

A second related problem involves the inappropriate placement of patients in the criminal justice system. Although Steadman and Ribner's (1980) study of criminal offenders in New York State concludes that deinstitutionalization practices and revisions in mental health commitment codes probably have not altered the composition of prison populations appreciably, Stelovich's (1980) study in Massachusetts concludes that there is a "population of deinstitutionalization patients, who, lost to follow-up [drift] into the legal system and [land] in prison." Whitmer's (1980) observations in California concur with the latter view. In any case, a number of writers (Anonymous 1979; Kaufman 1980; Kihss 1980; Modlin 1979; Nunes 1980; U.S.G.A.O. 1979) appear to agree that psychiatric services in prisons are generally less than optimal, and the implication is clear that at least some of the more seriously psychiatrically ill inmates would profit from more appropriate placement in service settings where levels of psychiatric care are more consistent with their needs.

Robbins and associates (1978) assert that the number of patients who lack a place in the mental health system appears to be increasing as the result of deinstitutionalization practices. To the extent that this observation is accurate, the provision of services to patients who represent placement difficulties is a systems problem of the first order.

Writing in a systems frame of reference, Bradley (1976) shows that deinstitutionalization involves both program development objectives, such as establishing a system of community-based care, and program termination objectives, such as phasing out institutional care. The two objectives need not necessarily be effected simultaneously, and it is possible to vary the speed and completeness with which each is implemented. But because strong partisan views have prevailed, and because economic resources are scarce, these two potentially separable processes have become linked, and scholars like historian David Rothman are quoted as saying that " 'there is good reason to believe that deinstitutionalization and state mental hospitals cannot coexist' " (Sargent 1980). The implication is clear that disengagement from institutional care must be total and immediate if deinstitutionalization efforts are to meet with success.

Systems theory would permit the theoretical and practical separation of these two policy objectives, so that priorities could be set and intermediate goals could be effected. In fact, Bradley (1978) provides a most insightful discussion of the steps that must be followed in making critical choices in the formulation of public policy. "Since all ends and needs are not equal or equally met," she writes, "these choices must be among competing priorities and should be closely tied to political and fiscal exigencies. . . . [A plan for effecting changes in policy] when viewed in this light forms the impetus for change and bridges the gap between ideology and implementation" (p. 52).

In summary, deinstitutionalization planning involves the formulation of complex public policy decisions and implementation strategies. There is now a need to translate our technology, which is substantial, into systems-related action. It will take fundamental changes in attitudes and in funding practices to shift from the habit of looking at deinstitutionalization mechanistically toward a more molar approach. But this objective must be realized if the global needs of the chronically mentally ill are to be met, and if the serious problems that are now, unfortunately, so widely identified with the deinstitutionalization movement are to be eliminated.

REFERENCES

Anonymous. Mainstreaming. *Currents* 2, 9–14 (1977).

Anonymous. Prisoners seen needing better mental treatment. Washington *Post*, August 15, 1979.

Anonymous. An imperfect reform. Raleigh (N.C.) *News and Observer*, September 24, 1980.

Ashbaugh, J. W., and Bradley, V. J. Linking deinstitutionalization of patients with hospital phase-down: The difference between success and failure. *Hospital and Community Psychiatry* 30: 105–110 (1979).

Bachrach, L. L. *Deinstitutionalization: An Analytical Review and Sociological Perspective*. Rockville, Md.: National Institute of Mental Health, 1976.

Bachrach, L. L. Planning mental health services for chronic patients. *Hospital and Community Psychiatry* 30: 387–393 (1979).

Bachrach, L. L. Is the least restrictive environment always the best? Sociological and semantic implications. *Hospital and Community Psychiatry* 31: 97–102 (1980a).

Bachrach, L. L. Overview: Model programs for chronic mental patients. *American Journal of Psychiatry* 137: 1023–1031 (1980b).

Bachrach, L. L. Continuity of care for chronic mental patients: A conceptual analysis. *American Journal of Psychiatry* 138: 1449–1456 (1981).

Bachrach, L. L. Assessment of outcomes in community support systems: Results, problems and limitations. *Schizophrenia Bulletin* 8: 39–61 (1982).

Bachrach, L. L., and Lamb, H. R. Conceptual issues in the evaluation of deinstitutionalization, in *Innovative Approaches to Mental Health Evaluation*, W. Tash and G. Stahler, eds. New York: Academic Press 139-161 (1982).

Bassuk, E. L., and Gerson, S. Deinstitutionalization and mental health services. *Scientific American* 238: 46-53 (1978).

Bassuk, E. L., and Gerson, S. Chronic crisis patients: A discrete clinical group. *American Journal of Psychiatry* 137: 1513-1517 (1980).

Bean, J. F., Makowiecki, M. M., and Yessian, M. R. *A Service Delivery Assessment on Community Mental Health Centers: Executive Report.* Rockville, Md.: National Institute of Mental Health, 1979.

Bradley, V. J. Policy termination in mental health: The hidden agenda. *Policy Sciences* 7: 215-224 (1976).

Bradley, V. J. *Deinstitutionalization of Developmentally Disabled Persons: A Conceptual Analysis and Guide.* Baltimore: University Park Press, 1978.

Budson, R. D. Sheltered housing for the mentally ill: An overview. *McLean Hospital Journal* 4: 140-157 (1979).

Cannon, L., and Kotkin, J. Crisis grows in California mental hospitals. Washington *Post*, April 16, 1979.

Carpenter, M. D. Residential placement for the chronic psychiatric patient: A review and evaluation of the literature. *Schizophrenia Bulletin* 4: 384-397 (1978).

Christensen, R. Many states reviewing deinstitutionalization. Raleigh (N.C.) *News and Observer*, September 21, 1980.

Colen, B. D. Some outpatients come "home" to St. Elizabeths for Christmas holiday. Washington *Post*, December 30, 1977.

Cramer, P. K. Report on the current state of deinstitutionalization: Period of retrenchment. Commentaries on Human Service Issues (May 1978), Health and Welfare Council, Inc., Philadelphia.

Division of Biometry and Epidemiology. Data sheet on state and county mental hospital patients. National Institute of Mental Health, Rockville, Md. (1979, photocopied).

Division of Biometry and Epidemiology. Unpublished data. National Institute of Mental Health, Rockville, Md.

Dorwart, R. A. Deinstitutionalization: Who is left behind? *Hospital and Community Psychiatry* 31: 336-338 (1980).

Goldman, H. H., Gattozzi, A. A., and Taube, C. Defining and counting the chronically mentally ill. *Hospital and Community Psychiatry* 32: 21-27 (1981).

Governor's Task Force. Report on Mental Health. Raleigh, N.C. (September 1980, Draft report).

Gruber, L. N., Brown, A., and Mazorol, C. Ex-patient visitors to the hospital psychiatric unit. *Hospital and Community Psychiatry* 29: 731-734 (1978).

Halpern, J., Binner, P. R., Mohr, C. B., and Sackett, K. L. *The Illusion of Deinstitutionalization*. Denver, Col.: Denver Research Institute, 1978.

Hansell, N. Services for schizophrenics: A lifelong approach to treatment. *Hospital and Community Psychiatry* 29: 105-109 (1978).

Hayakawa, S. I. *Language in Thought and Action*, 3rd ed. New York: Harcourt, Brace, Jovanovich, 1972.

Hersch, C. Social history, mental health, and community control. *American Psychologist* 27: 749-754 (1972).

Holder, H. D. Accountability and Productivity in a System of Services for Chronic Patients. Presented at the 29th Institute on Hospital and Community Psychiatry, San Francisco (October 1977).

Johnson, P. J. *Community Support Systems for the Mentally Ill: A Study of the General Public, Mental Health Workers, and Board Members in Leon County, Florida, 1979-1980*. Ph.D. Dissertation, Florida State University School of Social Work (June 1980).

Kennedy, J. F. Message from the President of the United States to the 88th Congress. Document No. 58. Washington (February 5, 1963).

Kihss, P. City jails seek to prevent suicides. New York *Times*, October 23, 1980.

Kotkin, J. Governor Brown is sued over confinement of mental patients. Washington *Post*, February 14, 1979.

Kramer, B. A., and Rubinson, E. A study of former mental patients who returned to visit the ward on which they were hospitalized. *Psychiatry* 41: 302-307 (1978).

Lamb, H. R. The board and care home wanderers. *Archives of General Psychiatry* 37: 135-137 (1980).

Lamb, H. R., and Goertzel, V. The long-term patient in the era of community treatment. *Archives of General Psychiatry* 34: 679-682 (1977).

Langsley, D. G. The Community Mental Health Center: Does It Treat Patients? Presented at the 32nd Institute on Hospital and Community Psychiatry, Boston (September 1980).

Link, B., and Milcarek, B. Selection factors in the dispensation of therapy: The Matthew effect in the allocation of mental health resources. *Journal of Health and Social Behavior* 21: 279-290 (1980).

Mansfield, S. The neon havens of last resort. Washington *Post*, September 29, 1980.

Marmor, J. The relationship between systems theory and community psychiatry. *Hospital and Community Psychiatry* 26: 807-811 (1975).

Miller, J. G. Beware the "experts" on mental health. Washington *Star*, September 18, 1977.

Minkoff, K. A map of chronic mental patients, in *The Chronic Mental Patient*, J. A. Talbott, ed., 11-37. Washington: American Psychiatric Association, 1978.

Miser, H. J. Operations research and systems analysis. *Science* 209: 139-146 (1980).

Modlin, H. C. The Mentally Ill Inmate. Presented at the Annual Meeting of the American Psychiatric Association, Chicago (May 1979).

Moos, R., and Igra, A. Determinants of the social environments of sheltered care settings. *Journal of Health and Social Behavior* 21: 88-98 (1980).

Moran, A. E. Psychiatric bed needs: Quantifying the impact of alternative services. *Journal of Medical Systems* 4: 9-26 (1980).

Neill, J. R. The difficult patient: Identification and response. *Journal of Clinical Psychiatry* 40: 209-212 (1979).

Nunes, D. Little care available for mentally ill in D.C. jail. Washington *Post*, June 12, 1980.

Omang, J. Entry of handicapped children into schools brings problems. Washington *Post*, January 14, 1979.

Panzetta, A. F. The concept of community. *Archives of General Psychiatry* 25: 291-297 (1971).
Peele, R., and Keisling, R. Commitment to Freedom. Presented at Meetings of American Academy of Psychiatry and the Law, Chicago (September 1980).
Peele, R., and Palmer, R. R. Patient rights and patient chronicity. *Journal of Psychiatry and Law*: 59-71 (Spring 1980).
Pepper, B., Edmonds, J., Goldberg, W., and Grabel, H. 1,000 "Chronics" in Community Mental Health Center Treatment: Theory and Practice. Presented at the Annual Meeting of the American Psychiatric Association, San Francisco (May 1980).
President's Commission on Mental Health. *Report to the President from the President's Commission on Mental Health*, Vol. 1. U.S. Government Printing Office, Washington (1978).
Rich, S. Figures show end of era in social-program growth. Washington *Post*, February 14, 1979.
Robbins, E., Stern, M., Robbins, L., and Margolin, L. Unwelcome patients: Where can they find asylum? *Hospital and Community Psychiatry* 29: 44-46 (1978).
Robins, E. Diagnosis and chronic mental illness. *Psychiatric Quarterly* 50: 166-177 (1978).
Rosenblatt, A., and Mayer, J. E. Patients who return: A consideration of some neglected influences. *Journal of the Bronx State Hospital* 2: 71-81 (1974).
Salzman, E. Examining California's mental health. *California Journal*: 231-233 (July 1975).
Sargent, M. Deinstitutionalization and state mental hospitals: We can't have both —historian. ADAMHA *News*, August 8, 1980.
Scherl, D. J., and Macht, L. B. Deinstitutionalization in the absence of consensus. *Hospital and Community Psychiatry* 30: 599-604 (1979).
Shore, M. F., and Shapiro, R. The effect of deinstitutionalization on the state hospital. *Hospital and Community Psychiatry* 30: 605-608 (1979).
Silverman, M. Beyond the mainstream: The special needs of the chronic child patient. *American Journal of Orthopsychiatry* 49: 62-68 (1979).
Simon, W. B. On reluctance to leave the public mental hospital. *Psychiatry* 28: 145-156 (1965).
Smith, C. A., and Smith, C. J. Learned helplessness and preparedness in discharged mental patients. *Social Work Research and Abstracts* 14: 21-27 (1978).
Smith, W. G., and Hart, D. W. Community mental health: A noble failure? *Hospital and Community Psychiatry* 26: 581-583 (1975).
Spiegel, D. E., and Keith-Spiegel, P. K. Why we came back: A study of patients readmitted to a mental hospital. *Mental Hygiene* 53: 433-437 (1969).
Steadman, H. J., and Ribner, S. A. The Mentally Ill in Local Jails: New Claims Versus Old Problems. New York State Department of Mental Hygiene, Bureau of Special Projects Research, Albany (May 1980).
Stelovich, S. From the hospital to the prison: A step forward in deinstitutionalization? *Hospital and Community Psychiatry* 30: 618-620 (1979).

Stern, R., and Minkoff, K. Paradoxes in programming for chronic patients in a community clinic. *Hospital and Community Psychiatry* 30: 613-617 (1979).

Stratas, N. E., and Boyd, C. The chronic patient: A systems approach in North Carolina, in *Chronic Mental Patients: Treatment, Programs, Systems*, J. A. Talbott, ed. New York: Human Sciences Press (1981).

Stratas, N. E., Bernhardt, D. B., and Elwell, R. N. The future of the state mental hospital: Developing a unified system of care. *Hospital and Community Psychiatry* 28: 598-600 (1977).

Sullivan, R. Hospital forced to oust patients with psychoses. New York *Times*, November 8, 1979a.

Sullivan, R. Hospitals will gain by cutting bed use. New York *Times*, December 31, 1979b.

Talbott, J. A. Toward a public policy on the chronic mentally ill patient. *American Journal of Orthopsychiatry* 50: 43-53 (1980).

Task Panel on Deinstitutionalization, Rehabilitation and Long-Term Care. Report. In President's Commission on Mental Health, *Report to the President from the President's Commission on Mental Health*, Vol. 2, 356-375. U.S. Government Printing Office, Washington (1978).

Teltsch, K. Young terminal patients to get a loving hospice. New York *Times*, April 10, 1980.

U.S. General Accounting Office. *Returning the Mentally Disabled to the Community: Government Needs To Do More*. U.S. Government Printing Office, Washington (1977).

U.S. Government Accounting Office. *Prison Mental Health Can Be Improved by Better Management and More Effective Federal Aid*. U.S. Government Printing Office, Washington (1979).

Whitmer, G. E. From hospitals to jails: The fate of California's deinstitutionalized mentally ill. *American Journal of Orthopsychiatry* 50: 65-75 (1980).

Witkin, M. J. Provisional patient movement and selective administrative data, state and county medical hospitals, inpatient services by state: United States 1976. *Mental Health Statistical Note* No. 153 (August 1979).

Witkin, M. J. Trends in patient care episodes in mental health facilities, 1955-1977. *Mental Health Statistical Note* No. 154 (September 1980).

Wolfensberger, W. The principle of normalization and its implications to psychiatric services. *American Journal of Psychiatry* 127: 291-297 (1970).

Zusman, J., and Lamb, H. R. In defense of community mental health. *American Journal of Psychiatry* 134: 887-890 (1977).

CHAPTER 2

PRESERVING CHRONIC PATIENTS' ASSETS FOR SELF CARE

ERNEST M. GRUENBERG
JANET ARCHER

The automobile production line increases worker productivity by fragmenting a complex task into very simple elements, each elementary task being performed by one worker in a routine way. This production-line device has proved enormously valuable in manufacturing large numbers of identical products, put together from identical components. Instead of making each worker a highly specialized technical expert, however, it makes him a highly specialized non-expert—that is, an operator who can learn his simple task in a short time. The workers thus become readily interchangeable and the product correspondingly impersonal. For many tasks, this method of organizing work is efficient and effective. But treating a chronic mentally ill person—preserving his functional assets in accordance with the present state of our knowledge, deciding when he is ready to leave the hospital and deciding when he needs hospitalization once again—is not such a task.

INTEGRATION VS. FRAGMENTATION

"While one person holds the needle and another moves the thread, before the needle's threaded the patient will be dead."

In contrast to the unified inpatient and outpatient services that chronic mental patients need, the current direction of policy has been to add on more and more treatment elements and more and more treatment personnel—community general hospital psychiatric units, mental health center outpatient units, nursing homes, halfway houses, quarterway houses, patient advocates, patient management teams, psychologists, sociologists and social workers. Each of these has a contribution to make, but shifting the responsibility from one clinical setting to another and from one category of treatment personnel to another simply adds to the selective ignorance with which each of these personnel approaches the patient's problems and increases the patient's frustration. If implemented, the recent recommendation of the President's Commission on Mental Health (1978) for a system of case managers—to provide the "human link" to ". . . assist in assuring continuity of care and of a coordinated program of services"—would, at best, make it easier for the patient to cope with the fragmented services available to him. It would do nothing to reduce that fragmentation, and is certainly no substitute for the inpatient-based unified clinical team with systematic access to the community that is most beneficial to chronic seriously mentally ill patients.

Conventionally, a condition is called "chronic" because it lasts a long time. By contrast, acute conditions are short-lived. Some acute conditions kill quickly, such as the plague, cholera or some severe heart attacks. Some lead to quick spontaneous recovery, such as the common cold. Others are cured quickly: for instance, some cases of depression and most cases of pneumonia or appendicitis. Chronic conditions, then, are those for which we have no effective curative treatment, and whose sufferers neither die quickly nor recovery quickly.

In general, the technology of specific treatments for chronic mental disorders is not highly complicated. Since our treatments do not terminate these disorders, our greatest resource is personal attention and judgment, not impersonally performed functions. The special knowledge that the clinical worker really needs in order to help each patient to the maximum extent possible is knowledge regarding the particular person who is ill and the particular world in which he is living.

Fragmenting the treatment of a person who has a chronic mental disorder among a large number of people who are either filling super-skilled specialized roles or executing routine maneuvers is inappropriate to the nature of the work that needs to be done for the patient because we cannot predict what task will need to be performed during the next period of time. There are patients who are going to be dependent on psychiatric care for many years; today we cannot predict with confidence whether an individual patient in crisis will restitute quickly or slowly, whether he will restitute almost completely or only partially. And for the restituted patient, we cannot predict whether or when he will relapse.

Hence, any given therapeutic program for a particular patient with a chronic disorder concentrates on making the best of an inadequate treatment job. We know, however, that if the patient's assets are built on throughout every stage of the process, and if all of the family's and community's assets are strengthened in their ability to help the patient function, in the long run fewer patients will become severely disabled. We can be successful at least in keeping bad from becoming worse.

Because the techniques for doing this were learned in the context of organizing psychiatric care for patients in government mental hospitals, many of them are imperfectly or incompletely understood by today's clinician, who for the most part has been trained in university and community-based clinics, which until very recently treated patients with mental disorders less severe than those served by the state mental hospitals (Gruenberg 1967a). As a broader variety of mental health workers, psychiatrists and other physicians become familiar on a firsthand basis with the problems of chronic severe mental disorders, our knowledge is bound to grow. New treatment techniques for dealing with these chronic mental disorders will undoubtedly develop. This article attempts to summarize for these practitioners the current state of our knowledge, which is based on previous experience and studies regarding the nature of chronic mental disorders, and the techniques now available for providing useful treatment. We begin by describing the evolution of the concept of social breakdown syndrome, the set of patterns of disability secondary to chronic mental illnesses and the techniques by which chronic forms of this syndrome can be prevented. We then discuss some of the ways in which the present organization of services for chronic mentally ill people fails to make use of these important principles.

CHANGES IN PATIENTS' BEHAVIOR FOLLOWS CHANGES IN ORGANIZING PSYCHIATRIC SERVICES

Before World War II the majority of patients admitted to a mental hospital were expected to remain for a long period, if not for life. In the hospital many were found mute and withdrawn, they neglected their personal appearance, were incontinent, had uncontrollable emotional outbursts or exhibited senseless and uncommunicative talking.

Some patients were controlled by camisoles and confined behind locked doors. Custodial functions dominated mental hospital operations (Deutsch 1948). "Aftercare" was given to patients "on parole" who showed promise of recovery sufficient to hope that they could be discharged within six months or a year (Kramer et al. 1955).

Between the end of the War in 1946 and the introduction of the first ataractic drug, chlorpromazine, in 1955, three British mental hospital directors, Macmillan, Rees and Bell, began to humanize the atmosphere in their hospitals by systematically removing physical restraints, locked doors and involuntary hospitalization. They rediscovered what Pinel and Tuke had learned a century and a half before —that patients could be held safely responsible for their own conduct (Deutsch 1937, 1944; Bockoven, 1972). They also found that patients could be cared for outside of the hospital even though they were not fully recovered. They established extended outpatient and consultation services in the fabric of community life and adopted a relaxed approach to rehospitalization on very short notice. Hence, Macmillan, Rees and Bell transformed "aftercare" into long-term care in the community, interrupted by short-term episodes of hospitalization when needed in periods of crisis (Gruenberg 1974a). The same clinical team of psychiatrists, nurses, social workers and attendants took responsibility for patients during both community and hospital phases of care. The three mental hospitals, serving well-defined populations, carried the direction of change so far that their medical staffs were soon devoting half of their time to patients who were living outside of the hospital. Patients rarely stayed more than two or three months following admission, and despite a greatly increased admission rate, their hospital censuses were falling during the same period when mental hospital censuses were rising elsewhere (Milbank Memorial Fund 1958).

By the time the programs had reached that point, patient's behavior as a whole had taken on an unexpected, different appearance. Not only did long-term hospital cases recover many social abilities, but among new cases, disturbed behavior improved quickly after admission and withdrawal rarely occurred. Chronically disturbed and chronically withdrawn behavior could no longer be regarded as an inherent, unavoidable consequence of serious mental illness, but had to be viewed, to a large extent, as a product of the interaction between the disease, the individual and his social environment (Gruenberg 1969). These improvements were observed in patients with a wide range of mental disorders; in fact, Macmillan's community care program at Mapperley Hospital was begun for geriatric patients and only later was extended to schizophrenics and other nongeriatric patients (Macmillan and Shaw 1966; Macmillan 1958).

These psychiatrists' reports of how they had converted mental hospital practices into a new model of care and treatment were looked on with suspicion by colleagues familiar with the intractable nature of long-term mental patients. But a committee of New York State hospital directors who traveled to Britain to study these pioneering programs returned convinced that the new community-care, open-hospital pattern was a forerunner of what mental hospitals should become if the symptomatic relief provided by the new psychopharmaceuticals was to be used constructively (Hoch et al. 1957; Milbank Memorial Fund 1960). By the early 1960s, many state mental hospitals in the U.S. were operating as "open hospitals," and some were providing comprehensive services to most of their patients in the community (Milbank Memorial Fund 1962).

These changes in the U.S. represented a reformed use of very good government mental hospitals. They were initiated by mental hospital directors who were well-trained psychiatrists, having risen to high rank in a competitive system of government medicine. At the time they began their reforms, they were receiving almost all their patients on involuntary certificates, and all the wards of their hospitals were locked. The directors were administratively and legally responsible for the care and treatment of all the patients certified to their care. They slowly and courageously lowered the frequency with which they used the enormous powers they then had. They used their autonomy to *not* lock up all their patients, to release patients early in the course of recovery and to see them as outpatients at home—*before* admission. As will be discussed later, mental hospitals no longer have these powers.

The term "social breakdown syndrome" was first used by an American Public Health Association committee (1962) to describe the secondary syndrome of withdrawal and/or disturbed behavior that seriously interferes with personal and social functioning, the chronic forms of which became less common following the introduction of new systems of delivering psychiatric services. The recognition that much disability associated with chronic mental illness might be prevented with treatment practices designed to maximize the preservation of patients' personal and social assets led the APHA committee to identify the chronic social breakdown syndrome (SBS) as a major public health priority.

The SBS concept was operationalized in the first systematic test of the new principles of organizing psychiatric services in Dutchess

County, New York, after a transformation of psychiatric services similar to that achieved by Macmillan, Rees and Bell was inaugurated there in 1959. In order to test whether the reorganized services were responsible for lowering the frequency of chronic SBS (episodes of SBS lasting more than one year), a separate service for Dutchess County residents was organized at Hudson River State Hospital to provide services of humane, open hospital care, combined with early discharge of patients to the community under supervision by the same hospital team. Readmissions to hospital for short stays were encouraged in periods of crisis in the course of the disorder (Hunt et al. 1961).

The research showed that the reforms at least halved the number of new cases of chronic SBS (episodes persisting for more than 12 months), starting each year, representing an annual savings of at least 75 years per person of chronic severe disability for each 100,000 population receiving the unified, comprehensive services. Rates of recovery from an SBS episode fall with the square of time; hence, a case that has lasted four weeks is four times more likely to recover in the next week than a case that has lasted eight weeks. The reforms lowered the frequency of chronic SBS by increasing the probability of terminating acute episodes within a few weeks. But the Dutchess County unit was no more effective in rehabilitating cases of SBS that did become chronic than were the specialized continued treatment services being provided to the other patients in Hudson River State Hospital (Gruenberg 1966; Gruenberg et al. 1969).

This practical demonstration, confirmed by evaluation research, made possible a fuller elaboration of the SBS concept and a more complete understanding of how the new way of organizing psychiatric services lowered the frequency of chronic SBS (Gruenberg 1967b, 1967c, 1969, 1972, 1974a, 1975).

THE SOCIAL BREAKDOWN SYNDROME: A SET OF FALLING DEFENSES

The ways in which a person becomes disabled in the presence of a mental disorder are best seen as a set of falling defenses against impaired functions. People with organic syndromes, for example, have an impaired ability to integrate the conflicting signals coming from the environment into a coherent picture of what is demanded of them in such a way that they can adequately respond to those demands. People with functional mental disorders are also impaired in important functions, and this makes them vulnerable to social breakdown syndrome. Because vulnerability of individuals to the social breakdown syndrome has not been investigated systematically, our notions of what makes people vulnerable are only loosely formulated. This represents an important area for future research to which contemporary clinicians can expect to make useful contributions.

The set of disablement patterns comprising the social breakdown syndrome is limited. These patterns tend to be forms of withdrawing from some aspects of life, or rebelling against some aspects of life. Although SBS episodes can be mild, moderate or severe, the manifestations are remarkably similar regardless of the type of mental disorder, its course or severity. But episodes of disablement can run an entirely different course from that of the underlying disorder. In this way, SBS in a person with a chronic mental disorder is similar to cardiac decompensation in a person with chronic heart disease; it has its own consequences and its own dynamics of continuation, progression or restitution to previous functioning without a cure of the underlying condition.

Today, only a small proportion of the people clinicians see with social breakdown syndrome are in their first episode. However, it is important to keep in mind that there are first episodes of SBS and that this is a group of special interest.

The social breakdown syndrome has a variable duration, lasting from minutes to decades. Over 90% of SBS episodes are acute; they terminate within weeks. But about 10% of SBS episodes become chronic (last for more than a year), representing wasted lives and a heavy burden to the patient, the family and the community. The following discussion of the pathogenesis of SBS (discussed more fully by Gruenberg 1969, 1974a, 1980) illustrates how a humane, unified inpatient and outpatient service can at least halve the frequency of chronic SBS in the community it serves.

Terminating an SBS Episode

The social breakdown syndrome seems to emerge as a result of a spiraling crescendo of interactions between the patient and the people in his immediate social environment. The setting requires a discrepancy between what a person can do and what he is expected to do. At that moment, he becomes more dependent upon current cues from the environment regarding himself, his values and his customary ways of dealing with life. This type of situation occurs very commonly for everyone. It is a precondition for constructive changes in attitude and behavior which, when the environment is suitable, leads to corrective modification of functioning. That is one way in which we learn. But if the discrepancy is not eliminated by improved performance, or by a reduced demand, or by an explanation that relieves the person of responsibility for meeting the demand, an SBS episode is likely to begin. He tends to make random movements in response to misinterpretations of the nature of the task, or to misunderstood clues from the environment as to how to deal with the problem. His unsatisfactory attempts to rectify the situation arouse fears or resentment, further putting him out of touch with the people around him. This produces a more urgent feeling of need to modify his behavior to satisfy increasingly urgent demands. But his response to this still more tense situation results in still more misunderstanding and hostility. The human response to maintain situations of tension is to attack or withdraw—fight or flight. If this process of action-reaction continues, the result can be a highly explosive manifestation of aggression and hostile behavior, or a progressive withdrawal from interaction and from usual roles and functions.

Sometimes the process is stopped at this point because the patient's social support network reexamines the task situation (at work, in studies, in housekeeping, or whatever) and finds a way to redefine what is expected in a way that he can accept. But often, the disruptive or withdrawn functioning becomes an indication to others that the individual has become "incapable of caring for himself" or is "a danger to self or others," and they seek a clinician's attention. In fact, most admissions to mental hospitals are associated with an episode of social breakdown syndrome.

With good clinical services, most episodes of SBS terminate very quickly. The key to quick termination of an SBS episode depends on organizing a rapid relevant response to the early signs of disrupted personal and/or social functioning. This requires a long-term treatment relationship, even though great intensity of attention is rarely needed. When the current crisis is defined in terms of a specific problem that the clinician will handle, with the patient's active participation, a quick resolution of the crisis can be expected. The availability of acute treatment protects the patient's social support systems in times of crisis by helping to prevent family and friends from developing rejecting attitudes towards the patient and his illness. The tendency to deteriorate in personal and social functioning is greatly reduced if the patient's fulfillment of ordinary roles is systematically preserved. This is best facilitated by maintaining patients in their community life as much as possible. However, a brief hospitalization is often indicated; many SBS episodes terminate within minutes of admission to a good open hospital with sympathetic personnel and appropriate preadmission care. This is not the universal response, but it is very common. It is not due to drugs, because often these have not yet been administered; it is most likely due to the dramatic initiation into the sick role which serves as an explanation to the patient for his sense of failure in managing his own life.

Although it is not generally looked on in this way, it might be helpful for the clinician to think about the authority that his position represents. Whether he sees the patient in hospital or in the office setting, by accepting the patient's and his relatives' or friends' claims that he is in trouble and has a disorder, the clinician quickly identifies him as a sick person and places him in the sick role as described by Parsons (1951) and others. This may be the clinician's most powerful tool at this point, because a sick person is not expected to do the things that a healthy person is expected to do and hence is excused of task performance failures.

The clinician should take a meticulous present-illness history to discover what the person was attempting to do when his behavior began to deteriorate. Generally, the individual (or the family member who accompanies the patient) can describe the situation in which the troubled mental state started. The clinician should do everything possible to help those who accompany the patient to reformulate their expectations of his performance without losing their respect for him or harming his self-respect. Too often, clinicians regard life stresses and problems as irrelevant to the symptoms, and so do family members and patients unless such problems are brought to their attention. That is why, presently, our clinical records do not indicate the circumstances in which patients first began to feel troubled and unable to deal with life; thus we have little systematic knowledge of the precise situations in which SBS develops.

Perpetuating SBS

We know what features of good clinical attention and services prevent chronic disability. We also know some ways that inadequate care and services can perpetuate it. Involuntary admission to a hospital can intensify feelings of inadequacy and self-rejection, especially when those closest to the family join with the community, via a formal commitment mechanism, to certify the individual as incompetent. Once in the hospital, locked doors, excessive or unnecessary restraint and sedation undermine the patient's self-respect and his assets for self-care.

But overprotective treatment can be as bad as, or even worse than, inhumane treatment. An overly sheltering treatment environment can perpetuate an SBS episode and hence encourage chronic disability by relieving the patient of responsibility for self-care and autonomous functioning at the price of being identified as having a condition which makes his own impulses, thoughts and speech largely irrelevant to any practical activities of daily life. By restricting visits and by discouraging the family's interest in the patient's progress, it can encourage his isolation from community ties. In such a restrictive, isolated environment, the patient comes to identify with the long-term patient role, and whatever his former capacities were, his ability to carry out ordinary social exchange and work tasks decreases and becomes awkward from disuse.

The clinical staff can undermine the patient's assets for self-care by exaggerating the seriousness of his condition. Many clinicians are tempted to do this, either because they will get credit for a therapeutic miracle in the event that the patient improves, or because they want to protect themselves from later criticism if the patient fails to improve or deteriorates even more. The staff must resist such temptations if they are to be as effective as possible for their patient. It is quite easy to express one's uncertainty about a prognosis clearly enough to protect oneself against later fault finding if things turn out poorly, without emphasizing or predicting in an ominous tone of voice that things are going to get worse. The clinician should set as short a time period for the sick role as possible in the minds of the patient and those who are close to him. When an SBS episode terminates in a hospitalized patient, the staff should define the patient as having recovered from the symptoms that led to his institutionalization, and they should immediately plan and implement his discharge. In the best situation, that same hospital staff will continue to care for the person as an outpatient, so they are, in effect, discharging him to themselves, and hence can readmit him if their fears that he is not ready to leave should prove justified.

ABANDONMENT IN THE NAME OF "DEINSTITUTIONALIZATION"

The systematic evaluations of the Dutchess County reforms that showed that much chronic SBS is preventable were evaluations of a *unified*, hospital-based community care service. This stands in sharp contrast to the highly fragmented proliferation of services now serving the chronic seriously mentally ill population. It cannot be assumed, therefore, that patients being released shortly after hospital admission under today's "deinstitutionalization" policies are functioning at much higher levels than during earlier years. Many may be. But many may be functioning with the same types and severity of symptoms as their predecessors, but in different locations.

Abandoning patients in the name of "deinstitutionalization" is a new stage in the natural history of the chronic social breakdown syndrome. It is the result of practices that have developed only in the last decade. These people are to be seen in clusters in the community: in single-person-occupancy hotels which cater to former mental hospital patients, in "halfway houses," and sometimes wandering the streets in the slums of our large cities (Group for the Advancement of Psychiatry 1978). There is sometimes systematic community resistance to the presence of these individuals, but there is also systematic resistance on the part of mental health officials to rehospitalizing them. Administrative rules have been substituted for clinical judgment as to who should be released from the mental hospital. These administrative rules tend to be dominated by a need to gain administrative credit for a lower hospital census and for "phasing out the state mental hospital."

Elsewhere, we have discussed the social forces that led to these practices (Gruenberg and Archer 1979). But it is necessary here to point out that "deinstitutionalization" practices are associated with the removal of a responsible government institution, the responsible state mental hospital. Whatever their faults, state mental hospitals up until recent times were designated by law, and were operated in practice as a last line of resource for people in trouble. With the exception of some particularly violent, criminally inclined patients who could sometimes be sent to special institutions for the criminally insane, state mental hospitals rarely had the option of referring their patients elsewhere for care. The emphasis on treatment in the changed state mental hospitals has implicitly left the responsibility for chronic care of incurable mental patients untended to, and has given the hospitals the privilege—and in some states the obligation—of discharging patients for whom modern psychiatric treatment could not expect to produce dramatic benefits. These patients have been abandoned by the medical care system which previously existed, and they are the greatest challenge facing psychiatric services today.

The path leading to the demise of state responsibility for the seriously mentally ill and the current crisis of abandonment was paved with good intentions. Tragically for the seriously mentally ill, the current policies underlying the pattern of abandonment are based on erroneous interpretations of what patients need and what our current techniques can produce to help people with serious mental disorders. These interpretations have been systematically encouraged by a general crisis in government and social policy. The fashion has been for "cost-benefit" reasoning, dramatic efforts to reduce operating budgets and the shifting of responsibilities away from one element of government to another. Many of these errors are shared by both the advocates and the opponents of "deinstitutionalization." In the remainder of this chapter, we shall discuss some important principles of good patient care that are often ignored or distorted in the present discussions of the crisis of abandonment.

The Unified Clinical Team

In psychiatry today, chronic patients suffer most from our tendency to keep inpatient and outpatient staffs separate, and to move the patient from one clinical team to another when the locus of treatment needs to be changed. Many crucial decisions must be made on a "try-and-see" basis. In such cases, those who do the "trying" ought also to be able to "see." If the person who decides to send a patient home is different from the person who sees the result, neither is able to learn from the decision that has been made.

The unified clinical team, which continues to take responsibility for a set of patients during both inpatient and community phases of care, is a crucial feature of a service's ability to organize a rapid relevant response to an acute episode of SBS. A unified clinical service can serve only a small area. Short channels of communication and familiarity with local community resources and personnel are needed. A big staff for a big area does not work (Hunt et al. 1961). Even the best community mental health center is not equipped to provide the type of long-term psychiatric attention that is most beneficial to chronic seriously mentally ill patients, even if it has a close, cooperative relationship with an inpatient service. One acknowledgment of the difficulties that can ensue is Panzetta's (1971) description of the Temple University Mental Health Center in Philadelphia: "Outpatient staff tended to see the patient as having been rushed out of the hospital without adequate treatment or preparation. The inpatient staff tended to see the outpatient staff as disorganized and unwilling to follow up on patient needs." This is not surprising to anyone who has had experience trying to organize psychiatric services for the severely ill psychiatric patient. Obviously, what is needed is a unified clinical team, to take responsibility for conducting aftercare and followup after its own decision to release. If these same team members also continue the treatment of the same patient after readmittance within the inpatient service, they will not have any grounds for feeling that someone else has failed the patient. They will learn to respond realistically to what they can do for their patients.

Ataractic Drugs

The ataractic drugs have remarkable and unanticipated properties. But their value is currently overemphasized in American psychiatry, and their toxic effects are underestimated (Crane 1974). These drugs are often misprescribed and misperceived because their prescribers tend to have limited knowledge of the ways in which service organization affects patient functioning and the course of psychotic episodes. Some see drugs as suppressing symptoms, analogous to the way Dilantin suppresses epileptic convulsions. Others see the role of these drugs as analogous to that played by insulin for diabetics—a compensator for some metabolic defect, and thus not only warding off immediate symptoms but retarding disease processes, thereby reducing the frequency of complications.

No such simple models for understanding the action of these drugs emerges, however, when one observes their effects in psychotic episodes. It is clear that they do not function as simple suppressors of troublesome behavior, even though patients who receive such medications do exhibit such behavior less often than do control patients (Pasamanick et al. 1967). But patients who have been admitted to open wards after emergency consultation in the community, and who receive appropriate personal attention so as to gain their cooperation in treatment, also exhibit fewer of these behavior patterns than patients who are brought by force into the hospital, with no effort to explain what is being done for them (Macmillan 1958). When humane and understanding, flexible psychiatric service goes along with the use of drugs, even better results follow (May 1975).

In the predrug period, some community care programs were able to produce results for entire communities that were similar to those now attributed to the new drugs. And deterioration appears to have continued unabated into the drug era whenever no concomitant change has occurred in service organization (Smith et al. 1965). We know that these helpful drugs potentiate anaesthesia, without themselves producing it (Caldwell 1970). Hence, clinical units can think of the ataractics as facilitators of efforts to preserve the patient's self-caring abilities, his ability to cooperate in treatment, and his socially organized attempts to maintain his assets.

Early Release Requires Easy Readmission

Reforms that transformed many mental hospitals from primarily long-term institutions into hospitals in which an increasing proportion of beds were occupied by short-term crisis admissions (a median of two weeks) were common between 1955 and 1965. This progressive reorganization was accompanied by a rising readmission rate. But the shortened average length of stay led to a net drop in the number of beds occupied. So the hospital census count dropped. During that period, a falling mental hospital census was a fairly reliable index of a mental hospital that was moving forward. But "deinstitutionalization" policies, substituting the index for the desired phenomena, tried to find ways to make the census drop faster. This makes about as much sense as a child trying to push an automobile speedometer needle to make the car go faster. A falling census that occurs after the introduction of a progressive reform of community care, combined with short-term hospitalization as needed, is accompanied by a rising readmission rate, because a responsible policy of early release requires a policy of easy readmission. Early release from the hospital with continuing responsibility for patient care in the community requires a readiness to readmit when hospitalization is needed again (Milbank Memorial Fund 1958). To refuse readmission to patients who are released before they are fully recovered is to abandon responsibility for them.

Benefits of Short-Term Hospitalization

The observation that inpatient care, especially long-term inpatient care, can undermine the patient's ability for self-support is analogous to the cardiologists' discovery that excessive bed rest is bad for most patients. It can produce an atropy of disuse. Cardiologists, however, have not refused bed rest to cardiac patients. Yet many mental health policy makers actually deny, both implicitly and explicitly, the therapeutic values of even short-term hospital care. In fact, short-term hospitalization can, as described earlier, prevent long-term institutional placements by speeding the process of resolving a crisis in the course of the disorder, and by providing relief admissions. It is helpful to group the indications for short-term hospital treatment under seven headings (Gruenberg 1974b).

1. *Safety.* This indication is the legal justification for involuntary commitments. It is a good indication for admitting a patient to the hospital when no other safe location for care exists. Because most patients with this indication today will accept hospitalization voluntarily if a little work is done to reduce their fear of the hospital, and because an excessive preoccupation with safety can be harmful to patients, at least one of the other six benefits can and should be emphasized in any decision to hospitalize a patient.

2. *Diagnosis.* Certain diagnostic procedures, some of which require close observation on a 24-hour basis, are done more safely in a hospital. Psychiatric diagnosis can also be hastened by a short-term hospital admission. Diagnosis includes an appraisal of the patient's condition and familiarization with the patient's personal characteristics. Rapidity in appraising the patient accelerates the speed with which the optimal treatment plan is formulated.

3. *Treatment.* As with diagnosis, use of the hospital for treatment is indicated to facilitate a rapid, relevant response to the presenting crisis. Treatments such as ECT are safer, and the speed with which higher doses of dangerous drugs can be safely achieved is greater in hospital than out. Retraining is also a form of treatment, and the hospital can provide intensive retraining programs unequalled outside.

4. *Asylum.* A protective, nurturing environment isolated from the patient's life situation provides a "retreat" from life's stresses when they become overwhelming. In the hospital, the patient has the opportunity to remobilize his resources and assets in a context away from needs for immediate responses to demands which overwhelm him.

5. *Burden Sharing.* The tendency to deteriorate in personal and social functioning is greatly reduced if the patient's fulfillment of ordinary living roles is systematically preserved. This is best facilitated by maintaining patients in their community life as much as possible.

However, modern community care always places some burden on families or neighbors who are generally willing to accept the troubles. But if the burden becomes too prolonged, or is too limiting on the lives of other household members, their attitude toward the patient is likely to become more negative (Morris 1977–78). Once rejection towards the patient occurs, it is almost impossible to reverse. If the hospital defines its relationship as one of burden sharing, it can make itself available to provide relief admissions for short periods, and hence prevent rejection by families and friends.

6. *Insight*. If the patient is to use the clinician's help constructively, it is necessary that he accept the patient role. A brief hospitalization can sometimes help resistant patients accept their need for aid more quickly than any other method. The switch from the normal person overwhelmed by insoluble conflicts and life problems to the patient on whom altered expectations are placed can, in itself, reduce tension sufficiently to terminate an episode of SBS.

7. *Partnership*. Patients with chronic severe mental disorders must be told that their future depends largely on what they do for themselves, but that there is a role for clinical help and that it will be made available fully. Some patients have strong needs to test out the boundaries of this partnership; they go through periods when they fear that they will fall apart unless they can be hospitalized. Early in the course of their care, and sometimes later, they will present themselves for admission in such a state. Sometimes it is wise to admit them, for a short time only, simply to assert the hospital's availability in time of need.

Chronic SBS in the Community

Although the belief that all SBS episodes are caused by mental hospitals may be comforting to administrators hoping to lower state mental hospital budgets, it has no basis in reality, and it justifies the damaging practice of discharging unrecovered patients into communities without providing continuing inpatient services. About half of the savings in chronic SBS that occurred in Dutchess County when good community care programs were introduced were due to a quick termination of social breakdown syndrome episodes which began outside of hospitals (Gruenberg 1977). Hence, only about half of the SBS cases that became chronic in Dutchess County could be attributed to an overly restrictive hospital environment. Today, with "deinstitutionalization" and greatly reduced hospital censuses, this percentage may well be lower.

Today we understand very well the ways in which bad hospital care can foster chronic deterioration. In fact, the many compassionate, vivid accounts of how this occurs (e.g., Barton 1959; Goffman 1961) have diverted investigator's attention away from studying those features in the family, in the community and in nonstate mental hospital institutional settings (e.g., nursing homes) that give rise to and foster chronic sociogenic disability. There is an urgent need for systematic investigation of the development of chronic social breakdown syndrome in community settings.

CONCLUSION

It is important to remember that the techniques we have described in this paper are methods for preserving patients' assets for self-care. Their success lies not in rehabilitating patients who have become chronically disabled, but in preventing disability from becoming chronic. And even with the best organization of psychiatric services that we know how to provide, we cannot prevent all cases of chronic SBS. In caring for patients with conditions that threaten severe functional disability, we are trying to provide clinical assistance with only limited treatment techniques, in a state of knowledge that leaves us unable to make a detailed prognosis on a case-by-case basis. Under these conditions, we have learned that if we adopt an attitude of acting on our best hopes, backed up with readiness to act if our worst fears become justified, our patients do less badly than if we permit ourselves to act on our fears without giving hope a chance.

While the above formula may strike the reader as more like a sentiment extracted from the final paragraph of a minister's sermon than a scientific assertion, the simple fact is that regardless of such emotional reverberations, it is the best summary of the principles behind the community care of the severely ill mental patients that can be made in the light of today's knowledge, and is based on empirical data and not on sentiment. It might be observed that in practice, when caring for patients in this type of situation, the clinician would much rather feel capable of being able to definitively sort those patients who will do well on release from those who must be kept in the hospital. Emotionally it is much harder to accept the suspended judgment it is necessary to exercise: each next step in the care of a patient must be taken with a readiness to have it succeed, together with a preparedness to have it fail.

REFERENCES

American Public Health Association. *Mental Disorders: A Guide to Control Methods.* New York: American Public Health Association, 1962.

Barton, R. *Institutional Neurosis.* Briston: John Wright & Sons, Ltd., 1959.

Bockover, J. S. *Moral Treatment in Community Mental Health.* New York: Springer, 1972.

Caldwell, A. E. *Origins of Psychopharmacology. From CPZ to LSD.* Springfield, Ill.: Charles C. Thomas, 1970, p. 136.

Crane, G. E. Two decades of psychopharmacology and community mental health: Old and new problems of the schizophrenic patient. *Transactions of the New York Academy of Sciences* 36: 644-657 (1974).

Deutsch, A. *The Mentally Ill in America.* Garden City, N.Y.: Doubleday, Doran, 1937.

Deutsch, A. The history of mental hygiene, in *One Hundred Years of American Psychiatry.* New York: Columbia University Press, 1944.

Deutsch, A. *The Shame of the States.* New York: Harcourt, Brace and Company, 1948.

Goffman, E. *Asylums.* New York: Doubleday and Company, Inc., 1961.

Group for the Advancement of Psychiatry. *The Chronic Mental Patient in the Community.* New York: Mental Health Materials Center, 1978.

Gruenberg, E. M. Editor. Evaluating the Effectiveness of Mental Health Services. *Milbank Memorial Fund Quarterly*, Vol. 44 (no. 1), part 2 (1966).

Gruenberg, E. M. Psychiatric progress and the universities. *American Journal of Orthopsychiatry* 37: 645-650 (1967a).

Gruenberg, E. M. Can the reorganization of psychiatric services prevent some cases of social breakdown syndrome?, in *Psychiatry in Transition, 1966-67*, A. B. Stokes, ed. Toronto: University of Toronto Press, 1967b, pp. 95-109.

Gruenberg, E. M. The social breakdown syndrome—Some origins. *American Journal of Psychiatry* 124: 1481-1489 (1967c).

Gruenberg, E. M. From practice to theory: Community mental health services and the nature of psychoses. *Lancet* April 5: 721-724 (1969).

Gruenberg, E. M. The social breakdown syndrome and its prevention. In *American Handbook of Psychiatry*, Vol. 2, G. Caplan, ed. New York: Basic Books, 1974a, pp. 448-463.

Gruenberg, E. M. Benefits of short-term hospitalization, in *Strategic Intervention in Schizophrenia: Current Developments in Treatment*, R. Cancro, N. Fox, and L. E. Shapiro, eds. New York: Behavioral Publications, 1974b, pp. 251-259.

Gruenberg, E. M. New methods for assessing the effectiveness of psychiatric intervention, in *American Handbook of Psychiatry*, Vol. 6, D. Hamburg, ed. New York: Basic Books, 1975, pp. 791-810.

Gruenberg, E. M. Community care is not deinstitutionalization, in *New Trends of Psychiatry in the Community*, G. Serban, ed. Cambridge, Mass.: Ballinger, 1977, pp. 257-264.

Gruenberg, E. M. Chronic disabilities of the mentally disordered. (Unpublished manuscript, 1980).

Gruenberg, E. M. and Archer, J. Abandonment of responsibility for the seriously mentally ill. *Health and Society* 57(4): 485-506 (1979).

Gruenberg, E. M., Snow, H. B., and Bennett, C. L. Preventing the Social Breakdown Syndrome, in *Social Psychiatry*, F. C. Redlich, ed. Baltimore: Williams & Wilkins, 1969, pp. 179-195.

Hoch, P. H., Hunt, R. C., Snow, H. B., Pleasure, H., O'Neil, G. J., Terrence, C. F., and Beckenstein, N. Observations on the British "open" hospitals. *Mental Hospitals* 8: 5-15 (1957).

Hunt, R. C., Gruenberg, E. M., Hacken, E., and Huxley, M. A comprehensive hospital-community service in a state hospital. *American Journal of Psychiatry* 117: 817-821 (1961).

Kramer, M., Goldstein, H., Israel, R. H., and Johnson, N. A. *A Historical Study of the Disposition of First Admissions to a State Mental Hospital.* Public Health Monograph No. 32, Washington, D.C. (1955).

Macmillan, D. Hospital-community relationships, in *An Approach to the Prevention of Disability From Chronic Psychoses.* New York: Milbank Memorial Fund, 1958, pp. 27-50.

Macmillan, D. and Shaw, P. Senile breakdown in standards of personal and environmental cleanliness. *British Medical Journal* 2: 1032-1037 (1966).

May, P. New models for continuity of care: What are the needs? *Hospital & Community Psychiatry* 26: 599-601 (1975).

Milbank Memorial Fund. *An Approach to the Prevention of Disability from Chronic Psychoses.* New York: Milbank Memorial Fund, 1958.

Milbank Memorial Fund. Reports on group visits to Great Britain's community-based open mental hospitals, in *Steps in the Development of Integrated Psychiatric Services.* New York: Milbank Memorial Fund, 1960.

Milbank Memorial Fund. *Decentralization of Psychiatric Services and Continuity of Care.* New York: Milbank Memorial Fund, 1962.

Morris, R. Integration of therapeutic and community services: Cure plus care for the mentally disabled. *International Journal of Mental Health* 6: 9-26 (1977-78).

Panzetta, A. F. *Community Mental Health. Myth and Realities.* Philadelphia: Lea and Fegiger, 1971, p. 133.

Parsons, T. *The Social Systems.* Glencoe, Ill.: The Free Press, 1951.

Pasamanick, B., Scarpitti, F., and Dinitz, S. *Schizophrenics in the Community.* New York: Appleton-Century-Crofts, 1967.

President's Commission on Mental Health. *Report to the President*, Volume I. U.S. Government Printing Office, Washington, D.C. (1978).

Smith, T. C., Bower, W. H., and Wignall, C. M. Influence of policy and drugs on Colorado State Hospital population. *Archives of General Psychiatry* 12: 352-362 (1965).

CHAPTER 3

SOCIAL NETWORKS AND THE LONG TERM PATIENT

MURIEL HAMMER

I. INTRODUCTION

There has been a general concensus over many years that social relationships constitute a major area of difficulty for psychiatric patients. Only recently, however, has there begun to be an interest in studying the systematic properties of these social relationships as structured *networks* of connections, and in the implications of these network properties for the course of illness and for treatment.

There is not yet sufficient knowledge of the sets of social relationships, or "social networks," of psychiatric patients, or of the processes involved in social networks more generally, for one to be able to "prescribe" the social needs of psychiatric patients in the community. It is clear nonetheless that any form of treatment (or neglect) has an impact—generally unintended and unremarked—on the structure of the patient's social relationships, and it may be wise to become aware of these effects and consider them explicitly. As a very simple example, if a patient is to receive medication at a clinic, then whether the patient comes for it twice a week or once a month, and whether the clinic also has other, informal social facilities, will not only affect the likelihood of the patient continuing to come for the medication, but will also affect the likelihood of the patient forming relationships with other people at the clinic—which will in turn have some effects on the patient's other relationships. More significantly, when a patient is encouraged to learn a trade, or to join a church group, or to share an apartment, the full range of probable impacts on the patient's previous and potential new social connections and their interrelationships is never genuinely assessed.

While the bases for such assessments are not yet adequately developed, what is known can be taken into account; and with some attention explicitly focused on these social impacts, we may be able to learn considerably more about them.

What I propose to do here, then, is to discuss some of the characteristics of social networks generally, and of the social networks of psychiatric patients more specifically, with some indication of the ways these might enter into our considerations in planning the treatment of patients in the community.

We might, however, first ask, who are we talking about? Who are the chronic psychiatric patients in the community, where and with whom do they live, how do they spend their time, what happens to them over the course of time? And what can we draw from our incipient knowledge of social network processes that may bear on this?

While certain statistical and clinical generalizations can be made about chronic psychiatric patients, it should be clear from the start that any such generalizations will be false and potentially misleading for some proportion of that population. Many patients are poor, urban, relatively uneducated and from low status ethnic backgrounds; but others may be rich, suburban or rural, highly educated and drawn from the dominant subculture. Patients typically have considerable difficulty coping with schools, jobs and other demands; but some are highly competent and successful. Psychiatric problems may be long-term and fairly constant or recurrently episodic. For those who are hospitalized, perhaps half are discharged to live with parents or a spouse, and half to a variety of other arrangements, including other relatives or friends, supervised homes and unsupervised hotels (see, e.g., Blumenthal et al. 1982).

Recognizing that the range of economic, social and personal characteristics of chronic psychiatric patients is extremely broad, one may still emphasize certain patterns, partly because they are more pervasive, partly because they seem to require more attention. It is commonly the case that chronic psychiatric patients are economically dependent, relatively inept at self-care and socially unskilled (Strayer and Keith 1979). Psychiatric patients tend to spend time with fewer people than is normal for others in the society, and to spend less time, on an average, even with the people they do see (Silberfeld 1978). The relatively low amount of social interaction probably contributes to the generally poor development of basic social skills in psychiatric patients.

The complex codes of social behaviors and meanings—predominantly not explicit or conscious—that people in a society acquire as they grow through infancy, childhood and adulthood require considerable practice, with ongoing monitoring and modification, if they are to be used smoothly with the variety of people and for the variety of situations in which people normally operate. It is characteristic of chronic psychiatric patients that the smooth use of appropriate social codes was never acquired, or has deteriorated through insufficient or distorted practice, or has been modified in problematic ways (Gruenberg 1967; Mosher and Menn 1978; Makiesky-Barrow and Gutwirth in press; Test and Stein 1978).

The most basic potential contribution to the functioning of the chronic psychiatric patient that might be made through enhanced social networks is the improvement of these micro-level social skills. Since these are called for in every aspect of life, it would not be too extreme to expect that if such improvement could be achieved, it would contribute to improved coping in every area, including the economic.

II. SIZE, STRUCTURE AND FUNCTIONS OF SOCIAL NETWORKS

Social Networks: Size and Structure

I will begin with some very broad discussion about the size, structure and functions of social networks generally, before considering some of the evidence on the relationship of networks to health, and some specific implications for chronic psychiatric patients.

A social network consists simply of a set of individuals and a set of social connections linking them. These can be looked at in the same way as an engineering diagram with points and connections. A network is not conceptually specific to human beings or even to organisms—which incidentally permits the use of certain analytic methods from other fields, like mathematics and engineering—although some of the properties of social networks may be found to be specific to human beings.

The selection of the set of points, or set of individuals to be analyzed, and of the criteria for what constitutes a connection, can proceed from a number of different perspectives. One could, for example, take a location like a school, with all the individuals who are in that school, and include either all the contacts that take place among those individuals or some selected kinds of contacts among them. Or one could take an event, such as a political candidacy or an episode of illness, and consider all the individuals involved in that event and the connections among them. Most of the research on social networks has dealt with what is typically called the personal network, which starts from some individual, the focal individual, and moves out from that individual either to all contacts or to some predefined set of contacts, such as kin or colleagues or neighbors or people seen at least twice a week. For any particular focal individual, the total set of contacts would include such people as other household members, neighbors, people at school or at work, several sets of kin for most people, friends, mechanics, doctors, librarians, the grocer, and such persons as the neighbors of the focal individual's brother—whom the focal individual may occasionally see when visiting the brother—or friends of the focal individual's neighbor—who are occasionally seen when they visit. These are all people whom the focal individual has direct contact with, although many of them may be connected to the focal individual only through slight acquaintanceship.

There are no fully satisfactory estimates of how large an individual's total set of direct contacts may be, but such networks are probably on the order of several hundred to two thousand individuals at a particular point in time, and, extended back through time, considerably larger than that (Boissevain 1974; Hammer 1980; Pool and Kochen 1978). If one moves out from the focal individual not only to the people he or she knows directly, but to people with whom there may be indirect exchange through personal links (second-order contacts), the size of the set expands geometrically. For example, if an acquaintance of my sister wants a recommendation for a psychiatrist or an anthropology course, that information may be mediated through my sister, from me, to her acquaintance. Thus, the extent of the connections that are relevant, even though they are not all direct, would include the thousand or so people an individual knows directly and the thousand or so people each of them knows directly.

Since it is obviously not feasible to collect data on perhaps a million people in each individual's first- and second-order network, it is necessary to place some limits on the sets of contacts that will be included in any social network study. However, as I will try to indicate below, it is important that one not remain bound by the same restrictive definitions, since the initially excluded sets of people may turn out to be consequential. For example, we may limit our initial network definition to include only the people a focal individual knows directly and sees frequently, on the grounds that these are the people who are most significant. For many purposes this may be valid; but we will have omitted (1) people seen infrequently, who provide a person with new sources of information and viewpoints that may not be available through one's familiars; and (2) friends of friends, who are both a pool of people with whom one is likely to form relationships and a direct influence on the people one regularly interacts with.

For the immediate personal network—the people a person interacts with fairly often and regularly—which is the kind of network that has been most extensively studied, there does by now seem to be some generality in the findings on network size and structure for normal individuals. My own data are from London, New York and a rural area in Vermont; and there are data from Edinburgh (Cubitt 1973), Malta (Boissevain 1974) and several places in Africa (Kapferer 1973; Sutton 1979). To the extent that the material reported in different studies is comparable, the sizes of the most immediate networks seem to be within a rather narrow range. For individuals who are considered "close" by the focal individual, the data from these sources indicate an average of about 8 or 9 people, with a range of only about 6 to 12 for most of the data. If you extend this to include other individuals with whom a person has fairly frequent regular contact, there again seems to be a certain consistency: in my data with few exceptions the range is from 20 to 60 people, and the means for different samples are about 30 to 40, which are about the same as those reported in other studies.

In addition to size, there appears to be some generality in the findings to date on certain structural features of these networks. The 40 or so connections of a focal individual typically constitute five to six clusters of about 5 to 8 individuals who are almost all connected with each other as well as with the focal individual; and there are some, but far fewer, connections between individuals from different clusters. Overall, of the 780 theoretically possible connections among 40 individuals, one typically finds that about 20% are actual connections. Most of these connections are clustered into five or six sets; but perhaps a quarter of them connect people from different clusters. Thus, for example, there may be a cluster of close kin who are connected with each other, and a cluster of workmates who are connected with each other, of whom perhaps one or two are also connected with someone in the kin cluster.

The implications of this kind of structure for social feedback to the participants warrant careful investigation: within a cluster, all or almost all possible channels of communication are available, and information from any source can potentially be validated or modified by any other source. Furthermore, the existence of multiple clusters provides multiple responses to one's behavior, multiple views that can reinforce or modify each other. As will appear later, this feedback structure seems typically not to be available (at least in this society) to chronic psychiatric patients, whose networks are more likely to consist of a single cluster—possibly mediated through a single major connection—or of no cluster, but a scattering of individuals not connected with one another (Hammer 1981).

For the immediate personal network of 30 to 40 individuals, we find so far for normal individuals no consistent differences based on age, sex, class, ethnicity or rural-urban residence. (Although our suburban informants do seem to have slightly larger networks, they still tend to be in the same range.) However, studies specifically designed to investigate such differences are quite recent, and the existence of such systematic differences cannot yet be ruled out (Cubitt 1973, 1978; Polgar 1979; Walker 1978). For the total network—including people known only slightly or seen infrequently, in addition to the regular immediate network of about 40 people—there are fewer data to call on. Our own estimate is on the order of 1,000 people, which is similar to the estimates arrived at by two other studies (Hammer 1980; Boissevain 1974; Pool and Kochen 1978). For this larger network, however, the available data suggest substantial class differences, with blue-collar workers having far fewer people they see infrequently than white-collar workers, who in turn have smaller networks of acquaintances than do professionals (Pool and Kochen 1978; Walker 1978). While these infrequently seen or slightly known people are not likely to be of much use in helping with a sick child or doing the household chores, they do constitute potential sources of information and routes of connection that may by quite important when a person needs a job, a school, a doctor, a person to chat with or perhaps a contact in a new community.

All of these networks of people—those a person is close to, the slightly larger immediate network and the total network—can be considered first-order connections, since they are all direct. For certain purposes, however, we might limit the first-order network to those who are seen fairly regularly—typically about 40 people. The first-order connections of those 40 people—that is, the people *they* see fairly regularly—would then be one's second-order connections, although some of these people might be one's own acquaintances. (For example, my sister's friends are part of her immediate network and would be second-order connections for me, although some are also my acquaintances.) People who are second-order connections to each other are still sources of information and possible recommendations on such varied things as movies or apartments or jobs or doctors or bargains or political candidates. This is somewhat more true if they are directly acquainted, but it is still true if they are not. Equally significantly for our purposes here, these second-order connections are the ones whose opinions, demands and so on most directly affect one's own immediate connections. For example, a friend's opinions may well affect a person's behavior towards a spouse or a boss or another friend.

Functions of Social Networks

Thus, one important function of networks is that they are transmission paths. They mediate everything in the society, including official information. For example, our information on which schools or hospitals are good, or how to qualify for food stamps, tends to be mediated through either direct or indirect personal connections. We may get certain kinds of information from public media or from calling an official agency, but we tend either to get it initially or to evaluate and verify it from what some personal source tells us about it. We are not only transmission paths for information; we are also transmission paths for all kinds of behavior patterns, including things like food and drinking habits, and for viruses and other infectious agents.

Another function of networks might be conceived of as a "cushioning" function. Actually, this is the one that has received most attention in the health literature—the notion that networks provide social supports which can buffer the effects of stress. For example, someone to care for a child who is ill can intervene so that a working mother can keep her job; or a sufficient social support system can provide a loan of money for a mortgage in a bad period so that one can keep one's home; or the emotional trauma of some distressing event can be somewhat mitigated by having supportive people to talk to.

A third critical function of the social network is its influence on the formation and modulation of one's behavior. This is perhaps most significant in the initial formation of behavior, although it continues throughout life. I suggested earlier that characteristically, psychiatric patients tend not to have adequate command of the complex cultural codes governing every level of social behavior. In some cases, one may suppose, such command was never acquired. Although there is little direct evidence of the social variables necessary to such acquisition, there can be no question that differences in social exposure are relevant. The very young child learns the language that will be spoken, the dialect of that language, the ways of relating to people and virtually everything that he or she knows from the people around. These patterns are very likely to be different if there are many people around or few; if there are the same people repeatedly or a number of different people; if there are other children around, and if they are the same age or older or younger.

Social Networks and the Development of Social Skills

There are virtually no data on the social networks of young children, or on their consequences for the acquisition of social skills. Our preliminary work (Hammer and Gutwirth 1979) on several presumably normal infants shows an impressive range of contacts even in the first year of life, with clusters consisting of household members, father's kin, mother's kin, parents' friends, older siblings' friends, neighbors, and some additional people such as a couple of the mother's work contacts, a grandmother's friends, an aunt's neighbors. At this young age (the infant's first year), peer contacts may be minimal, but there are numerous contacts with older children. Lewis and Feiring (1979) report for the networks of three-year-olds an average of about six frequent peer contacts in addition to the child's relatives and almost all of the mother's important contacts. S. Salzinger et al. (1975) find, also for children about age 3, that those with more peer interaction tend to have relatively more communicative speech; and a study in Hungary (Hollos 1977) reports more sophisticated pronominal usage for children with more social contacts.

Apart from these few findings, we can make certain tentative inferences from a variety of indirect sources, such as a number of primate studies on isolation from the mother or from peers, or some of the studies of institutionalized infants, or the effects of twinning on language development. (Twins, and even more so triplets and quadruplets, have somewhat retarded language development (Bates 1975), perhaps because the structure of their social feedback system is somewhat deviant from that of single children.) One recent primate study is of particular interest here (Suomi 1979). Physical arrangements were designed for young rhesus monkeys which either intensified or inhibited the amount of peer contact in middle infancy. When the animals from the two contrasting settings were later brought into contact with each other, those reared in the high-peer-interaction setting were invariably dominant over the others. In addition, the high-peer-interaction monkeys were markedly less vulnerable than the others to depression during and after the stress of temporary isolation. Note that these results are controlled by the differing amounts of peer interaction engendered by the experimental conditions, and thus not initially inherent in the individual monkeys. Note, too, that neither group of animals was *deprived* of peer contact during rearing; the physical conditions simply *encouraged* more peer contact in one group than in the other.

Based on the primate work, the limited data on children and the evidence of early social restrictedness for certain psychiatric patients (Gittelman-Klein and Klein 1969), one may hypothesize that for some patients, early social experiences may not have provided the foundations for adequate acquisition of social skills. Others seem to have experienced a deterioration of such skills, either through the social distortions engendered in large institutions (Gruenberg 1967) or through a relative lack of social practice as a result of having comparatively few social contacts (Silberfeld 1978; Mechanic 1978; Grierson and Green 1979). We cannot say what levels of varied social feedback are necessary to the modulation of one's behavior; nor is it likely that the same levels are appropriate to all people. But below some minimum, the ability to function socially is disrupted. There is in fact some reason to speculate that schizophrenic patients—who are a considerable proportion of chronic psychiatric patients—may require *more* social input for the modulation of behavior than normal adults do, though they typically elicit less (K. Salzinger and Pisoni 1958, 1960, 1961; Beels 1979).

III. SOCIAL NETWORKS AND HEALTH

Social Networks and Health: Conceptual Models

As noted above, most of the available material on the impact of social networks on health conceptualizes the relationship as a buffering one—that is, that the network has the capacity to intervene and offset some of the impact of other conditions. In the studies I will refer to below, the work on depression in young mothers appears to follow a more direct causal model. It may be useful here briefly to sketch out several kinds of models of the ways in which social networks may have an impact on health—causal, mediating, buffering or more generally moderating.

In a causal model, some network characteristic is purported to have a direct effect on some health-related outcome. I mentioned before primate work on the effects of early isolation from the mother or from peers, both of which have impacts on subsequent social behavior and subsequent health. The study cited above by Suomi (1979), which shows a direct effect on vulnerability to depression of the early experimental manipulation of peer contacts in rhesus infants, provides a clearer example of a causal model than is readily available from human studies. In human work studies on the association of depression with significant social losses, or with a general contraction of social contacts, seem also to follow a causal model (e.g., Paykel 1974).

Another model involving social networks that may be of less interest here is a biosocial model, with social networks providing routes for the spread of an infectious agent, the spread of nutritional habits, the spread of drug and alcohol habits, the spread of information (Coleman et al. 1957; Kandel 1974; Greenwald et al. 1979). Depending on emphasis, this model may be viewed as either causal (with emphasis on the transmission routes) or mediating (with emphasis on what is being transmitted).

The model of networks as mediating rather than causing a health condition sees the network as affecting the likelihood of occurrence of various health-relevant events or conditions—the loss of one's home, or poverty, as well as infectious agents or drug use. For example, the probability of becoming a heavy drinker or drug user is obviously affected by the patterns of use mediated by one's social connections; and somewhat less obviously, the probability of obtaining or keeping one's home may depend on whether one's network can mediate a source of money (jobs, loans, etc.) for dealing with the rent or the mortgage payment.

The network may also make an event like losing one's home more or less serious by "buffering" the effects. If you do lose your home, will you have a place to live; or if you lose your spouse, will you have people to see; if you lose your job, are there people who can tide you over (a buffering role) or connect you with another job (a mediating role)?

The networks may, more generally, have a complex moderating effect on developments in the individual's life. If, for example, an individual has, for whatever personal reasons, some tendency to withdraw, he or she may simply become more and more isolated if involved in a rather loose and brittle network; whereas in a strongly interconnected network, the connections with the individual may not become severed despite the individual's attempted withdrawal.

Finally, the network plays a role in how its members directly treat the patient and in the choice of other sources of treatment. Given that a person has psychiatric symptoms, he or she may go to a psychiatrist, to a clinic, to a church, to a spirit cult, to friends (Garrison 1977). The selection of where one goes with the problem is very largely a function of one's network.

It is obvious that the causal, mediating, buffering and other moderating models are not totally separate—for example, with respect to the transmission of an infectious agent, the network could be considered mediating or causal. But these rough conceptual models may set a framework for the findings I will refer to shortly. Something about the networks may in and of itself lead to or mitigate against a psychiatric condition; or some event or life condition with a psychiatric risk may be more or less likely to occur in different networks; or some event or life condition may occur which one kind of social network will handle differently from another, and the outcome of these two will be different psychiatrically for the focal individual; or the focal individual may have some psychiatric condition which gets handled differently by different networks, and the life course of that psychiatric condition may be quite different.

Evidence of the Impact of Social Networks on Health

To set the psychiatrically relevant network studies in a broader health context, a few nonpsychiatric findings should be mentioned here. The most general indication of the impact of social contacts on health is provided by a recently published study of mortality from 1965 to 1974 in Alameda County, California. Berkman and Syme (1979) analyzed social and health data on a population sample of 4,700 men and women aged 30 to 69 and found consistently lower mortality rates for people with many social contacts than for those with few social contacts. These differences remained when controlled for social class, types of health care used, health condition at the start of the study period and a number of other variables; the findings held for both men and women, and in all age categories, with the relative risks for different subgroups ranging from about 2 to about 4.5.

There are several studies which indicate that a combination of stressful life events and "psychosocial assets" (which include network-related variables) is related to a variety of health conditions. One study (Nuckolls et al. 1972) of 170 army wives found that in the presence of a high number of stressful events before and during pregnancy, women with high psychosocial supports had only one third the rate of complications of pregnancy experienced by women with low psychosocial supports. Comparable health differences in relation to psychosocial supports have been reported for asthma (de Aranjo et al. 1973) and angina pectoris (Medalie and Goldbourt 1976), as well as for the health consequences of unemployment due to a factory shutdown (Gore 1973). Pilisuk and Froland (1978), in reviewing a number of studies of social contact patterns and health, cite positive findings in a wide range of health conditions.

Several more psychiatrically oriented studies have examined the importance of having a close confiding relationship as a buffer against the possible psychiatric consequences of stressful events. The presence of a confidant for people undergoing stress has been found to be associated with lower rates of psychiatric disorder (particularly depression) among women (Brown et al. 1975; Miller and Ingham 1976) and among the elderly (Lowenthal and Haven 1968).

In the Miller and Ingham (1976) study, it was also found that women with many casual friends had lower symptom levels than those with few friends. Results for men were similar but weaker. Several other studies have found lower rates of psychiatric symptomatology for people with strong social supports (e.g., Myers et al. 1975; Andrews et al. 1978). Brown et al. (1977) found that women with weaker social supports were more subject to depression, but less subject to anxiety, than women with stronger (more integrated) social supports. This finding warrants further discussion, and I will return to it later since it is indicative of the kinds of cautions that are called for in considering the possible social needs of patients in the community: "more" is not necessarily "better" for all purposes.

High rates of depression have been found among mothers of young children (Brown et al. 1975; Richman 1976), and several writers have emphasized a relative lack of social contacts for these women (Gavon 1966; Weissman and Paykel 1974). Our own data (Hammer et al. in press) as well as findings reported by Pool and Kochen (1978) and by Szalai (1972) suggest that while the network size as such is not typically diminished for these women, frequency of contact or amount of time spent with people may be markedly lower—as it seems to be more generally for people who are not employed.

The Pool and Kochen (1978) data show, for example, that while housewives may see 10 people as often as twice a week, working men and women typically see several times that number. Szalai (1972) reports that nonworking mothers spend less than half the number of hours a day in the company of adults other than the spouse than do employed men and women.

Paykel (1974) has found that events involving "exits" from the social field are strongly associated with depression. He estimates a sixfold increase in risk of depression for persons experiencing such events—e.g., death of a close family member, divorce, a family member leaves home. The data on mothers of young children suggest that the risk of depression associated with social "losses" may not require dramatic exit events: the day-to-day relative sparseness of social contacts experienced by many nonworking mothers may have a comparable impact.

Finally, there are several recent studies of the social networks of schizophrenic patients (Garrison 1978; Pattison et al. 1975; Sokolovsky et al. 1978; Cohen and Sokolovsky 1978; Tolsdorf 1976). The main findings have to do with size, the pattern of clustering of the connections, the content and directionality of the relationships, and the effects on relapse. Tolsdorf (1976), in a study of schizophrenic patients at their first admission to the psychiatric ward of a veteran's hospital, found that while their networks were somewhat smaller than those of a comparable nonpsychiatric sample, they were not significantly so. Other studies (Sokolovsky et al. 1978; Pattison et al. 1975; Garrison 1978), mainly of chronic patients, typically find very small networks. Without longitudinal studies, it is impossible to say whether these different findings reflect a fundamental difference in the samples studied, or a tendency for those patients who initially have the smallest networks to become the chronic patients, or a tendency for patients to lose network connections as they become more chronic (Grierson and Green 1979). With respect to the clustering of connections, Tolsdorf's data suggest unusually high clustering among the kin of these early schizophrenic patients, and relatively little clustering among their nonkin contacts, compared to nonpsychiatric patients. Pattison et al., for samples with more chronic psychotic patients, report a pattern of a single, tightly interconnected cluster of close kin; and the data of Sokolovsky et al. on chronic schizophrenic patients in SRO hotels suggest a scattering of contacts with no clusters. Both Tolsdorf and Sokolovsky et al. report relatively few reciprocal relationships, and relatively few relationships that have more than a single content area. Sokolovsky et al. further report that these variables are associated with the likelihood of relapse. I will try below to utilize some of what we are beginning to know about the normal operation of social networks to interpret these findings.

IV. SOME NETWORK PROPERTIES AND THEIR IMPLICATIONS

Methodological Orientation

Before turning to a more careful examination of the ways networks operate, or of their possible implications for chronic psychiatric patients, I would like simply to mention one methodological consideration. I think there is a tendency in applied fields such as the medical to use a kind of tunnel-vision approach—that is, one focuses on a disorder and on some hypothesized factor that may affect it, then tries to make a quick index of the factor and find out if it is or is not significantly associated with the disorder. Basic examination of how that hypothesized factor operates in its own domain is not part of such an approach.

To take an analogy, there is no question now of the relevance of genetics to many medical conditions; but without what most health institutions would consider rather far-fetched research—that is, studying green and yellow sweet peas and winged and wingless fruit flies, about whose health most of us care very little—we would not know enough about genetics to apply it to health. Note that for most considerations an organism does not have good or bad genes; it has genes that are more or less well adapted to the life conditions of the organism. These life conditions may shift, which would alter the goodness or badness of the set of genes. There are some genetic structures that are not viable or that produce defects in functioning in any potentially available environment, but for many genes this is not the case.

Similarly, for the most part I think it is not appropriate to conceptualize in terms of good and bad network characteristics: let me refer back to the example from Brown's study (1977) of the socially well-integrated individuals who were protected from depression but were more subject to anxiety, and vice versa. There may be some network characteristics that are pathogenic in any social environment, but more generally different network structures will probably have different adaptive properties, with different positive and negative potentials for the individuals involved (Wellman and Leighton 1978; Hirsch 1979). I think these network properties must be studied for their range of effects (not limited to health conditions) in order for us to be able to understand how they may operate with respect to health conditions that we may be interested in.

Structural Supports Among Social Connections

Let me turn now to examine one basic network parameter, the strength of structural supports among social connections, and try to relate it, in terms of its significance for the persistence or severance of relationships, to some of the findings on schizophrenia. In addition to the recent studies cited above, a variety of kinds of evidence over the years points to relative social isolation for schizophrenic patients (although there may be some argument about whether this isolation precedes or is a consequence of illness). I should make it clear that I am interested here not in the psychological processes that may be involved, but in the network processes. These are outside the focal individual, and certain general network processes seem relevant.

Figure 1 shows a diagram of a fairly typical normal personal network limited to people seen fairly often and regularly. The central dot with a circle around it is the focal individual, and the other dots are people the focal individual sees fairly often or considers close. Each of these individuals is by definition directly connected to the focal individual. (For diagrammatic simplicity, these lines of connection are therefore not shown.) No longer by definition, but empirically, there are also a large number of connections among these individuals, and they tend to be clustered. There are about six clusters in this diagram, showing heavy interconnectedness within a cluster, and some cross-cluster connections. The next diagram (Figure 2) shows the network of an individual who was part of a normal community sample but was hospitalized for schizophrenia within the year after the time that this network was plotted. In terms of size, his network is rather on the low side, but there are seemingly normal individuals who have networks this small. More importantly, his connections do not form a number of clusters: there is one cluster and a number of scattered individuals with virtually no connection to each other.

In normal networks, there are virtually no unsupported connections—that is, there is rarely a connection with an individual who is not also connected to some other individuals that the focal individual is connected to. By contrast, in the network of the man subsequently

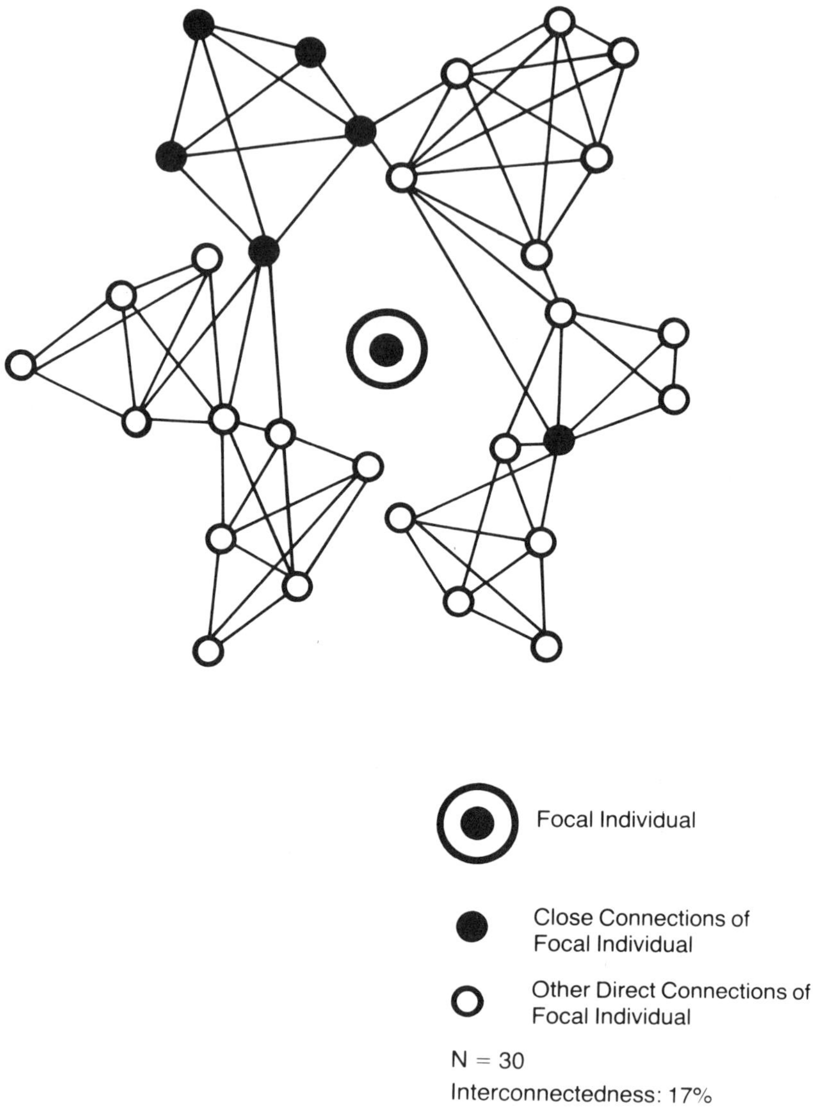
Focal Individual
Close Connections of Focal Individual
Other Direct Connections of Focal Individual
N = 30
Interconnectedness: 17%

Figure 1

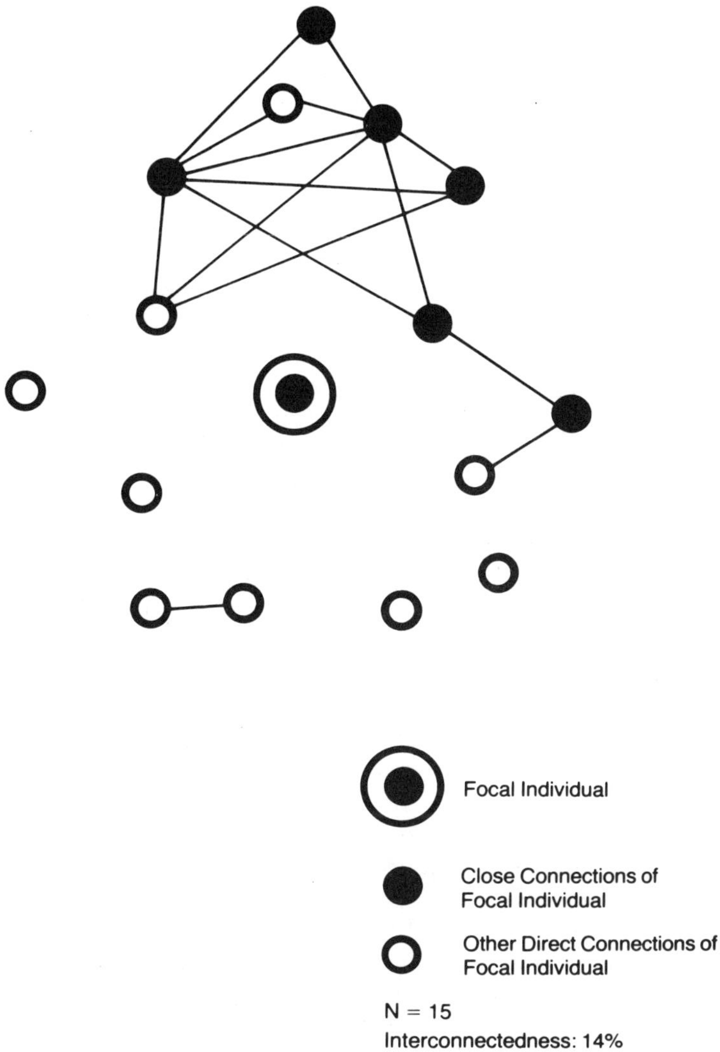
Focal Individual
Close Connections of Focal Individual
Other Direct Connections of Focal Individual
N = 15
Interconnectedness: 14%

Figure 2

diagnosed as schizophrenic, there are four individuals he is connected to who are not connected to anyone else he knows; there is one pair who are connected only to each other; and then there is one cluster of individuals. In fact, this network is even less clustered than it appears, since the focal individual was actually connected to most of the individuals in the cluster primarily through one individual in that cluster, who was a close neighbor. The other individuals in the cluster were people he saw through this one main friend. Shortly after this time, he and his friend moved to separate places, at which time the focal individual's connections to that entire cluster ended, except for occasional contact with the main friend. No direct connection was retained to any of the others in that cluster; and all but one of the additional scattered connections were also severed. The one remaining connection was to a geographically distant relative with whom he continued to be in touch.

This example is in many ways a reflection of the more general findings in studies of schizophrenic patients. The network is fairly small, though not necessarily outside the normal range. The clustering of connections in the network is unlike that of normal networks, with many scattered connections unsupported by links among those connections. In addition, many connections, although they involve direct contact, are basically mediated through a single close connection.

The point to be made here, based on data from psychiatric patients and from normal individuals, is that unsupported connections tend not to persist. In a study I did a number of years ago of schizophrenic patients at Bellevue (Hammer 1961, 1963–4), one of the variables considered was the connectedness of the individuals whom the patient was closest to. Figure 3 shows a number of possible ways that the patient might be linked with other people he or she is close to. The patient may be directly connected to two (or more) individuals who are connected to each other (and then connected indirectly to others through them), as against being connected to individuals who are not connected to each other, and therefore the connections to those individuals do not support each other. This is the basic distinction in the diagrams: on the left, the individuals the patient is closest to are connected to each other, and therefore involve supported connections in the structural sense; on the right, the individuals the patient is closest to are not connected to each other, and these are therefore unsupported connections.

In this study of the 55 patients in the sample, about half had connections like those on the left of Figure 3, and about half like those on the right. Of those with supported connections, all but one set of

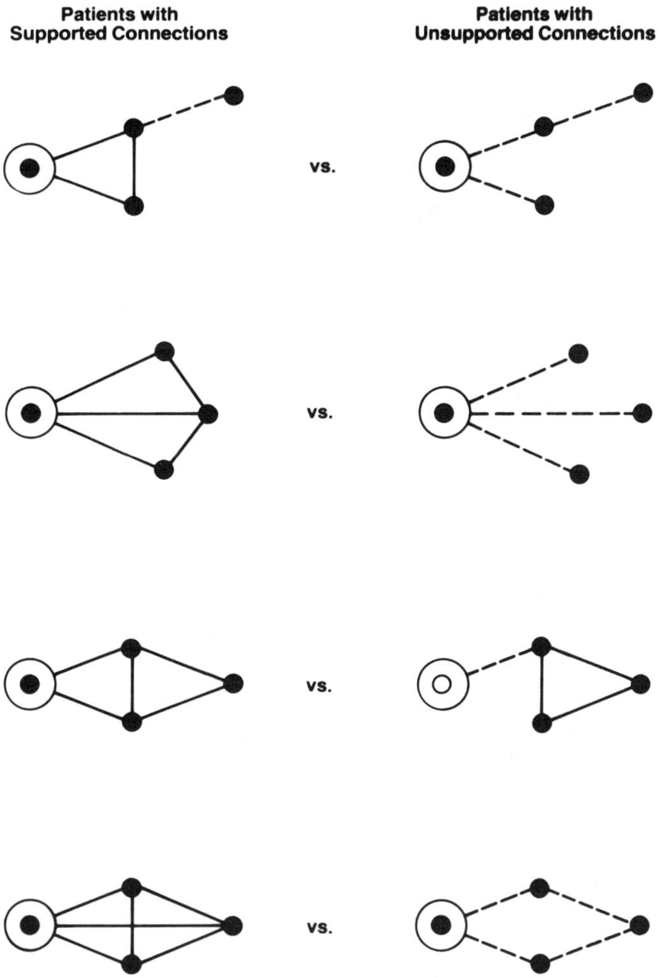
Patients with
Supported Connections
Patients with
Unsupported Connections
vs.
vs.
vs.
vs.

Figure 3

connections persisted through the stress of the period just prior to and during hospitalization; of those with unsupported connections (like those on the right), half had connections that were severed by the time of hospitalization. This is independent of sex and independent of ethnicity, since both groups included Black and Jewish men and women. I should point out here that this finding is probably not attributable to greater network deviance for those patients with unsupported connections: while there is a tendency in normal networks for a focal individual's close connections to know each other, it is by no means aberrant to find that among the closest connections of a normal focal individual, some are not connected to each other (Hammer 1980).

Let me turn now to our findings on structural supports in the networks of normal individuals, and the possible implications for these patterns in schizophrenia. We have data for three locality-based networks, each at two points in time (Hammer 1979-80); data from one of these networks are shown in Figure 4. Given the distribution of connections at the first point in time, one may consider not only who is directly connected to whom, but how many common connections each pair of individuals has—that is, how many individuals have direct connections with both members of the pair.

If you compare all possible pairs in terms of the number of common connections at Time 1, you find a direct linear relationship between the number of common connections at Time 1 and the likelihood that the pair will be directly connected at Time 2. That is, the particular connections grow out of the surrounding connections. This is true both for pairs whose members were directly connected with each other at Time 1 and for pairs whose members were not directly connected with each other at Time 1. Taking the inverse of this for the directly connected pairs at Time 1, the probability that their connection will be severed by Time 2 is again a linear function of the number of common connections at Time 1—less than 20% of connected pairs with many common connections (7-9) fail to persist to Time 2, as compared with almost 60% of those with few common connections (1-3).

This finding holds for normal individuals in three different networks, one of which is a church group, one of which is a local hangout at a doughnut shop and one of which is a factory; and they are from different parts of the world, two in New York and one in Africa (Hammer 1979-80). This seems to be a very strong trend: regardless of any other characteristics of the people or what they are doing, those connections that lack common supporting connections will probably not persist.

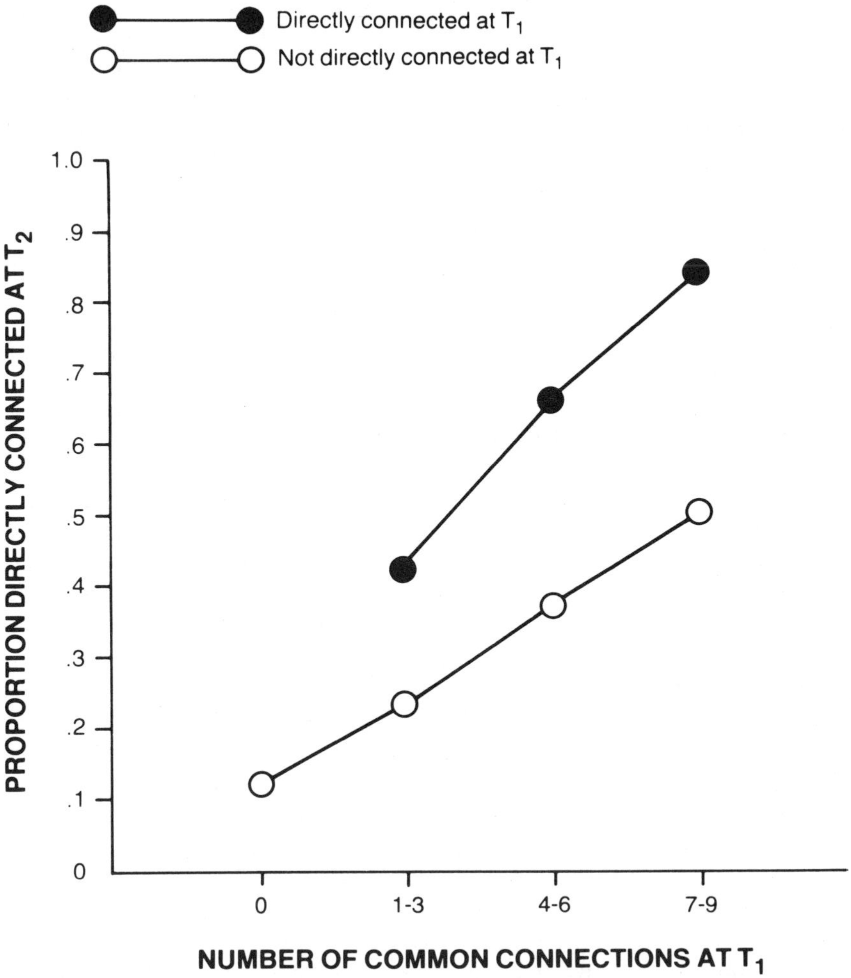

NOTE: This figure is based on data presented in Kapferer (1972).

Figure 4

Thus, if we come back to consideration of schizophrenic individuals, it seems likely that one of the ways in which the schizophrenic patient's network becomes depleted is that it lacks sufficient cross-connectedness among the individuals in the network to assure the maintenance of connections. It would be interesting also to relate this to social "losses" in relation to depression. One would expect that the loss of someone from one's network, through death or for any other reason, would have much more profound impact if one's other relationships depended to a marked extent on that person. For example, a woman with a network of connections primarily in common with her husband would presumably be far worse off at her husband's death than a woman whose important connections also included connected sets of people at her own job and a connected set of neighbors whom she knew better than her husband did (see also Hirsch in press).

Social Class Variants

One may also try to relate these cumulative processes of formation, maintenance and severance of connections to such large-scale variables as migration and class status, which show strong (though complex) epidemiological associations with psychopathology (Hammer et al. 1978). There is little data yet available on such things as class differences in social networks. In fact, as indicated earlier, the size and the clustering pattern for immediate personal networks seems quite similar. However, the Pool and Kochen (1978) data on the size and frequency distribution of larger direct personal networks (including acquaintances as well as people who are known well) is suggestive. Their approach was to have a number of people keep track in detail of everyone they saw or spoke to on the phone or got mail from during a 100-day period. Figure 5, which is based on their data,* shows that in terms of the number of people who are seen fairly frequently, there is virtually no difference between white-collar and professional workers. The blue-collar workers, on the other hand, see a very large proportion of the network quite frequently. For example, though they have smaller networks overall, they see

**The estimates I have calculated should be considered as very rough indications of possible trends. The Pool and Kochen data—drawn largely from the work of Gurevich (1961)—were collected for other purposes and are on a very small number of individuals (N=28) who were not selected to represent the populations from which they were drawn. In addition, the data presented are not complete and do not permit precise computations. The trends, however, are consistent with some other reported findings (Szalai 1972; Walker 1978).*

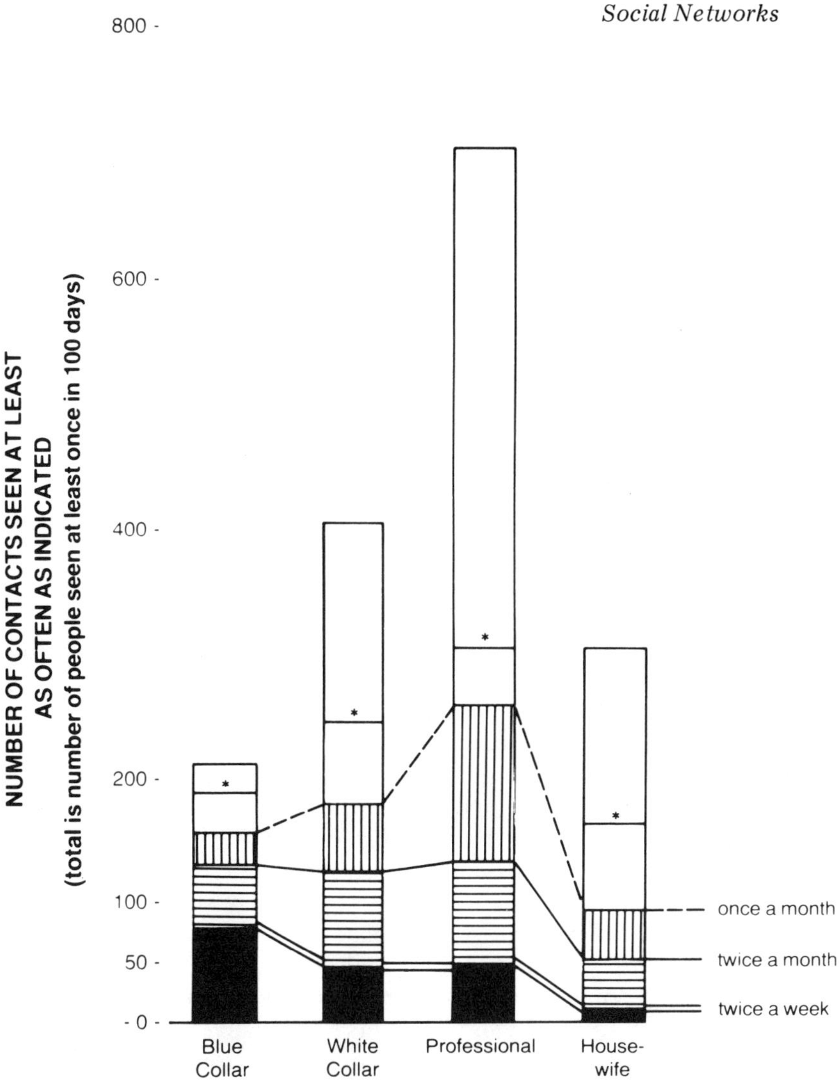

**The uppermost part of the bar represents people seen only once in 100 days.*

NOTE: This figure is based on data presented in Pool and Kochen (1978).

Figure 5

twice as many people as often as twice a week, compared to the white-collar or professional workers. But there are relatively few people they see infrequently. At the other extreme, for professionals, there is a very large number of people whom they see as little as once during the 100 days in which they kept a record. If you consider the upper end of these bar graphs, the professionals see almost half of their total reported network only once during that period. Similarly, although for smaller total networks, housewives and white-collar workers see almost half of their total networks once only; whereas the blue-collar workers see a relatively small number and small proportion that infrequently.

Let us consider a few possible implications of this. The blue-collar workers would seem to have a very solid, steady, regular network. They do however seem at a disadvantage if anything comes along to disrupt their normal situation—if for some reason they have to move or leave a job, they have very little in the way of a network extending out on which they can draw. For the professionals, there is a rather large network—one would have to project that "once-only" in 100 days to a substantially larger number who might be seen other parts of that year, or who might not be seen that year but are still known and potential contacts. If a professional moves, even a considerable distance, it may well be that there is some contact there to move to. Extended out to second-order contacts—people to whom one has access through a personal link—the other professionals known to the focal one have similarly large networks, so that connections one step removed should be a huge number.

In addition, the patterns of socializing that go along with seeing people virtually all of whom are familiars help to develop skills that are rather different from those called for in relating to new situations where almost everyone is unknown to you. Professionals (and to a lesser extent other middle class workers) typically have to acquire some of these more mobile socializing abilities in the ordinary course of their living and work patterns. In moving to new situations, they therefore have these social skills as habits, whereas the stable blue-collar worker, having had less occasion to acquire a different set of skills, is then at a disadvantage. This is of course speculative at this point, but it is perfectly researchable, and could potentially cast light on some of the reasons for higher rates of psychopathology associated with lower class status and with certain patterns of migration (Murphy 1977; Hammer et al. 1978).

Effects of Duration of Connections

Some further characteristics of social network processes may be useful to consider here. The first of these is another aspect of a cumulative process. The extent to which the individuals composing a network are connected to each other increases regularly over time (Hammer and Schaffer 1975). Thus, any network, or part of a network, which consists of relationships of long duration is likely to show interconnected clusters, and this is less often true for contacts of short duration. Duration of contacts also affects "multiplexity"—the degree to which a relationship has multiple content areas (Fitzgerald 1979); and it is associated with reciprocity of relationships, with nonreciprocal ties occurring often in the early phases of friendship formation (Hallinan 1978). Thus, if we return to a consideration of the findings discussed above for schizophrenic patients—relatively sparse connections among the nonkin members of their networks, relatively few multiplex relationships and relatively low reciprocity—we find from studies of normal network processes that the duration of network connections is relevant to the aberrant findings reported for the networks of schizophrenic patients.

Network Boundedness and Reciprocity of Connections

A major distinction that would appear in any typology of networks would have to do with relative boundedness. The personal networks we have emphasized are structurally unbounded: we set a practical limit, based on distance or frequency or some other criterion, but the nature of the network (first-order close or regular or total contacts, second-order contacts, third-order and so on) is unbounded. But there are also structurally bounded networks of which the locality-based sets (such as a small factory or a church group) we discussed earlier are an example. These two network types are participated in by the same people—that is, a given individual who works in a factory or attends a church group also has an "open" personal network. Nevertheless, these network types have different relational properties. For example, connections in open networks tend overwhelmingly to be reciprocal, at least in the sense that if A names B as a connection, B is very likely to name A as a connection. In contrast, in a bounded network, a substantial proportion of the relationships are nonreciprocal, since in a group setting many interactions are of unequal salience to the participants. (If A is talking to B, C and D, A's participation is more salient to B, C and D than B or C or D is individually to A—Hammer, ms.)

By tentative inference, if a schizophrenic patient is encouraged to participate in bounded groups in order to increase the patient's sociability in a comparatively undemanding mode, there is a danger of encouraging increasing proportions of nonreciprocal relationships in his or her network.

Summary

There are several ways in which the social network may be relevant to health in general and to mental health in particular. It is clearly relevant to the way in which the individual is treated once that individual becomes psychiatrically ill, in terms of people's knowledge about facilities and in terms of the degree to which the individual will be taken care of by personal contacts. It may also be relevant in terms of mediating the occurrence of health-relevant events, or of buffering the impact of various sources of stress on a vulnerable individual. It may affect the likelihood of illness or the severity of illness; and it may be relevant independently as a causal factor in the way it affects the person's life style, the amount of satisfaction a person has in the way he or she lives, and the feedback system in which the person is involved, which helps that person to moderate and coordinate his or her own behavior in ways which will fit the social requirements.

Social networks have their own properties, quite apart from an individual's input. Some people may be more gregarious than others, some people may know more people because they are involved in more activities. But beyond this, the networks that one is involved in have their own properties—they expand and they contract in accord with the characteristics of their own structure. Furthermore, there are certain regularities of size for at least the most immediate network that seem to cut across very wide social differences. The size of the total network appears to differ for different social groups, and this again has its implications for the individuals involved in the network.

Network processes involve certain cumulative features: reciprocity of relationships, multiplexity and interconnectedness are all in part a function of duration. The likelihood of connections persisting through time is also a function of the number of supporting links adjacent to that connection. And different types of networks, such as bounded and open networks, have different structural properties, with different implications for the component relationships.

V. IMPLICATIONS FOR TREATMENT

It is clear that despite increasing evidence of the impact of people's social networks on their functioning in many areas, attempts to help chronic patients to modify their patterns of social contact call for extreme caution. (Such caution is called for in all therapy—such as in the use of drugs—but that is not the subject of this paper.) Any alteration has multiple effects, and we do not yet know enough to predict them. In addition, as indicated earlier, differences in network characteristics need not be uniformly "good" or "bad," but may be one or the other (or neither) under different conditions or possibly for different people. Loss or severe restriction of social contacts may elicit depression (Paykel 1974); but involvement in highly integrated social networks may lead to increased anxiety (Brown et al. 1977). Wing (1978) noted, for schizophrenic patients, that lack of social stimulation produces apathy, but that "overstimulation" may trigger florid symptoms.

In addition to what may be considered the more technical reasons for caution—our limited knowledge in this area—it is important to bear in mind ethical issues which will only be partly resolved by increased knowledge. The manipulation of social relationships may have instrumentally beneficial consequences; but relationships are not merely instrumental, and the noninstrumental ways in which they are valued must be respected. For example, the honoring of confidentiality, the recognition of a sense of privacy, will at times conflict with obtaining or using the personal information necessary to a network intervention; but without strict concern for these ethical demands, the therapist is likely to contribute more to the dehumanization of the patient than to the patient's social functioning.

Nonetheless, given the critical importance of the social functioning of chronic patients—both for themselves and for those directly and even indirectly connected to them—one must make some cautious attempts in this direction. From what was discussed earlier, several suggestions can be derived for further exploration.

If connections are to persist, they need to support each other. For those chronic patients whose contacts are mainly with separate individuals not related to each other, it may be worth investigating some combination of three possible interventions: can several of these individuals be brought into meaningful relationship with each other? can the patient be brought into relationship with several of the other connections of one of his or her main contacts? can the patient's relationships with a more connected set be strengthened or initiated? Single connected sets, however, do not seem to provide sufficient feedback or satisfaction, and care should be taken to encourage more than one cluster of connections (see Hirsch in press).

The use of groups to foster more social contacts may well be on the wrong track, unless these are used as starting points for the development of more open network connections (e.g., Budson and Jolley 1978). Our limited evidence suggests that groups tend quite normally to have more asymmetry of relationships than do open networks, and increasing the asymmetry in the chronic patient's set of connections is probably not the right direction of change.

A major asymmetry noted for many patients (Kostant et al. 1979; Hammer 1961) is the encapsulation of the network in someone else's —the patient's set of contacts being largely mediated through one major contact, often a spouse or a mother. It may be possible to modify this encapsulation by helping to develop a few of those relationships more directly; or by helping to develop a set of relationships separate from that mediator. (This may be one important extra benefit in holding a job.) One approach to modifying this encapsulation insists on complete (if temporary) severance of certain dominant connections, while intervening actively to help create other connections (Stein and Test 1978). Significantly, the Stein and Test approach provides the patient with a team of people (rather than a single therapist) available around the clock and available to the patient in the contexts in which the patient functions, rather than in a disconnected office. Whatever else their approach may accomplish, they are providing the patient with a connected cluster, not mediated through a single individual, in addition to other connections that the patient may maintain or form.

The building of social networks is not a quick process even for normally adept people. It is important to be aware that many patients may need continuing input from a staff over many years (Beels 1979; Makiesky-Barrow and Gutwirth in press), though this "staff" may consist of community people who are not professionals (Weinman and Kleiner 1978).

One further use of social networks in community-based psychiatric programs is not concerned with social intervention as such, but with improving the effectiveness of these programs in reaching the relevant people. A substantial number of psychiatric patients have little or no contact with programs designed for them (Makiesky-Barrow and Gutwirth in press). While there are a number of factors contributing to this, two are based on inadequate communication—patients may not know what programs exist; and programs may be ignorant of patients' needs and opinions. Informal social networks can potentially provide the most effective routes for the transmission of such information, in both directions; but these networks are listed in no directory and can only be uncovered by direct community research.

What I have so far said views the patient in the classic way as the recipient of treatment. It does seem to be possible that some benefits can be achieved in this way. But a patient is part of a community of people, all of whom have social relationships, some of them with patients. It may prove more productive to examine what characteristics of the social relationships in a community enhance or diminish their availability, in the "natural" course of events, to people with special needs. Two very different sources of information support the view that our communities are so structured that many people find their social ties to be inadequate: a good deal of nontechnical writing, both fiction and social commentary, has been saying this for some years and seems consistent with survey data (Wellman 1979); and the finding that schizophrenic patients seem to have much better prognoses in non-Western-industrial cultures (Waxler 1979; World Health Organization 1979) is at least plausibly a function of social patterns involving large extended family and friendship networks of long duration that appear to be quite persistent—e.g., in Nigeria (Sutton 1979). While there is no easy formula for doing so, it seems entirely appropriate that community oriented mental health care should devote some substantial energy to the community, rather than more narrowly and exclusively to the patient in the community. I do not mean to suggest that it is within the province—or the ability—of mental health programs to reorganize society (see Borus 1975; Roche report 1980); but it does seem both necessary and possible to develop approaches that nonetheless go beyond an exclusive focus on identified patients.

Finally, to return to the point with which I started, while the social networks of psychiatric patients in the community seem clearly to be important, one cannot yet "prescribe" which specific interventions would most effectively modify them. However, whether deliberately or not, any treatment program necessarily involves some manipulation of the patient's social network, and it may be as well to do so consciously, and to monitor the consequences. What might be worth emphasizing at this time is that those who are responsible to the patients and the communities should make themselves much more aware of the probable impacts of any course of treatment on the patient's set of social connections, keep track of them and contribute to increasing our knowledge of the relevant processes.

REFERENCES

Andrew, G., Tennant, C., Hewson, D. M., and Vaillant, G. Life event stress, social support, coping style, and risk of psychological impairment. *J. Nerv. Ment. Disease* 166: 307-316 (1978).

Bates, E. Peer relations and the acquisition of language, in *Friendship and Peer Relations*, M. Lewis and L. A. Rosenblum, eds. New York: Wiley, 1975, pp. 259-292.

Beels, C. C. Social networks and schizophrenia. *Psychiatric Quarterly* 51: 209-215 (1979).

Berkman, L. F., and Syme, S. L. Social networks, host resistance, and mortality: a nine-year follow-up study of Alameda County residents. *Am. J. Epid.* 109: 186-204 (1979).

Blumenthal, R., Kreisman, D., and O'Connor, P. A. Return to the family and its consequence for rehospitalization among recently discharged mental patients. *Psychol. Med.* 12: 141-147 (1982).

Boissevain, J. *Friends of Friends*. New York: St. Martin's Press, 1974.

Borus, J. F. Issues critical to the survival of community mental health. *Am. J. Psychi.* 135(9): 1029-1035 (1978).

Brown, G. W., Bhrolchain, M. N., and Harris, T. Social class and psychiatric disturbance among women in an urban population. *Sociology* 9: 225-254 (1975).

Brown, G. W., Davidson, S., Harris, T., MacLean, U., Pollack, S., and Prudo, R. Psychiatric disorder in London and North Uist. *Soc. Sci. Med.* 11: 367-377 (1977).

Budson, R. D., and Jolley, R. E. A crucial factor in community program success. *Schizophrenia Bulletin* 4(4): 609-621 (1978).

Coleman, J., Katz, E., and Menzel, H. The diffusion of an innovation among physicians. *Sociometry* 20(4): 253-270 (1957).

Cubitt, T. Network density among urban families, in *Network Analysis Studies in Human Interaction*, J. Boissevain and J. C. Mitchell, eds. The Hague: Mouton, 1973, pp. 67-82.

Cubitt, T., Friends, neighbors and kin; development of social contacts with special reference to stages in the life cycle and class factors. *Connections* 1(3): 42 (1978).

de Aranjo, G., van Arsdel, P., Holmes, T. H., and Dudley, D. L. Life change, coping ability and chronic intrinsic asthma. *J. Psychosom. Res.* 12: 359-363 (1973).

Fitzgerald, M. The content and structure of friendship: An analysis of the friendships of urban Cameroonians. *Connections* 2: 100-101 (1979).

Garrison, V. Doctor, Espiritista, or Psychiatrist? Health-seeking behavior in a Puerto Rican neighborhood of New York City. *Medical Anthro.* 1(2): 65-180 (1977).

Garrison, V. Support systems of schizophrenic and non-schizophrenic Puerto Rican migrant women in New York City. *Schizophrenia Bulletin* 4(4): 591-596 (1978).

Gavon, H. *The Captive Wife: Conflicts of Housebound Mothers.* London: Routledge and Kegan Paul, 1966.

Gittelman-Klein, R., and Klein, D. Premorbid social adjustment and prognosis in schizophrenia. *J. Psychi. Res.* 7: 35-53 (1969).

Gore, S. *The Influence of Social Support in Ameliorating the Consequences of Job Loss.* Ph.D. dissertation, Univ. of Pennsylvania (1973).

Greenwald, P., Rose, J. S., and Daitch, P. B. Acquaintance networks among leukemia and lymphoma patients. *Am. J. Epid.* 110: 162-177 (1979).

Grierson, S. B. and Green, B. C. The effects of psychiatric hospitalization: a social network analysis. *Am. Psychol. Assoc.*, New York (1979).

Gruenberg, E. The social breakdown syndrome—some origins. *Am. J. Psychi.* 123: 1481-1489 (1967).

Gurevich, M. *The Social Structure of Acquaintanceship Networks.* Cambridge, Mass.: MIT Press, 1961.

Hallinan, M. The process of friendship formation. *Social Networks* 1: 193-210 (1978).

Hammer, M. An analysis of social networks as factors influencing the hospitalization of mental patients. Ph.D. Dissertation, Columbia University, *Dissertation Abstracts International.* Ann Arbor, Michigan: University Microfilms (No. 61-3383) 1961.

Hammer, M. Influence of small social networks as factors on mental hospital admission. *Human Org.* 22: 243-251 (1963-64).

Hammer, M. Social supports, social networks, and schizophrenia. *Schizophrenia Bulletin* 7(1): 45-57 (1981).

Hammer, M. Social access and the clustering of personal connections. *Social Networks* 2: 305-325 (1980).

Hammer, M. Predictability of social connections over time. *Social Networks* 2: 165-180 (1979-80).

Hammer, M. Direct and indirect connections in two types of social network. (ms.).

Hammer, M., and Gutwirth, L. Some preliminary data on the social networks of parents and infants. Amer. Anthro. Assoc., Cincinnati (1979).

Hammer, M., and Schaffer, A. Interconnectedness and the duration of connections in several small networks. *Am. Ethnologist* 2(2): 297-308 (1975).

Hammer, M., Makiesky-Barrow, S., and Gutwirth, L. Social networks and schizophrenia. *Schizophrenia Bulletin* 4: 522-545 (1978).

Hammer, M., Gutwirth, L. and Phillips, S. L. Parenthood and social networks: A preliminary view. *Soc. Sci. Med.* (in press).

Hirsch, B. Psychological dimensions of social networks: a multimethod analysis. *Am. J. Community Psychol.* 7: 263-277 (1979).

Hirsch, B. Natural support systems and coping with major life changes. *Am. J. Community Psychol.* (in press).

Hollos, M. Comprehension and use of social rules in pronoun selection by Hungarian children, in *Child Discourse*, S. M. Ervin-Tripp and C. Mitchell-Kernan, eds. New York: Academic Press, 1977.

Kandel, D. Inter- and intragenerational influences on adolescent marijuana use. *J. Soc. Issues* 30(2): 107-135 (1974).

Kapferer, B. *Strategy and Transaction in an African Factory*. Manchester: Manchester University Press, 1972.

Kapferer, B. Social network and conjugal roles in urban Zambia: a reformulation of the Bott hypothesis, in *Network Analysis: Studies in Human Interaction*, J. Boissevain and J. C. Mitchell, eds. The Hague: Mouton, 1973, pp. 83-110.

Kostant, E., with Fishman, J., Garrison, V., Rabin, A., and Watson, A. M. *A Special Kind of Help*. Mental Health Association of Essex County (1979).

Lewis, M., and Feiring, C. The child's social network: social object, social functions, and their relationship, in *The Child and Its Family*, M. Lewis and L. A. Rosenblum, eds. New York: Plenum Publishing Corporation, 1979.

Lowenthal, M. F., and Haven, C. Interaction and adaptation: intimacy as a critical variable. *Am. Soc. Rev.* 33: 20-30 (1968).

Makiesky-Barrow, S., and Gutwirth, L. Community treatment as the least restrictive alternative, in *Patient Rights and Patient Advocacy: Issues and Evidence*, B. L. Bloom and S. J. Asher, eds. Community Psychology Series (in press).

Mechanic, D. Alternatives to mental hospital treatment: a sociological perspective, in *Alternatives to Mental Hospital Treatment*, L. I. Stein and M. A. Test, eds. New York: Plenum Press, 1978.

Medalie, J. H. and Goldbourt, U. Angina pectoris among 10,000 men: II. Psychosocial and other risk factors as evidenced by a multivariate analysis of a five year incidence study. *Am. J. Med.* 60: 910-921 (1976).

Miller, P. Mc C., and Ingham, J. G. Friends, confidants and symptoms. *Social Psychi.* 11: 51-58 (1976).

Mosher, L. R. and Menn, A. Z. Lowered barriers in the community: the Soteria model, in *Alternatives to Mental Hospital Treatment*, L. I. Stein and M. A. Test, eds. New York: Plenum Press, 1978.

Murphy, H. B. M. Migration, culture and mental health. *Psychol. Med.* 7: 677-684 (1977).

Myers, J. K., Lindenthal, J. J., and Pepper, M. P. Life events, social integration and psychiatric symptomatology. *J. Health Soc. Beh.* 16: 421-427 (1975).

Nuckolls, K. B., Cassel, J., and Kaplan, B. H. Psychosocial assets, life crisis and the prognosis of pregnancy. *Am. J. Epid.* 95: 431-441 (1972).

Pattison, E. M., de Francisco, D., Wood, P., Frazier, H., and Crowder, J. A psychosocial kinship model for family therapy. *Am. J. Psychi.* 132: 1246-1251 (1975).

Paykel, E. S. Life stress and psychiatric disorder: applications of the clinical approach, in *Stressful Life Events: Their Nature and Effects*, B. S. Dohrenwend and B. P. Dohrenwend, eds. New York: Wiley, 1974, pp. 135-149.

Pilisuk, M., and Froland, C. Kinship, social networks, social support, and health. *Soc. Sci. Med.* 12B: 273-280 (1978).

Polgar, S. K. Menopause: Factors affecting social redefinition and support systems. *Am. Anthro. Assoc.*, Cincinnati (1979).

Pool, I. de S., and Kochen, M. Contacts and influence. *Social Networks* 1: 5-51 (1978).

Richman, N. Depression in mothers of preschool children. *J. Child. Psychol. and Psychi.* 17: 75-78 (1976).

Roche Report. The realm of mental health: discriminating mandate from myth. *Roche Report: Frontiers of Psychiatry* 10(1): pp. 1 & 6 (1/1/80).

Salzinger, K., and Pisoni, S. Reinforcement of affect responses of schizophrenics during the clinical interview. *J. Abn. Soc. Psychol.* 57: 84-90 (1958).

Salzinger, K., and Pisoni, S. Reinforcement of verbal affect responses of normal subjects during the interview. *J. Abn. Soc. Psychol.* 60: 127-130 (1960).

Salzinger, K., and Pisoni, S. Some parameters of the conditioning of affect responses in schizophrenic subjects. *J. Abn. Soc. Psychol.* 63: 511-516 (1961).

Salzinger, S., Patenaude, J. W., and Lichtenstein, A., A descriptive study of the effects of selected variables on the communicative speech of preschool children. *Annals of the N.Y. Acad. Sci.* 263: 114-131 (1975).

Silberfeld, M. Psychosocial symptoms and social supports. *Soc. Psychi.* 13: 11-17 (1978).

Sokolovsky, J., Cohen, C., Berger, D., and Geiger, J. Personal networks of ex-mental patients in a Manhattan SRO hotel. *Human Org.* 37(1): 5-15, (1978).

Stein, L. I., and Test, M. A. An alternative to mental hospital treatment, in *Alternatives to Mental Hospital Treatment*, L. I. Stein and M. A. Test, eds. New York: Plenum Press, 1978.

Strayer, R. G. and Keith, R. A. An ecological study of the recently discharged chronic psychiatric patient. *J. of Community Psychol.* 7: 313-317 (1979).

Suomi, S. Diminishing vulnerability to social incompetence through early peer play. *Am. Psychol. Assoc.* New York (1979).

Sutton, C. Personal communication. (1979).

Szalai, A., ed. *The Use of Time*. The Hague: Mouton and Co., 1972.

Test, M. A., and Stein, L. I. Training in community living: research design and results, in *Alternatives to Mental Hospital Treatment*, L. I. Stein and M. A. Test, eds. New York: Plenum Press, 1978.

Tolsdorf, C. C. Social networks, support, and coping: an exploratory study. *Family Process* 15(4): 407-418 (1976).

Walker, R. L. Social and spatial constraints in the development and functioning of social networks: A case study of Guildford. *Connections* 1(3): 45-48 (1978).

Waxler, N. E. Is outcome for schizophrenia better in non-industrial societies? The case of Sri Lanka. *J. Nerv. Ment. Disease* 167: 144-158 (1979).

Weinman, B., and Kleiner, R. J. The impact of community living and community member intervention on the adjustment of the chronic psychiatric patient, in *Alternatives to Mental Hospital Treatment*, L. I. Stein and M. A. Test, eds. New York: Plenum Press, 1978.

Weissman, M., and Paykel, E. *The Depressed Woman: A Study of Social Relationships*. Chicago: University of Chicago Press, 1974.

Wellman, B. The community question: the intimate networks of East Yonkers. *Am. J. Sociol.* 84: 1201-1231 (1979).

Wellman, B., and Leighton, B. Networks, neighborhoods and communities. Research Paper #97, Centre for Urban and Community Studies, Toronto (1978).

Wing, J. K. Social influences on the course of schizophrenia, in *The Nature of Schizophrenia: New Approaches to Research and Treatment*, L. C. Wynne, R. L. Cromwell, and S. Matthysse, eds. New York: Wiley, 1978, pp. 599-616.

World Health Organization. *Schizophrenia An International Follow-up Study.* New York: Wiley, 1979.

CHAPTER 4

PROBLEMS IN PROVIDING EFFECTIVE CARE FOR THE CHRONIC PSYCHIATRIC PATIENT

IVAN BAROFSKY, Ph.D.
CATHERINE E. CONNELLY, D.N.Sc.

INTRODUCTION

A critical question for any provider dealing with the chronic psychiatric patient in the community is whether the patient will follow advice or requests made of him or her. The public, in general, suspects that the psychiatric nature of the person's dysfunctions will lead to noncompliance and a lack of effective management of the patient when in the community. This chapter deals with this issue by focusing on one aspect of this complex problem: medication compliance.[1] Even limiting the discussion to this one issue, however, raises a variety of questions. For example:

- What is the rate of medication noncompliance by the chronic psychiatric patient in the community?
- Is this noncompliance rate different than that for patients prescribed other medications?
- Does medication noncompliance result in an increase in relapse and/or rehospitalization rate?
- What factors determine the noncompliance rate of the chronic psychiatric patient in the community?
- What factors determine relapse of the chronic psychiatric patient in the community and how is this related to compliance behavior?

It was quickly discovered that the available literature does not provide adequate answers to all these questions. To provide such information required that this chapter be more data oriented and analytic than would be expected of other chapters in this book.

Quantification, it can be argued, is especially necessary in addressing problems in a field characterized by chronicity and palliative treatment. This is due to special difficulties inherent in sustaining each member of the treatment team in the face of the frustrations of ongoing illness. In this situation it is easy for the clinician to point an accusing finger at the supposed uncooperativeness of the patient to account for recurrent illness. There are two common misconceptions in regard to the treatment of the chronic psychiatric patient. First, that he is uniquely medication noncompliant due to the psychiatric nature of his condition. Second, that he primarily relapses explicitly due to this medication noncompliance. In fact, the psychiatric patient is no less compliant in taking his medications that any other type of patient; furthermore, relapse is not necessarily caused by medication noncompliance. Actually, a measurable relapse rate occurs in spite of, and in the face of, medication compliance, This clearly suggests that it is not the compliance behavior of the patient which alone or uniquely accounts for relapse. Rather, one of the significant causes must be identified as being the limited efficacy of the medications themselves. As will be shown, a whole host of variables, outside stresses included (Table VII), can contribute to relapse in spite of ongoing medication compliance. Thus, the patient's uncooperativeness should not be simplistically blamed for his own relapse.

A therapeutic regimen consists of a wide range of activities (from providing living facilities to providing drugs), each of which may be evaluated as "effective" if its implementation results in the achievement of certain therapeutic goals. These goals may be either curative or palliative depending on the illness and the treatment options. Treatment goals are curative when the application of specific measures corrects the underlying pathology resulting in the alleviation of symptoms and the end of the need for further treatment. In contrast, palliative treatment controls symptoms but does not usually alter the pathological state or dysfunction. Effective care for palliative treatment programs, therefore, is measured by the degree to which symptoms are controlled. A third type of care involves persons who lack some of the elements required for independent living, and who also require palliative treatment. Effective care for these patients, who will most likely receive their care in an institutional setting, will also be evaluated differently. Psychiatric patients may receive each of the types of care, but effective care for the chronic psychiatric patient in the community would ordinarily only involve evaluation of palliative care.

Table 1 Providing Effective Care for the Chronic Psychiatric Patient in the Community: Structural Variables, Process and Outcome Measures

Structural Variables	Process Measures	Outcome Measures
Patient Characteristics Health Care System Variables Situational Determinants	Interpersonal Relationships Participation Pattern — Medication Compliance —Appointment Keeping Social Functioning	Medical Status Psychiatric Status — Relapse Rate — Hospitalization Rate — Length of Community Stay Functional Status

Table 1 summarizes an analytic model which includes the elements involved in providing care for the chronic psychiatric patient in the community. The model is similar to that used to evaluate the quality of provider-based medical care (e.g., Donabedian 1978). It differs from this model in the unit of analysis, which is broader than commonly used, and which includes "situational factors" as a structural variable. By including "situational factors" as a structural variable, we are acknowledging that the unique sensitivity of the psychiatric patient to over- or understimulation in social situations has an organic base and can be an overriding determinant of the care the patient receives. The model rests on the assumption that the outcome of the therapeutic encounter depends on what the patient brings into the situation (whether extended or recent in history) and characteristics of the health care system, as mediated by a variety of specific processes that describe the care process itself. Clearly, the care provided a patient is effective if it maximizes the medical, psychiatric and functional status of the patient.

A review reveals three broad sets of studies, each of which measures some aspect of effective care (Table 1). Included are:

A. studies which relate patient characteristics (such as age, sex or race), health care system variables (such as a physician's attitude toward drugs, the care setting, etc.) or situational determinants (such as a life crisis) to a patient's participation pattern (appointment keeping, medication compliance),

B. studies which measure how the patient's participation pattern (such as failure to take medication) contributes to his/her psychiatric status; and

C. studies which predict the patient's psychiatric status on the basis of various structural variables (e.g., age as a predictor of hospitalization rate).

The maximum information about the quality and nature of care a psychiatric patient receives in the community would be provided if both Type A and Type B studies were performed on the same sample of patients. Unfortunately, this is rarely true. Instead, inferences from the literature will most often have to be drawn on the basis of uncorrelated studies.

The plan for this chapter is to discuss what is known about compliance behavior for a specific group of patients, outpatients schizophrenics prescribed phenothiazines, and to assess the contribution of this behavior to problems in providing effective care. We will start with a review of some of the issues involved in measuring noncompliance and then summarize what is known about Type B, A and C studies in that order. What we will learn is that the mechanics of providing care (which can range from insuring that a patient keeps an appointment or takes a medication, to managing a community's response to the presence of the chronic patient) is just one factor—along with such factors as the efficacy of the treatment options (do the drugs work?) and the nature of the dysfunction (a thought disorder)—which determines the clinical status of the chronic psychiatric patient in the community. Effective care, it will be suggested, will depend on an adequate assessment of the determinants of the patient's behavior, the constraints a treatment's efficacy places on the therapeutic options and the modifiability of the natural history of the illness.

THERAPEUTIC COMPLIANCE OF THE CHRONIC PSYCHIATRIC PATIENT IN THE COMMUNITY

Therapeutic compliance refers to a class of behaviors that reflects the patient's participation in the process of care. What is common to all such behaviors is that they have implicitly or explicitly been labeled by a provider as essential for effective treatment. Thus, a patient not taking all their prescribed oral medications, a patient not faithfully attending a clinic to receive a long-acting phenothiazine or a patient not keeping all appointments for psychotherapy sessions are examples of behavior which could adversely impact the clinical status of the patient. However, the threshold for this adverse impact very often is not known or can vary sufficiently among individuals, so that less than 100% compliance may occur without clinical significance (Gordis 1976; Sackett 1976). For the psychiatric patient this issue reaches an extreme, since it is possible to have a sample of psychiatric patients who are effectively not receiving therapy, due to noncompliance, in which some will fare well in the community while others will relapse and be rehospitalized (see below).

The request by a provider for compliant behaviors can also be looked upon as a stage in the development of the interpersonal relationship between the patient and provider (Barofsky 1978). At first a provider requests that a patient comply, but compliance can develop into the patient adhering to patient-provider agreed-to goals, or the patient can negotiate components of a therapeutic alliance. While such changes in the quality and nature of the interpersonal relationship between provider and patient do occur, it is also true that most relationships start with the request for compliance.

The need to comply is also a part of the social-functioning process. Thus, the patient must learn the rules and regulations of the community, residence or work site so that his/her behavior will not deviate from the norm. Not complying with these rules can limit the opportunities that the psychiatric patient has to function in such social situations.

Compliance issues, therefore, are part of each dimension of the process of providing care. We will limit our discussion to the patient's participation in his/her treatment regimen only for the sake of convenience and not because a discussion of compliance issues in interpersonal relationships or social functioning are of any less importance. It is also true that most of the available data deals with medication compliance and appointment-keeping behavior, and significantly fewer studies have been reported dealing with other aspects of the care process.

MEDICATION NONCOMPLIANCE BY THE CHRONIC PSYCHIATRIC PATIENT IN THE COMMUNITY

The phenothiazines include a wide variety of drugs that have been shown to control psychotic symptomatology (see the Chapter by Baldessarini in this book). Appendix A summarizes research studies in English published since 1960, from which it was possible to calculate the noncompliance rate of psychotic outpatients prescribed phenothiazines. Appendix A also reflects a history of the development of methods of providing care for the chronic psychiatric patient in the community. For example, in most early studies patients received only oral drug preparations, whereas today most studies compare self-administration of oral medication with provider-administered long-acting phenothiazines (LAPs),[2] or compare LAPs of different chemical composition. In early studies patients were usually prescribed an oral medication and sent into the community with the expectation that their family or formal psychotherapy would provide the needed support for the patient. Today it is common for patients on LAPs to attend special clinics and to participate in the wide range of social therapies (clubs, sheltered workshops, etc.) available in the community (Hogarty et al. 1979). By using LAPs and social therapies, it is also becoming increasingly feasible to treat acute, as well as chronically ill, patients in the community. Thus, the practice of institutionalizing a patient until an acute illness is under control is becoming less common (Goldstein et al. 1978).

The studies summarized in Appendix A also reflect a progressive development and maturation of the research methodology used in various studies. Studies in the early 1950s and 60s were predominantly followups of small-scale trials, in which comparisons of groups or methods of controlling bias were seldom used. These studies were followed by the so called "mirror image" studies (Denham and Adamson 1971; Gottfries and Green 1974; Polonowita et al. 1976) which measure change by comparing the patient's clinical history before and after introduction of a new drug or procedure. Blackwell and Sheppard (1968), however, have pointed out the significant limitations in drawing inferences from these types of studies. More recently, studies have been reported where samples of patients were first stabilized, either in the community or as inpatients, and then randomly assigned to alternative drug treatments (Hirsch et al. 1973; Hogarty et al. 1979; Schooler et al. 1980).

Even though the studies listed in Appendix A are limited to the same type of subjects (schizophrenics) receiving the same class of drugs (phenothiazines) in the same situation (as outpatients), differences in how the patients were cared for and the experimental design used are sufficient to make these studies quite dissimilar. To bring some order to the assessment of these data will require the application of specific criteria. For example, some investigators (e.g., Haynes et al. 1976) suggest that a study be rated in terms of the extent it possesses characteristics indicative of an adequate experimental design. This information could then be used as an index of the adequacy of the study, and inferences based on the study would

Table II Outpatient Attrition as a Function of Patient and Physician Decisions During Different Phases of an Experimental Study*

	Patient Eligibility Phase	Chronic Treatment Phase
Physician Decisions	Lack of Drug Effectiveness Side Effects Suicides/Death	Relapse or Rehospitalization Side Effects Suicides/Death
Patient Decisions	Refused to Participate in Study	Moved Away
	Refused Treatment (Appear for, continue, complete)	Refused Treatment (Appear for, continue, complete)

*Calculation of noncompliance rate did not include patients whose eligibility was established while the patient was an inpatient. The relapse rate, for experimental studies, was usually based on the chronic treatment phase of the study.

be qualified accordingly. An alternative method would restrict inferences to specific groups of studies that have common characteristics (e.g., relapse rate would be described as a function of the research method used: followup studies, mirror-image studies, experimental studies). The data reported in these studies would be reevaluated with noncompliance rates now being calculated on the basis of common criteria applied across studies. Both of these procedures were adopted in the present paper.

Reading the papers in Appendix A quickly reveals that many studies measure patient attrition rather than noncompliance. Table II describes reasons for patient attrition as a function of the phase of an experimental study and the individual making the decision. Noncompliance, as used in this report, is a *voluntary* decision of an outpatient receiving a phenothiazine.[3] Thus, studies whose estimates of noncompliance include in the denominator counts of patients who died, relapsed or were dropped from the study because of drug side effects would provide an inaccurate reflection of a patient's decisions. For this reason each study was carefully reviewed and only measures of noncompliant behaviors (Table II) were included in rate estimates. These estimates included both the eligibility and chronic treatment phase of a study, if both phases occurred when the patient was an outpatient (see Appendix A).

A method of calculating noncompliance rates which would take advantage of most of the available data would be an actuarial life-table analysis. In this type of analysis the number of patients at any one moment who can be noncompliant are used to calculate the current noncompliance rate. Thus, the numerator and the denominator are both adjusted as attrition occurs, independent of the reason for the dropout. The application of this analysis rests on the assumption that noncompliance will remove the patient from the eligible pool of compliant patients. Unfortunately, the nature of noncompliance in most clinic situations makes this decision a complicated one. For example, some patients may fail to initiate their prescribed regimen (e.g., fail to make an original purchase of their medication, or fail to return for their first injection of an LAP after returning to the community), some patients may fail to continue after having initiated their therapy (e.g., patients who decide not to refill a prescription or return for a visit to a psychotherapist), and some patients may comply with some but not all aspects of the prescribed regimen (as would occur if a patient took 3 of 4 prescribed pills per day). Thus, patients who refuse to participate in the study, who move or who fail to initiate some aspect of their regimen could all be labeled as noncompliant. Noncompliance (or nonparticipation), therefore, is a collection of specific behaviors that have the common characteristic of reflecting discordance between the patient and provider. Any particular measure of noncompliance could vary in the number of behaviors that can be included, and this will effect the probability of demonstrating noncompliance. A review of Appendix A reveals that not one study has used a life-table analysis to measure "the survival" of compliance, and only 3 studies measure the survival of the patient in the community (del Giudice et al. 1975; Hogarty et al. 1979; Schooler et al. 1980).

a. What Is the Rate of Medication Noncompliance by the Chronic Psychiatric Patient in the Community?

The data in Appendix A can be summarized in terms of drug preparation used (oral versus long-acting phenothiazines) and social support provided. Patients who were prescribed LAPs were considered to have received social support—primarily because their maintenance on therapy was the responsibility of a particular provider (e.g., the visiting nurse) who ensured that the patient had the regular opportunity to receive medication. Whether the patient actually received support during these sessions was not always stated, although it was clear that this type of support was considered part of a well-run clinic (e.g., Hiep and Marriott 1976). In contrast, the patients prescribed

Table III Mean Percent Noncompliance Rate as a Function of Social Support and Phenothiazine Drug Preparation[1]

	Social Support			
	Minimal	Programmed		
Drug Preparation		Psychotherapy	Clinic	
Oral	46.7(13)*	40.2(3)	47.2(4) (44.9)	46.3
LAP[+]	x	23.0(1)	17.2(25) (17.2)	17.2
	46.7	20.6		27.7

*Weighted mean (Number of studies). The 46 studies included 2,757 patients.
[+]Long-acting Phenothiazines
[1] A Kruskal-Wallis one-way analysis of variance confirmed that the ranking of the percents varied significantly as a function of the 3 cells ($H=8.6$, $P<.02$). A multiple comparison test revealed that the Oral-Minimal Support group differed significantly from the LAP-Programmed Support group. (Hollander and Wolfe 1973).

an oral preparation usually had little contact with a provider when they ingested their medications, even though they may have been monitored by a provider on a regular basis. For this reason patients prescribed oral, self-administered medications were considered to be receiving minimal social support. If a patient was prescribed an oral medication but attended a clinic on a regular basis specifically for medication monitoring or specifically for psychotherapy, then the patient was classified as receiving programmed social support.

Table III summarizes the data from 46 separate studies that were available in the 36 reports summarized in Appendix A. Noncompliance rate was calculated for each study in the manner described above. Inspection of the table reveals that there have been no reports of studies in which patients have self-administered an LAP. The reader will be able to inspect Appendix A and identify the individual studies referred to in the remaining 3 cells.

Inspection of Table III reveals that the average noncompliance rate was higher for studies in which patients received oral as opposed to LAPs and minimal as opposed to programmed social support. A nonparametric analysis of variance (Kruskal-Wallis) revealed that the rankings of the percents in the 3 cells varied significantly, while a multiple comparison test confirmed that the Oral-Minimal Support Group differed significantly from the LAP-programmed Support Group. To conclude from this that LAPs can reduce noncompliance, however, would be premature, since the analysis of noncompliance behavior presented (Table II) indicates that the opportunities for noncompliance for patients taking an oral medication (refuse to participate, purchase drug, take all of drug, take some drug) are significantly greater than for patients prescribed LAPs (in which appointment keeping and compliance are confounded). This difference alone could account for differences in noncompliance rate for the two regimens.

Overall, the noncompliance rate for the chronic psychiatric patient in the community has been found to average 27.7%, with noncompliance rate varying as a function of social support (46.7% for minimal social support and 20.6% for programmed social support). These data are quite comparable to that found for other drugs (Barofsky 1976). For example, Barofsky found that noncompliance rate for antituberculosis drugs was 44.1% for 14 studies that provided minimal social support and 23.4% for 3 studies that provided programmed social system, while noncompliance rate for antiepileptic drugs was 45.1% (4 studies) and 20.0% (3 studies) for minimal and programmed social support. A similar 2:1 ratio in noncompliance rate as a function of social support was found for antihypertensive agents but not for antianxiety drugs. These data provide the appropriate comparison with which to evaluate the noncompliance rate observed with the schizophrenic patient, and they support the proposition that the noncompliance rate of the schizophrenic is no different than found for patients with medical problems.

b. Does Noncompliance Increase the Relapse and/or Rehospitalization rate?

Not all patients who relapse are hospitalized and not all patients who are rehospitalized have relapsed. For example, if a patient's psychosis is of such a nature that his/her family or community can tolerate and manage the individual, the hospitalization may not occur, while some patients are hospitalized for purely social reasons (such as to prevent them from being victimized, or as a result of family intolerance). Thus, both measures should be available to completely gauge the consequence of nonparticipation on a patient's psychiatric status (Type B studies).

Classifying a patient as having relapsed or suggesting that a patient be readmitted to a hospital is usually a decision made by a physician (Table II). In calculating the rate of these decisions, the question has to be asked as to what is the appropriate denominator. Should, for example, patients who leave the study catchment area be included in the denominator even though their relapse/rehospitalization rate may not be easily measured? The question being asked here is identical to that asked in estimating noncompliance rates (see above), and the approach to be used will be the same for both: studies will be grouped in terms of common characteristics, and the reported relapse rate for each study will be reviewed and recalculated in terms of specific criteria (see Appendix A). Relapse/rehospitalization rates will be calculated for only those patients who have the probability of relapsing (i.e., not patients who move or die), although it is recognized again that life-table analysis, if available, would provide the most complete estimate of the relapse rate. Since relapse/rehospitalization rate is being used here as a measure of efficacy, it is most appropriate to base estimates of rates, if available, on the chronic treatment maintenance phase of a study. The reason for this is that when the maintenance phase has started, the investigator has usually demonstrated that the study groups are comparable (i.e., are equally likely to relapse), and the question then becomes to what extent one drug treatment or another is more effective in preventing relapse (assuming two drugs are being compared).

Table IV summarizes those studies from Appendix A which provided both relapse/rehospitalization and noncompliance rates. Inspection of the table provides general support for the clinical impression that noncompliance and relapse or rehospitalization rates are systematically related. Calculation of a Spearman Rank correlation coefficient revealed an $r = 0.420$ (Siegal 1952), a correlation coefficient that was significant at the $P < .05$ level. A more critical method of measuring the relationship between relapse and noncompliance rates is to determine how many relapsers were noncompliant. Only 5 of the studies in Table IV make clear statements on this issue, and these studies involved only 24 of the 1,000 or more patients in the reported papers. Of these 24 relapsed patients, 17 were noncompliant (70.8%).

Three additional studies provide data on the relationship between noncompliance and relapse/rehospitalization rates, but these were not listed in Appendix A because they lacked one or more of the characteristics required for inclusion. Mason et al. (1963), for example, found that only 38% of a group of rehospitalized patients had evidence of regular chlorpromazine usage in their urine, whereas 29% had evidence of lower levels of drug usage and 33% no evidence of drug consumption. Reilly et al. (1967) interviewed schizophrenics

Table IV Relapse/Rehospitalization and Noncompliance Rate of Outpatients Prescribed Phenothiazines[1]

Type of Study	Study Number (Year)[2]		Relapse/ Rehospitalization Rate	Non-Compliance Rate	Proportion of Noncompliant Relapsers
Followup Studies	3.(1962)		16.2%(130)[3]	52.1%(121)[3]	—
	5.(1964)		21.0%(62)	61.2%(49)	—
	6.(1966)		47.0%(117)	54.2%(28)	—
	15.(1973)		10.3%(29)	53.6%(28)	2/3 persons
Mirror-Image Studies	9.(1971)		33.0%(102)	10.1%(69)	7/7 persons
	20.(1974)		34.0%	44.7%(47)	—
Experimental Studies	1.(1960)	A.	18.2%(55)	34.5%(55)	—
		B.	4.8%(62)	40.3%(62)	—
	7.(1968)		7.7%(13)	0.0%(12)	—
	10.(1971)		12.5%(24)	50.0%(20)	—
	12.(1971)	A.	35.0%(20)	71.4%(42)	—
		B.	35.0%(20)	10.0%(20)[4]	1/2 persons
	14.(1973)		12.5%(40)	23.3%(43)	—
	17.(1974)	A.	26.7%(15)	52.9%(17)	—
		B.	0.0%(14)	35.7%(14)	—
	21.(1975)		33.3%(15)	33.3%(15)	5/5 persons
	27.(1977)	A.	4.3%(23)	4.8%(21)	—
		B.	5.3%(19)	23.0%(13)	—
	29.(1978)		35.0%(20)	46.2%(13)	—
	30.(1978)		9.4%(96)	8.4%(95)	—
	32.(1979)	A.	28.6%(28)	30.0%(20)	—
		B.	21.0%(29)	47.8%(23)	—
	33.(1979)		49.5%(50)	13.0%(100)	—
			54.9%(55)		—
	35.(1980)	A.	35.7%(98)	39.7%(68)	—
		B.	27.1%(96)	35.5%(76)	—

[1] Relapse and rehospitalization were calculated for eligible sample of patients. The rate shown was the rehospitalization rate if both were available.

[2] The "Study Number" refers to the studies listed in Appendix A.

[3] Number in parenthesis refers to number of subjects.

[4] These data were calculated from a substudy of this report and consisted of relapse and compliance data collected only in the maintenance phase of the study.

(drug regimen not specified) at the time they were readmitted to the hospital. Including patients who claimed they stopped taking drugs due to side effects, they found that 63.5% (39/61) of the patients who relapsed were noncompliant. Hogarty et al. (1973) provides additional data, but unfortunately not in sufficient detail so that

Table V Mean Percent Relapse/Rehospitalization Rate as a Function of Social Support and Phenothiazine Drug Preparation[1]

	Social Support			
	Minimal	Programmed		
Drug Preparation		Psychotherapy	Clinic	
Oral	24.3(6)*	35.3(2)	29.7(3) (31.4)	26.9
Depot Injections[+]	x	5.3(1)	30.6(13) (29.8)	29.8
	24.3	30.2		28.4

[1]This summary does not represent the entire available literature but only those studies cited in Appendix A.

*Weighted mean (Number of Studies)

[+]Long-acting phenothiazines

compliance rates could be determined for each experimental condition. The patients received either a pharmacological or social work intervention, or both, but the compliance data were presented for only the drug/placebo groups. These data indicate that 86.7% of the patients who did not relapse took their drugs as prescribed, whereas only 45.4% of those who relapsed reported taking their drugs. A similar result was found for the patients who received placebo: 82.2% of the patients who did not relapse complied, whereas 53.1% of the patients who relapsed complied. Separate chi-square tests for drug and placebo treatments indicate that relapse rates varied significantly as a function of compliance behavior (Hogarty et al. 1979).

The data in Table IV, and the studies by Mason (1963), Reilly et al. (1967), and Hogarty et al. (1973) indicate that one half or more of each sample of relapsed/rehospitalized patients did not comply with their medication regimen.

Table V summarizes the relapse/rehospitalization rate as a function of type of medication and social support. Inspection of the table reveals that relapse/rehospitalization rate did not vary as a function of oral or LAP, or presence or absence of social support. This confirms, for a heterogenous sample of patients, what Schooler et al. (1980) have observed for a sample of compliant patients; namely, that the type of medication does not determine relapse/rehospitalization rate. It differs, however, from what Hogarty et al. (1979) observed, which was that social therapy and LAP resulted in a significantly lower relapse/rehospitalization rate than either oral therapy with or without social therapy, or LAP without social therapy.

Table VI Determinants of Noncompliance Behavior

Patient Characteristics	Health Care System Variables
Sociodemographic Variables:	Provider Characteristics
Age	Sociodemographic variables
Sex	Provider Attitude
Race	Interpersonal Skill
Education	Provider Decisions
Socioeconomic Factors	Referral
Marital Status	Establishment of Plan of Care
Occupation	Implementing Care
Psychosocial Variables:	Organizational Issues
Patient Attitudes/Behaviors	Philosophy/Policies
Family Attitudes/Behaviors	Milieu/Setting
Work Status	
Clinical History:	Situational Determinants
Age of Onset	Interpersonal Status/Family
Prior Hospitalization	Victimization
Drug History	Change in physical status
Disease Specific Factors:	Financial Reverse
Diagnosis	Occupational Disruption
Symptoms	Housing/Living Arrangements
Severity	

In answer to the question "does medication noncompliance increase the relapse and/or rehospitalization rate?" we can now state that the available data, however adequate, indicates that 50% or more of a sample of relapsed patients can be shown to be, or will report being, noncompliant. The significance of this observation is that this leaves a sizable proportion of patients who have relapsed but were compliant. Yet to be established is whether noncompliance precedes and precipitates a relapse, or whether noncompliance is just one element of an already established process leading to relapse. What can be said with confidence is that the simplistic view that a compliant patient will not relapse is untenable. These data suggest that compliance behavior is just one of several factors that will determine the effectiveness of the medication provided the chronic psychiatric patient in the community.

c. *What Factors Determine the Noncompliance Rate of the Chronic Psychiatric Patient in the Community?*

What patient characteristics, health care system variables and situational determinants predict that a patient will be noncompliant

(Type A studies)? Table VI lists some of the variables that have been associated with noncompliance. An extensive review of the relationship between these variables and compliance behavior, in general, is summarized in the studies of Blackwell (1976) and Sackett and his coworkers (Haynes et al. 1979). The present discussion, however, will consider the extent these variables predict noncompliance by the schizophrenic outpatient.

Since it is possible that investigators have not reported nonsignificant studies, or that very few studies have actually been done, the studies to be reviewed have to be considered a summary of the available literature rather than a critical analytic assessment of the role the variables may play in predicting noncompliance.

Sociodemographic Variables: Considered alone, there is little evidence that noncompliance and compliant outpatient schizophrenics differ in terms of age, sex and race (Table VII). A strong association seems to exist between whether the patient is married or is living with someone and the chance that he will take his medication (Table VII), although marital status doesn't seem related to the person's willingness to participate in a study (Schooler et al. 1980). Winkelman (1964) did find that factory workers (socioeconomic factors and occupation) tend to comply with their medication regimen less and relapse more than private practice patients. In general, marital status appears to be the sociodemographic variable most likely to be associated with the compliance behavior of the schizophrenic outpatients.

Psychosocial Variables: In contrast to sociodemographic variables, the individual's attitudes and the attitude and behavior of the patient's family are clearly implicated in the patient's compliance behavior (Table VII). Early studies (Michaux 1961; Raskin 1961; Richards 1964; Winkelman 1964) suggested that resistance to the acceptance of medication was associated with noncompliance behavior. Nelson et al. (1975) more recently found that if a patient accepted his illness he was more likely to comply with the medication regimen both in the hospital and as an outpatient. They also found that if a patient felt that the physician was interested in him, that his therapy worked and that the physician was competent, the patient was then more likely to be compliant. Bowden et al. (1980) found that patients who stopped attending therapy sessions were noncompliant with their medication regimen and tended to not accept their illness. Thus, the patient's attitude toward his medication and illness appears correlated with his medication compliance behavior.

Parke et al. (1962) observed that when drug administration was supervised by a family member or friend, a significantly larger

Table VII The Relationship Between Patient Characteristics, Health Care System Variables, and Situational Determinants and Noncompliance by the Schizophrenic Outpatient in the Community

Variable	Association with Noncompliance: Yes	Association with Noncompliance: No
A. Patient Characteristics		
Sociodemographic Variables		
Age	Bowden et al. (1980)	Raskin (1961); Renton et al. (1963); Willcox et al. (1965); Reilly et al. (1967); Nelson et al. (1975); Schooler et al. (1980)[1]
Sex	Bowden et al. (1980)	Renton et al. (1963); Willcox et al. (1965); Schooler et al. (1980)
Race		Schooler et al. (1980)
Education	Raskin (1961)	Willcox et al. (1965)
Socioeconomic Factors	Winkelman (1964)	Reilly et al. (1967); Nelson et al. (1975)
Marital and/or Domicilatory Status	Parkes et al. (1962); Renton et al. (1963); Willcox et al. (1965); Reilly et al. (1967); Nelson et al. (1975)	Raskin (1961); Schooler et al. (1980)
Occupation	Winkelman (1964)	Raskin (1961)
Psychosocial Variables		
Patient Attitudes/Behaviors	Michaux (1961); Raskin (1961); Richards (1964); Winkelman (1964); Nelson et al. (1975); Bowden et al. (1980)	Raskin (1961)
Family Attitudes/Behaviors	Parkes et al. (1962); Reilly et al. (1967); Brown et al. (1972); Vaughn and Leff (1976)	
Work Status	Schooler et al. (1967); Affleck et al. (1976)	Raskin (1961); Reilly et al. (1967)

Table VII (Continued)

Variable	Association with Noncompliance: Yes	No
Clinical Status	Bowden et al. (1980)	
Age of Onset	Bowden et al. (1980)	Renton et al. (1962); Schooler et al. (1980)
Prior Hospitalization	Reilly et al. (1967); Nelson et al. (1975)	
Drug History	Michaux (1961); Willcox et al. (1965); Irwin et al. (1971); Van Putten (1974); Nelson et al. (1975); Fallon et al. (1978)	Parkes et al. (1962)
Disease-Specific Factors		
Diagnosis	Reilly et al. (1967) Wilson and Enoch (1967)	Nelson (1975)
Symptoms	Raskin (1961); Reilly et al. (1967); Vaughn and Leff (1976); Van Putten et al. (1976); Bowden et al. (1980)	Raskin (1961)
Severity	Renton et al. (1963) Bowden et al. (1980)	Raskin (1961); Nelson et al. (1975); Schooler et al. (1980)
B. Health System Variables		
Provider Characteristics		
Sociodemographic Variables		
Provider Attitudes/Behavior	Haefner et al. (1960); Raskin (1961); Irwin et al. (1971); Nelson et al. (1975)	
Interpersonal Skill		
Provider Decisions		
Referral		
Plan of Care		

(continued)

Table VII (Continued)

	Association with Noncompliance	
Variable	Yes	No
Implementing Care	McClellan and Cowan (1970); Gold et al. (1976); MacPherson and Luterbach (1976)	
Organizational Issues		
Philosophy/Policies	Reilly et al. (1967); Serban and Thomas (1974); Cody and Robinson (1977); Davis et al. (1977)	
Milieu	Hare and Willcox (1967); Irwin et al. (1971); Bowden et al. (1980)	Hogerty et al. (1976)
C. Situational Determinants		
	Birley and Brown (1970); Leff et al. (1973)	

*The papers listed include those in Appendix A, with additional papers that dealt with the variable being considered but failed to meet the criteria established for inclusion in Appendix A.

[1] Eighty % of the patients who refused to participate (Table 9; Schooler et al. 1980) did so for their own reasons, whereas 20% did not participate because of a physician's objections.

[2] This study was based on inpatients.

proportion of patients were compliant. Reilly et al. (1967) found that patients whose families were accepting were proportionately more compliant than patients whose families indicated a lack of acceptance of the patient. Additional data on this issue come from the studies done by Wing and his coworkers in England (Brown et al. 1962, 1972; Leff 1978). They found that if a family expressed high emotion, particularly if directed to the patient, and if the patient did not take his medication, then the relapse rate of such patients was higher than that of patients who had the same type of family but who took their medication. This differential relapse rate as a function of drug compliance and high expressed family emotion was not found for the patients whose family members were low in their emotional expression. A patient could also avoid the adverse consequence of high emotional expression by reducing face-to-face contact with the family (Vaughn and Leff 1976).

The studies by Wing and his coworkers help us clarify the model presented in Table I. Their data suggest that the relationship among the components of the model (family attitude/behavior, medication compliance and relapse rate) is best described as conditional probability statements rather than as the linear model implied by Table I. The probability of relapse would, therefore, vary as a joint function of the probability that a patient was taking his medication and the probability that the family of the patient was critical of the patient. Of course, it would be expected that this model would still be applicable if the source of criticism were some other significant person (e.g., roommate, provider, etc.) to the patient. Drugs, from this analysis, function to reduce the responsiveness of the patient to social stimuli (Leff 1978).

Although work is a major psychosocial indicator of the clinical status of the schizophrenic outpatient, there have been very few studies relating the work history of a patient to his medication compliance behavior. The few studies reported do not provide clear evidence (Table VII), although occasional authors speculate that the attitude of coworkers or the patient's work situation contributes to noncompliance (e.g., Parkes et al. 1962).

Serban and Thomas (1974, 1980) report a study which is relevant to this discussion. However, they don't specify the drugs used by the patients or whether the noncompliant patient was the same person who failed to attend a clinic, or who was or was not working. What they found was that patients who were readmitted to the hospital were more noncompliant, both in terms of medication usage and of clinic attendance, and that they were less likely to have worked than patients who were not readmitted. The study demonstrates that work and compliance behavior covary, but it does not provide evidence that a causal relationship exists among the variables.

Brown et al. (1972), who did *not* find that relapse rate was related to medication compliance, did find that if a patient's relatives expressed high emotion, then it was also likely that the patient was not working, was exhibiting disturbed behavior and had relapsed. The direct correlation between work impairment and relapse rate, however, was less strong. Vaughn and Leff (1976), who successfully replicated the general findings of the Brown study but found that relapse rate varied with medication compliance, have not as yet reported the relationship between the patient's work status and medication compliance. Thus, the definitive study relating a patient's work status to his medication compliance and relapse rate has yet to be reported.

In summary, the available data is sufficient to indicate that the patient's attitude towards his illness or medication and the family's attitude and behavior towards the patient are adequate predictors of medication compliance behavior, whereas the data available on work status remains unclear.

Clinical Status: Prior hospitalization rate and drug history (including drug side effects), but not age of disease onset, appear to be correlated with noncompliance behavior (Table VII). Reilly et al. (1967) found that 62% of those patients who had been hospitalized four or more times were taking their medication, whereas only 36% of those who stopped their medication had been hospitalized as often. Nelson et al. (1975) essentially found the same thing; numerous prior hospitalizations were related to increased medication compliance.

A schizophrenic's drug history, particularly his or her history of experiencing drug side effects, appears to be correlated with medication noncompliance. The reader may view the studies listed in Table VII as an underestimate of the available literature, and from one perspective this is correct. For example, nearly all of the studies referred to in Appendix A discuss drug side effects (e.g., depression, extrapyramidal reactions) and could conceivably be included in Table VII. However, in most cases reading of the paper revealed that the physician responded to the patient's reports of side effects by removing the patient from the study. This was considered a physician decision (see Table II) even though the decision may have reflected the patient's "will." To determine the extent the patient participated in the physician's decision would require a detailed study of the role the patient plays in defining his/her own therapeutic regimen, data which was simply not available in these studies. The studies listed in Table VII represent studies in which the patient reported side effects and independently stopped taking his prescribed medication.

The precise relationship between drug side effects and compliance behavior is complex. For example, Willcox et al. (1965) and Irwin et al. (1971) report that a minimal number of side effects actually increased compliance, whereas Michaux (1961) found the exact opposite. Winkelman (1964) found that noncompliance increased with increasing frequency of drug side effects, while Van Putten (1974), Nelson et al. (1975) and Fallon et al. (1978) report that the incidence of noncompliance was significantly higher for patients who experienced side effects.

VanPutten and his coworkers (1974a,b,1976; 1981) studied the consequences of the side effects of the phenothiazines (oral and LAP) on a patient's compliance behavior in great detail. They found that 89% of the patients who chronically refused to take medications experienced extrapyramidal symptoms, while only 20% of the patients who took their medications reported such symptoms. The patient's response to these side effects, however, varied. One group was able to be pressured into taking an LAP, a second subgroup passively accepted their drugs as inpatients but refused to take the drugs as outpatients, a third group took less drugs than prescribed and a fourth group refused to take the drug, equating it to a poison. These various outcomes illustrate the fact that in clinical practice, as opposed to more tightly controlled conditions of an experimental study, a therapeutic regimen can be accommodated to the individual patient. A description of how these accommodations develop would, of course, provide insight into how a patient influences a physician's decision (see above).

One issue raised by these studies is that if 89% of drug-refusers (to generalize Van Putten's data) are suffering from side effects, to what extent is drug noncompliance voluntary? To answer this question an investigator would have to assess the frequency of reported side effects, independent of provider intervention, and determine the extent such side effects lead to medication noncompliance. The empirical question would be, "What is the probability that a patient would refuse to take his/her medication if the previous dose of the medication led to a side effect?" A study of this sort is, of course, technically quite difficult to do. What would be predicted, however, is that the probability of noncompliance following a drug side effect would vary among patients, and that for some patients (e.g., those patients who equate the drug with a poison), the relationship would be sufficient to suggest an involuntary or conditioned response, while for most others, the decision to be noncompliant would represent a voluntary decision based on the influence of a number of factors, including drug side effects. Data at the level of specificity required to answer this critical question has yet to be collected, but clearly would help determine the extent to which the drug-taking behavior of the patient is confounded by his thought processes.

It should be stated that Van Putten et al. (1976), although acknowledging the correlation between extrapyramidal symptoms and drug refusal, consider a patient's desire for the symptomatic consequences of noncompliance (i.e., grandiose thinking) a more powerful predictor of drug-taking behavior than the avoidance of neuromuscular dysfunction characteristic of extrapyramidal symptoms (see below). This view has not yet been supported by a different group of investigators.

A dimension of the drug-taking behavior of the schizophrenic outpatient, unexplored as of yet, is the compliance rate of patients prescribed antiparkinsonian drugs. It is well-known (see Chapter by Baldessarini) that the chronic administration of the phenothiazines, particularly the long-acting phenothiazines (LAPs), requires the concurrent administration of antiparkinsonian medications. The antiparkinsonian drugs offset the extrapyramidal symptoms that are produced by chronic drug administration. Although commonly prescribed, there was not a single report of compliance behavior for patients prescribed antiparkinsonian drugs in the paper reported in Appendix A. Since antiparkinsonian drugs are orally administered, simultaneous measures of compliance to LAPs and oral antiparkinsonian drugs in the same patient would provide an important opportunity to determine the factors that lead to medication noncompliance.

In summary, prior hospitalization and drug history are both adequate predictors of medication compliance behavior. To what extent the patient's decision to not comply is determined by drug side effects requires additional study.

Disease-Specific Factors: Only disease-specific symptoms, but not the diagnosis or the severity (as determined by a physician) of the dysfunction, appeared to predict medication noncompliance. The symptoms that were reported to be associated with medication noncompliance were hostility and aggression (Raskin 1961; Reilly et al. 1967) and grandiosity (Vaughn and Leff 1976; Van Putten et al. 1976). The observation by Wilson and Enoch (1967) and Reilly et al. (1967) that paranoid patients were also noncompliant is consistent with what was found for the symptoms of patients. In general, therefore, the suspicious patient who has clear indication of thought disturbance is most likely to be noncompliant. What remains to be determined is whether this suspiciousness was induced by drugs (e.g., extrapyramidal effects), by thought disturbances or by both. Noncompliance data collected as a function of diagnosis (e.g., paranoid, schizo-affective, hebephrenic, etc.) would help assess the relative contributions of drug side effects and specific thought disturbances to noncompliance behavior. Unfortunately, these data are not available.

Provider Characteristics: There is an adequate literature relative to the relationship between provider characteristics and patient compliance (particularly attendance at psychotherapy sessions; e.g., Baekeland and Lundwell 1975; Honigfeld 1967. Lorion 1974; Rickels 1968). This literature suggests that sociodemographic differences between the patient and provider, the provider's attitude particularly towards medications and the interpersonal skills of the provider can determine the patient's cooperativeness. Most of these data, however, have been collected for nonpsychotic patients, and the role of such nonspecific (actually nondrug-related) factors is less clear for schizophrenic outpatients (e.g., Cole et al. 1968).

What also seems to be reasonably well established is that the attitude of the provider can affect the medication compliance behavior of the schizophrenic outpatient. Medication compliance has been found to vary as a function of a provider liking the patient (Raskin 1961; Nelson et al. 1975), or believing in the efficacy of the medication (Irwin et al. 1971).

It is possible, as Irwin et al. (1971) has pointed out, that the differences in attitude may actually reflect differences in the amount of contact (frequency or duration) between the patient and physician and have little to do with the quality of their relationship. To what extent this accounts for the association between the providers attitude and the patient's compliance behavior has yet to be determined.

Provider Decisions: A potentially critical determinant of a patient's compliance is how well a provider makes decisions and implements a therapeutic regimen. The provider has to decide to refer a patient for appropriate services, decide on an appropriate drug regimen and dose, accurately modify a drug dose, provide for continuity of care, etc. Each of these factors can confound and contradict a patient's own efforts at self-management, contradictions which may lead to noncompliance. Again, however, we are faced with a gross lack of data on the specific issue—how does a provider's decision contribute to a schizophrenic patient's noncompliance with the medication regimen?

Table VIII summarizes estimates of the accuracy of a patient's and a physician's assessment of the drug-taking behavior of the patient. Thus, a patient or a physician was asked if the patient was taking a drug and a physical measurement (e.g., a urine analysis) was used to confirm these judgments. Inspection of the table reveals that estimates vary widely for both physician and patient, with modal values in the range of 40-50%. What Table VIII indicates is that neither the physician nor patient do very well when they have to judge the drug-taking behavior of the patient. An alternative explanation is that there is some limitation in the urine test for the drug or in the ability

Table VIII How Accurate Is the Patient or Physician in the Monitoring of a Patient's Drug-Taking Behavior

Patients Taking Drugs For:	Psychiatric Dysfunctions
I. Patient Estimates	
1. Park and Lipman (1964)*	59.8%
2. Rickles and Briscoe (1970)*	45.1%
3. MacPherson and Luterbach (1976)	38.8%
II. Physician Estimates	
1. McClellan and Cowan (1970)	80.0%
2. Gold, Nelson and Frazin (1976)	50.0%
3. MacPherson and Luterbach (1976)	30.2%

*Neurotic outpatients. All other studies deal with the schizophrenic outpatients.

of the patient to absorb the drug (Smith et al. 1979). This is unlikely, however, since all of these patients have been shown to respond to the drug before they become outpatients.

The significance of these data can be appreciated better by inspection of Table IX, where on the basis of an assessment of the patient's symptoms (Gold et al. 1976), the physician decided to change or not change the patient's therapy. The data summarized also indicates whether the patient was compliant at the time the patient's therapy was being evaluated. Inspection of the table indicates that of 30 patients whose clinical status was rated as worse, 21 were noncompliant and 9 were compliant. The psychiatrist changed the therapy in only 10 of 21 noncompliant patients, and none of the 9 compliant patients. Clearly, the provider's decision to change the patient's therapy was not a simple function of an exacerbation of symptoms. Consistent with this was the fact that the provider changed the therapy of 14 patients who experienced no change in symptoms. Also of interest was the fact that 14 patients, who on the basis of the physician's ratings improved, actually were noncompliant.

The decision-making process illustrated in Table IX was quite conservative, with only 15.7% of the entire sample having their therapy changed. If noncompliance with a drug regimen was the sole determinant of the symptom status of the patient, then about half of the patients should have had their therapy changed. This did not happen. Instead, Table IX suggests that 100% compliance may not be necessary for maintaining an adequate clinical status, that the clinical judgments of the provider may not be very precise, or that the drug therapy may be only one of several determinants (see above) of the

Table IX Comparison of Physician's Rating of Patient Symptoms as a Function of Physician Therapy Decisions and Patient Compliance (By Urinalysis)*

	No Change in Therapy		Change in Therapy		
Physician Assessment of Patient Symptoms	Compliant	Non-compliant	Compliant	Non-compliant	Total
Worsened	9	11	0	10	30
Unchanged	55	36	7	7	105
Improved	9	14	1	0	24
TOTAL	73	61	8	17	159

*From Gold, B. H., A. A. Nelson, and R. N. Frazin. Psychiatrists Assessment of Drug Default: Its Relationship to Their Treatment Activities. Presented at the American Pharmaceutical Association, April, 1976.

clinical status of the patient. Each of these issues make creditable the hypothesis that the provider's decision-making process may contribute to patient noncompliance.

Organizational Issues: Just as provider characteristics and decisions have been shown to be related to patient noncompliance, so too have the philosophy, policies and therapeutic milieu created by a health care organization been related to compliance behavior (Honigfeld 1964; Finnerty et al. 1973). We, however, are interested in the specific question of whether organizational issues effect the medication compliance behavior of the chronic schizophrenic patient in the community.

An organization's policy relative to a patient paying for the cost of his care has been shown to be related to compliance. Reilly et al. 1967 found that noncompliance was increased for veterans who had to pay for their own medication as compared to those who did not. Cody et al. (1977), who deliberately excluded veterans, found that noncompliance decreased when the patients had to pay for their medications. In a somewhat different study, Davis et al. (1977) found that schizophrenic outpatients who had to pay for their care tended to drop out of treatment more than similar private patients with affective disorders. Serbin and Davis (1974) found that 52% of all patients who relapsed were on welfare, while only 38% of those who did not relapse were on welfare. The implication of the data in the Serbin and Davis study (see Serbin 1980) is that somehow providing for a patient's costs increases their chances of relapsing. These studies don't permit a simple statement on what the relationship between cost and compliance is, but they do suggest that some relationship will exist. It is possible that the patients in these studies differed in terms of their expectations, both relative to the cause of their illness (e.g., the veterans may assume that their dysfunction is service-related and should be compensated) and to their role in its management, and that such differences are reflected in their response to having to pay for their therapy.

Obviously, there are other differences among institutions in philosophy and policy that can impact compliance behavior, and many of these are discussed in other chapters in this book.

The milieu or therapy setting (type of therapy, physical place, etc.) has an extended history of being associated with, and a determinant of, the therapeutic outcome of a drug (Sabshin and Ramot 1956; Honigfeld 1964; Rickels 1968). The therapy setting has also been correlated with compliance behavior of the chronic schizophrenic outpatient (Table VII). Hare and Willcox (1967), for example, found that noncompliance increased depending on whether the patients were inpatients, day patients or outpatients. Irwin et al. (1971) found essentially the same thing. On the other hand, Hogarty et al. (1976) did not find that major role therapy (provided by a social worker) significantly increased medication compliance. Bowden et al. (1980) did find that the therapy setting expected by patients was correlated with their continuation in therapy. The patients who did not continue in therapy were also more compliant, although the correlation between the patient's expectation and compliance behavior was not determined.

In general, it is clear that organizational issues will impact the medication compliance behavior of the patient, although this inference is mostly based on the data available from patient groups other than the chronic schizophrenic outpatient.

Situational Determinants: What are the immediately preceding events that precipitate medication noncompliance? A variety of types of life crises (Table VI) would be an appropriate answer (Dohrenwend and Dohrenwend 1980). The available data indicate that critical life events precede relapse by schizophrenic outpatients (e.g., Birley and Brown 1970; Leff et al. 1973), and that this association is mediated by medication noncompliance. The nature of the specific life event appears secondary to the fact that it precedes relapse by some extended time period (e.g., 3–5 weeks).

Do the data suggest that a life crisis is a necessary and sufficient precondition for noncompliant behavior? Unfortunately, there does not seem to be sufficient information to answer this question. To answer it, however, implies that a life crisis can be measured as an event separate from ongoing processes. For example, high expressed emotion by a patient's family was related to medication noncompliance and relapse (e.g., Vaughn and Leff 1976), but a specific example of such a relationship could also be the event precipitating relapse. The important question is, can an instance of expressed emotion, independent of a pattern of expressed emotion in the family, precipitate noncompliance behavior and relapse? There does not appear to be an answer to this question, at least for the chronic schizophrenic outpatient, although it is of fundamental importance for the design of intervention programs. What has been shown (see Chapter by Aguilera in this book) is that "crisis intervention" therapy can be an effective means of dealing with the consequence of a precipitating event.

Situational determinants of noncompliance behavior differ from the others listed in Table VI in that an acute occurrence may precipitate a relapse. Whether an acute occurrence is truly separable from long-term events or an artifact of the analytic process inherent in measurement is not clear (Brown et al. 1973a,b,; Dohrenwend and Dohrenwend 1980). We list them because the literature suggests that such a separation can be helpful, conceptually and in the design of interventions, but acknowledge their origins in the dynamics characteristic of the interpersonal relationship between patients and their providers, families and friends.

Summary: Table VII indicates that marital and/or domicilatory status, patient and family attitudes and behavior, prior hospitalizations, drug history, provider attitudes and behaviors, provider decisions, a health care organization's philosophy and policies, therapeutic milieu, and situational determinants are each related to noncompliance behavior by the chronic psychiatric patient in the community. The relative strength each of these factors has in predicting noncompliance is not known, but they do permit the statement that the psychiatric nature of the patient is only one of the determinants of medication noncompliance.

d. Prediction of Relapse by the Chronic Psychiatric Patient in the Community

Predicting if a chronic psychiatric patient in the community, taking a phenothiazine, will relapse (Type C Studies) has been the subject of extended study (e.g., Goldberg et al. 1977; May and Goldberg 1978; Strauss and Carpenter 1977). The task of identifying predictors, however, is as difficult and as complex as was discussed for noncompliance behavior, although the end point (relapse/rehospitalization) would presumably be a bit easier to measure. Since the cited literature adequately summarizes the available studies it does not seem necessary to repeat such a review here. Instead, this section of the paper will focus on issues that concern the prediction of both noncompliance and relapse.

As shown in Table VII, marital and/or domicilatory status was related to compliance behavior, and it also appears to be predictive of community survival (May and Goldberg 1978). Gittelman-Klein and Klein (1969), however, have shown that the association between marital status and relapse was almost totally accounted for by the patient's premorbid social adjustment. Those patients who tend to have a poor social adjustment before illness onset tend to remain single during illness, while those who had contact with their peers before illness onset had a significantly better chance of being married when ill. These data suggest that a major predictor of posthospitalization adjustment was the premorbid social adjustment of the patient. Whether the same relationship holds for medication compliance is not known (that is, whether social isolation prior to illness onset is related to medication noncompliance posthospitalization).

Premorbid factors also play a role in predicting a patient's response to drug. For example, Leff and Wing (1971) found that patients with good and poor prognostic indicators did poorer on drug than patients who were in the middle of the prognostic range. Consistent with this is the observation by May and Goldberg (1978) that there appears to be two subgroups of patients who ought not to receive drugs. One group consists of patients who do well in the community without drug, and the other consists of those who do poorly in general and who are not helped by drug. May and Goldberg (1978) also point out that it is now possible to identify these patients prior to drug exposure (see below). Whether these patients constitute a sizable proportion of the group of noncompliant patients is not known, but if confirmed, it would suggest that premorbid factors would be helpful in predicting medication noncompliance behavior.

If it is assumed that medication compliance leads to positive drug response (that is, the drug is effective and leads to a reduction of psychotic symptomatology) and a positive drug response facilitates adjustment to the community, then prediction of positive drug response should be a useful means of measuring medication compliance, as well as predicting community survival. Several procedures have been suggested for measuring a positive drug response. At the clinical level, May et al. (1976) and Van Putten and May (1977) have found that a single dose of a drug given early in the clinical history of the patient can predict the outcome of long-term drug administration. What they found was that if the patient's response to the test dose was euphoric, then the patient was more likely to show improvement in a wide range of measures, whereas a dysphoric response indicated a poor prognosis. Other measures that have been suggested as predictors of a positive drug response include electroencephalographic patterns (Itil et al. 1975) and drug side effects, particularly the development of fine motor inhibition (Haase and Janssen 1965).

Kolakowska et al. (1980) have approached this problem from a neuropharmacological dopamine-receptor-level level of analysis. Based on the available data, which indicate that the mechanism of action of antipsychotic drugs involves blockage of dopamine receptors and that one measure of dopamine blockage is plasma prolactin levels, Kolakowska et al. grouped patients according to their plasma prolactin levels and extrapyramidal responses to neuroleptic drugs. They then assessed whether this classification procedure led to the grouping of patients into homogeneous clinical entities (e.g., drug responders, remitters and resistant groups). In general, they found that their neuropharmacological classification system was clinically relevant, although they have yet to show that their system predicts the drug response of patients on chronic medication. Clearly, this approach to drug prediction will be of increasing use in the clinical management of the chronic psychiatric patient in the community, although at present the data supporting it are minimal.

The prediction of a drug response brings the topics of medication compliance and a patient's survival in the community together around a common issue. It also focuses attention on the social nature of drug therapy and the social significance of a palliative regimen. Stated another way, as long as most schizophrenia can't be cured (i.e., the underlying pathology remains unattended), and only its symptoms can be managed by chronic treatment, the outcome of such treatment will be socially determined, even when the therapy is effective.

SUMMARY

The purpose of this chapter was to identify some of the problems in providing effective care for the chronic psychiatric patient living in the community. The approach taken involved the discussion of one set of issues, issues that dealt with the determinants and consequences of medication noncompliance. Although limited in this way, it was still thought likely that related issues would be raised and that the outcome of the discussion would, in fact, be comprehensive. This appears to have been accomplished.

This paper had a second purpose, which was to determine the extent the available data justified limiting the therapeutic options for the chronic psychiatric patient. Thus, if the schizophrenic patient prescribed an oral phenothiazine was more noncompliant than the patient prescribed an LAP, a reason would exist for prescribing one regimen over another. The data summarized in Table III and V indicate that schizophrenic patients on oral medications were indeed more noncompliant than those prescribed LAP, but that this difference did not lead to a differential relapse rate. The significance of these observations is that the drug preparation used and compliance behavior are not the only determinants of relapse/rehospitalization rate.

As discussed, the evaluation of the relative effectiveness of the two drug preparations was confounded by the fact that each differed in terms of the opportunities provided for noncompliant behavior. For example, the task required of a patient prescribed an LAP is to attend a clinic where he accepts an injection of a drug. In contrast, a patient prescribed an oral phenothiazine has at least 3 times as many ways of being noncompliant. The patient may refuse to initiate the therapy, take it as often as prescribed or continue it. It is quite possible that if the observed noncompliance rates were adjusted for the opportunities for noncompliance, the resultant measures would not be significantly different (Table III).

The importance of these observations is that they provide a means of placing the popular argument for using LAP, for its efficacy and convenience, in a proper perspective. First, the data reviewed do not indicate that LAP are more effective in preventing relapse than oral medication (Table V); and second, that part of the convenience found in using LAP results from reducing a person's opportunities for noncompliance. Thus, the argument for using LAP or oral preparations comes down to deciding how much giving the patient the opportunity (freedom) to comply is in the interests of the chronic patient.

Table X summarizes some of the determinants of the community adjustment of the schizophrenic patient (Serban 1980). Prominent among these factors are representatives of the natural history of the illness—residual thought disturbances, lack of awareness and acceptance of illness, and impaired functional status. The extent that

Table X Determinants of the Community Adjustment of Schizophrenics*

Magnitude of Institutionally Induced Impaired Functional Status
Residual Thought Disturbance
Attitudes and Behavior of Family and Friends
Continued Medication Compliance
Patient's Awareness and Acceptance of Illness

*Adopted from Serban (1980)

these factors are present and characterize an individual will not only predict a patient's survival in the community, but will also be the basis upon which a provider makes decisions concerning the nature of the care a patient receives. If you add to this the fact that (drug) treatment, when effective, requires chronic administration, and the fact that patient management requires a level of patient monitoring that has not been achieved as yet, then you have defined the conditions within which effective care has to be established.

NOTES

1. We use the word compliance, as opposed to adherence or therapeutic alliance, because we believe it to be the most accurate descriptor of available alternatives for the issue we are discussing: medication compliance. This does not mean that we are promoting its usage or even suggesting that the coercion implicit in the word be the object of a clinician's activities. Instead, we use it because at some point the clinician can not avoid giving advice to the patient that the physician expects the patient to accept as being in his or her best interest. Thus, coercion is an unavoidable, almost existential, element in any doctor-patient relationship. The question asked in this paper is: does what we know about antipsychotic drugs, particularly the phenothiazines, permit the physician to advise the patient concerning drugs without also reflecting the limited efficacy of the available drugs; and does it permit the community to expect that adequate drug ingestion will control psychotic behavior.
2. Oral phenothiazines are usually short-acting and require repeated daily ingestion, whereas the long-acting phenothiazines (also referred to as depot injections) are intramuscular injections given once every 2 to 6 weeks.
3. The authors are aware of the arbitrariness of this definition and of the difficulty of inferring the voluntarism of a patient's decision from reading a paper. We felt more secure doing this, however, than basing our inferences on a collection of studies that used heterogenous criteria to define noncompliance. In either case, the best way to resolve the ambiguity that results from either type of secondary analysis is by a direct test of the inferences drawn. This, we believe, has been done and can be found in the literature (e.g., Schooler et al. 1980).

REFERENCES

Affleck, J. N., Burns, J., and Forrest, J. D. Long-term follow-up of schizophrenic patients in Edinburgh. *Acta Psychiatrica Scandinavica* 53(3): 227-237 (1976).

Baekeland, F., and Lundwall, L. Dropping out of treatment: a critical review. *Psychological Bulletin* 82: 738-783 (1975).

Barofsky, I., quoted in Huey, K. Special report: the chronic psychiatric patient in the community. Highlights from a conference in Boston. *Hospital and Community Psychiatry* 28: 283-290 (1977).

Barofsky, I. Compliance adherence and the therapeutic alliance: steps in the development of self-care. *Social Science and Medicine*, 12: 369-376 (1978).

Birley, J. L. T. and Brown, G. W. Crises and life changes preceding the onset or relapse of acute schizophrenia: clinical aspects. *British Journal of Psychiatry* 116: 327-333 (1970).

Blackwell, B. Treatment adherence. *British Journal of Psychiatry* 129: 513-531 (1976).

Blackwell, B., and Shepherd, M. Prophylactic lithium: another therapeutic myth? *Lancet* 1: 968-971 (1968).

Bowden, C. L., Starfield, L. S., and Adams, R L. A correlation between drop out status and improvement in a psychiatric clinic. *Hospital and Community Psychiatry* 31(3): 193-195 (1980).

Brown, G. W., Monck, E. M., Carstairs, G. M., and Wing, J. K. Influence of family life on the course of schizophrenic illness. *British Journal of Preventive and Social Medicine* 16: 55-68 (1962).

Brown, G. W., Birley, J. L. T., and Wing, J. K. Influence of family life on the course of schizophrenic disorders: a replication. *British Journal of Psychiatry* 121: 241-258 (1972).

Bucci, L., Fuchs, M., Simon, J., and Fink, M. Depot fluphenazine in the treatment of psychosis in a community mental health clinic. *Diseases of the Nervous System* 31: 28-31 (1970).

Carder, S. L., and Snibbe, J. Outpatient management of chronic schizophrenics with fluphenazine enanthate (Prolixin Enanthate): a clinical evaluation. *Current Therapeutic Research* 14: 589-598 (1973).

Carney, M. W. P., and Sheffield, B. F. Comparison of anti-psychotic depot injections in the maintenance treatment of schizophrenia. *British Journal of Psychiatry* 129: 476-481 (1976).

Case, W. G., Ryder, B. L., Dhopheshwarkar, V. P., Pereira-Ogan, J. A., and Rickles, K. Clomacran and Chlorpromazine in psychotic outpatients: a controlled study. *Current Therapeutic Research* 13: 337-343 (1971).

Chien, C. Drugs and rehabilitation in schizophrenia, in *Drugs in Combination with Other Therapies*, M. Greenblatt, ed. New York: Grune and Stratton, 1975, 13-34.

Chowdhury, M. E. H., and Chacon, C. Depot fluphenazine and flupenthixol in the treatment of stabilized schizophrenics: a double blind comparative trial. *Comprehensive Psychiatry* 21: 135-139 (1980).

Claghorn, J., Johnstone, E. E., Cook, T. H. and Itschner, L. Group therapy and maintenance of schizophrenics. *Archives of General Psychiatry* 31: 361-365 (1974).

Cole, J. O., Bonato, R., and Goldberg, S. C. Non-specific factors in the drug therapy of schizophrenic patients, in *Non-specific Factors in Drug Therapy*, K. Rickels, ed. Springfield, Ill.: C. C. Thomas, 1968.

Cody, J., and Robinson, A. M. The effect of low-cost maintenance medication on the rehospitalization of schizophrenic outpatients. *American Journal of Psychiatry* 134: 73-76 (1977).

Crawford, R., and Forrest, A. Controlled trial of depot fluphenazine in outpatient schizophrenics. *British Journal of Psychiatry* 124: 385-391 (1974).

Davis, K. L., Estess, F. M., Simonton, S. C., and Gonda, T. A. Effects of payment mode on clinic attendance and rehospitalization. *American Journal of Psychiatry* 134(5): 576-578 (1977).

Del Giudice, J., Clark, W. G., and Gocka, E. F. Prevention of recidivism of schizophrenics treated with fluphenazine enanthate. *Psychosomatics* 16: 32-36 (1975).

Dencker, S. J., Lepp, M., and Malm, U. Clopenthixol and flupenthixol depot preparations in outpatient schizophrenics. I. A one-year double blind study of clopenthixol decanoate and flupenthixol palmitate. *Acta Psychiatrica Scandinavica*. Supp. 279, 61: 10-28 (1980).

Denham, J., and Adamson, L. The contribution of fluphenazine enanthate and decanoate in the prevention of readmission of schizophrenic patients. *Acta Psychiatrica Scandinavica* 47: 420-430 (1971).

Dohrenwend, B. P., and Dohrenwend, B. S. Psychiatric disorders and susceptibility to stress, in *The Social Consequences of Psychiatric Illness*, Robins, L. W., Clayton, P. J., Wing, J. L., eds. New York: Brunner-Mazel, 1980.

Donabedian, A. The quality of medical care. *Science* 200: 856-864 (1978).

Donlon, P. T., Swaback, D. O., and Osborne, M. L. Pimozide versus Fluphenazine in ambulatory schizophrenics. A 12-month comparison study. *Diseases of the Nervous System* 38: 119-123 (1977).

Englehardt, D. M., Freedman, B. S. N., Glick, L. D., Hankoff, D. M., and Margolis, R. Prevention of psychiatric hospitalization with the use of psychopharmacologic agents. *Journal of the American Medical Assn.* 173: 147-149 (1960).

Fallon, W., Watt, D. C., and Shepherd, M. A comparative controlled trial of pimozide and fluphenazine decanoate in the continuation therapy of schizophrenia. *Psychological Medicine* 8: 59-70 (1978).

Finnerty, F. A., Show, L. M., and Himmelsbach, C. K. Hypertension in the inner city II: detection and follow-up. *Circulation* 47: 76-78 (1973).

Gittleman-Klein, R., and Klein, D. F. Marital status as a prognostic indicator in schizophrenia. *Journal of Nervous and Mental Disease* 147(3): 289-296 (1968).

Gold, B. H., Nelson, A. A., and Frazin, R. N. *Psychiatrists' assessment of drug default: its relationship to their treatment activities.* Paper presented at the annual meeting of the American Pharmaceutical Assn. Academy of Pharmaceutical Sciences, Economic and Administrative Science Section, New Orleans, 1976.

Goldberg, S. C., Schooler, N. R., Hogarty, G. E., and Roper, M. Prediction of relapse in schizophrenic outpatients treated by drug and sociotherapy. *Archives of General Psychiatry* 34(2): 171-185 (1977).

Goldstein, J. J., Rodnick, E. H., Evans, J. R., May, P. R. A., and Steinberg, M. R. Drug and family therapy in the aftercare of acute schizophrenia. *Archives of General Psychiatry* 34: 1169-1177 (1978).
Gordis, L. Methodologic issues in the measurement of patient compliance, in *Compliance with Therapeutic Regimens*, D. L. Sackett and R. B. Haynes, eds. Baltimore: Johns Hopkins Univ. Press, 1976.
Gottfries, C. G., and Green, L. Flupenthixol decanoate in treatment of outpatients. *Acta Psychiatrica Scandinavica* Supp. 255: 15-24 (1974).
Haase, H. J., and Janssen, P. A. J. *The action of neuroleptic drugs*. Chicago: Year Book, 1965.
Haefner, D. P., Sacks, J. M., and Mason, A. S. Physicians' attitudes toward chemotherapy as a factor in psychiatric patients' responses to medication.
Hare, E. H., Willcox, D. R. C. Do psychiatric in-patients take their pills? *British Journal of Psychiatry* 113: 1435-1439 (1967).
Haynes, R. B., Taylor, D. W., and Sackett, D. L. *Compliance in Health Care*. Baltimore: Johns Hopkins Univ. Press, 1979.
Hiep, A., and Marriott, P. Long-acting neuroleptics—a fairy story? *Nursing Times*, 863-866 (1976).
Hippius, H. Long-term pharmacotherapy of schizophrenia, in *Biological Treatment in Mental Illness*, M. Rinkel, ed. New York: Page, 1966, pp. 497-506.
Hirsch, S. R., Gaind, R., Rohde, P. D., Stevens, B. C., and Wing, J. K. Outpatient maintenance of chronic schizophrenic patients with long-acting phenothiazines: Double blind placebo trial. *British Medical Journal* 1: 633-637 (1973).
Hogarty, G. E., and Goldberg, S. C. Drug and sociotherapy in the aftercare of schizophrenic patients. *Archives of General Psychiatry* 28(1): 54-64 (1973).
Hogarty, G. E., Goldberg, S. C., Schooler, N. R., and Ulrich, R. F. Drug and sociotherapy in the aftercare of schizophrenic patients. *Archives of General Psychiatry* 31(11): 603-608 (1974).
Hogarty, G. E., Ulrich, R., Goldberg, S., and Schooler, N. Sociotherapy and the prevention of relapse among schizophrenic patients: an artifact of drug? in *Evaluation of Psychological Therapies*, R. L. Spitzer, and D. L. Klein, eds. Baltimore: Johns Hopkins Univ. Press, 1976.
Hogarty, G. E., Schooler, N. R., Ulrich, R., Mussare, F., Ferro, P., and Herron, E. Fluphenazine and social therapy in the aftercare of schizophrenic patients. *Archives of General Psychiatry* 36: 1283-1294 (1979).
Hollander, M., and Wolfe, D. A. *Nonparametric Statistical Methods*. New York: Wiley, 1973.
Honigfeld, G. Non-specific factors in treatment II. Review of social psychological factors. *Diseases of the Nervous System* 25: 225-239 (1964).
Irwin, D. S., Weitzel, W. D., and Morgan, D. W. Phenothiazine intake and staff attitudes. *American Journal of Psychiatry* 127: 1631-1635 (1971).
Itil, T. M., Marasa, J., Saletu, B., Davis, R. N., and Mucciaridi, N. Computerized E.E.G.: predictors of outcome in schizophrenia. *Journal of Nervous & Mental Diseases* 160: 188-203 (1975).
Johnson, D. A. W., and Freeman, H. Drug defaulting by patients on long-acting phenothiazines. *Psychological Medicine* 3: 115-119 (1973).

Keskiner, A., Holden, J. M. C., and Itil, T. M. Maintenance treatment of schizophrenic outpatients with a depot phenothiazine. *Psychosomatics* 9: 166–171 (1968).

Knights, A., Okasha, M. S., Allsalih, M., and Hirsch, S. R. Depressive and extra pyrimidal symptoms and clinical effects: A trial of fluphenazine versus fluphenthixol in maintenance of schizophrenic out-patients. *British Journal of Psychiatry* 135: 516–523 (1979).

Kolakowska, T., Gelder, M. G., and Orr, M. W. Drug-related and illness-related factors in the outcome of chlorpromazine treatment: testing a model. *Psychological Medicine* 10: 335–343 (1980).

Kolivakis, T., Azim, H., and Kingstone, E. A double-blind comparison of pimozide and chlorpromazine in the maintenance care of chronic schizophrenic outpatients. *Current Therapeutic Research* 16: 998–1004 (1974).

Leff, J. P. Psychophysiological monitoring of social and drug effects in schizophrenia, in *Depot Fluphenazines: Twelve Years Experience*, F. J. Ayd, ed. Baltimore: Ayd Medical Communications, 1978.

Leff, J. P. and Wing, J. K. Trial of maintenance therapy in schizophrenia. *British Medical Journal* 1: 599–604 (1971).

Leff, J. P., Hirsch, S. R., Gaind, R., Rohde, P. D., and Stevens, B. C. Life events and maintenance therapy in schizophrenic relapse. *British Journal of Psychiatry* 123: 659–660 (1973).

Lorion, R. Patient and therapist variables in the treatment of low income patients. *Psychological Bulletin* 81: 344–354 (1974).

MacPherson, A. S., and Luterbach, E. J. Mechanical aids to drug self-administration in psychiatric patients. Paper presented at the New England Conference on the Chronic Psychiatric Patient in the Community, Boston, November, 1976.

Mason, A. S., Forrest, I. P., Forrest, F. M., and Butler, H. Adherence to maintenance therapy and re-hospitalization. *Diseases of the Nervous System* 24: 103-104 (1963).

May, P. R. A., and Goldberg, S. C. Prediction of schizophrenic patients' response to pharmacotherapy, in *Psychopharmacology: a generation of progress*, M. A. Lipton, A. Di Mascio, and K. J. Killam, eds. New York: Raven Press, 1978.

McClellan, T. A., and Cowan, G. Use of antipsychotic and antidepressant drugs by chronically ill patients. *American Journal of Psychiatry* 126(12): 113–115 (1970).

Michaux, W. W. Side-effects, resistance, and dosage deviations in psychiatric outpatients treated with tranquilizers. *Journal of Nervous and Mental Diseases* 133: 203-212 (1961).

Nelson, A. A., Gold, B. H., Hutchinson, R. A., and Benezra, E. Drug default among schizophrenic patients. *American Journal Hospital Pharmacy* 32: 1237-1242 (1975).

Park, L. C., and Lipman, R. S. A comparison of patient dosage deviation reports with pill counts. *Psychopharmacologica* 6: 299-302 (1964).

Pinto, R., Baunerjee, A , and Ghosh, N. A double-blind comparison of flupenthixol decanoate and fluphenazine decanoate in the treatment of chronic schizophrenia. *Acta Psychiatrica Scandinavica* 60: 313-322 (1979).

Polonowita, A., and James, N. Mc I. Fluphenazine decanoate maintenance in schizophrenia: A retrospective study. *New Zealand Medical Journal* 83: 316-318 (1976).

Raskin, A. A comparison of acceptors and resistors of drug treatment as an adjunct to psychotherapy. American Documentation Institute Order No. 6647 ADI Auxiliary Publication Project, Library of Congress, Washington, D.C.

Reilly, E. L., Wilson, W. P., and McClinton, H. K. Clinical characteristics and medical history of schizophrenics readmitted to the hospital. *International Journal of Neuropsychiatry* 3: 85-90 (1967).

Renton, C. A., Affleck, J. W., Carstairs, G. M., and Forrest, A. D. A followup of schizophrenic patients in Edinburgh. *Acta Psychiatrica Scandinavica* 39: 548-581 (1963).

Richards, A. R. Attitude and drug acceptance. *British Journal of Psychiatry* 10: 46-52 (1964).

Rickels, K. *Non-specific factors in drug therapy*. Springfield: C. C. Thomas, 1968.

Rickels, K., and Briscoe, E. Assessment of dosage deviation in outpatient drug research. *Journal of Clinical Pharmacology* 10:153-160 (1970).

Rifkin, A., Quitkin, F., Rabiner, C. J., and Klein, D. F. Fluphenazine decanoate, fluphenazine hydrochloride given orally, and placebo in remitted schizophrenics. I. Relapse rates after one year. *Archives of General Psychiatry* 34: 43-44 (1977).

Routsonis, K. G., and Photiadis, H. The use of fluphenazine enanthate in psychotic patients. *Current Therapeutic Research* 15: 92-96 (1973).

Sabshin, M., and Ramot, J. Psychotherapeutic evaluation and the psychiatric setting. *Archives of Neurology & Psychiatry* 75: 362-370 (1956).

Sackett, D. L. The magnitude of compliance and non-compliance, in *Compliance With Therapeutic Regimens*, D. L. Sackett and R. B. Haynes, eds. Baltimore: Johns Hopkins Univ. Press, 1976.

Schooler, N. R., Levine, J., Severe, J. B., Brauzer, B., DiMascio, A., Klerman, G. L., and Tuason, V. B. Prevention of relapse in schizophrenia: An evaluation of fluphenazine decanoate. *Archives of General Psychiatry* 37: 16-24 (1980).

Serban, G. *Adjustment of schizophrenics in the community*. New York: Spectrum, 1980.

Serban, G., and Thomas, A. Attitudes and behaviors of acute and chronic schizophrenic patients regarding ambulatory treatment. *American Journal of Psychiatry* 131(9): 991-995 (1974).

Siegal, S. *Non-parametric statistics for the behavioral sciences*. New York: McGraw-Hill, 1956.

Smith, R. C., Crayton, J., DeKirmenjian, H., Klass, S., and Davis, J. M. Blood levels of neuroleptic drugs in non-responding chronic schizophrenic patients. *Archives of General Psychiatry* 36(5): 579-584 (1979).

Strauss, J., and Carpenter, W. T. Prediction of outcome in schizophrenia. III. Five year outcome and its predictors. *Archives of General Psychiatry* 34(2): 159-163 (1977).

Van Putten, T. Why do schizophrenic patients refuse to take their drugs? *Archives of General Psychiatry* 31(7): 67-71 (1974).

Van Putten, T., Mutalipassi, L. R., and Malkin, M. D. Phenothiazine-induced decompensation. *Archives of General Psychiatry* 30(1): 102–105 (1974).

Van Putten, T., Crumpton, E., Yale, C. Drug refusal in schizophrenia and the wish to be crazy. *Archives of General Psychiatry* 33(12): 1443–1446 (1976).

Vaughn, C. E., and Leff, J. P. The influence of family and social factors on the course of psychiatric illness. *British Journal of Psychiatry* 129: 125-137 (1976).

Willcox, D. R. C., Gillian, R., and Hare, E. H. Do psychiatric outpatients take their drugs? *British Medical Journal* 1: 790-792 (1965).

Wilson, J. D., and Enoch, M. D. Estimation of drug rejection by schizophrenic inpatients with analysis of clinical factors. *British Journal of Psychiatry* 113: 209–211 (1967).

Winkelman, Jr., N. W. A clinical and socio-cultural study of 200 psychiatric patients started on chlorpromazines 10½ years ago. *American Journal of Psychiatry* 120: 861–869 (1964).

APPENDIX A

Part I: *Method of Analysis of the Studies*

General Criteria: To be cited, a study had to include 10 or more outpatient schizophrenics who were prescribed phenothiazines. Each study was reviewed and classified according to specific criteria (see below). The summary statements with the codes provided should permit the reader to determine how noncompliance and relapse/rehospitalization rates were calculated. The drug used and sample size for each citation were also provided.

	Code
1. *Type of Study:*	A. Followup Study B. Mirror-Image Study C. Experimental Study (patients randomly assigned)
2. *Diagnostic Status:*	A. Acutely ill B. Stabilized C. Mixed patient group D. Not specified
3. *Data Source:*	A. Study starts immediately upon release of the patient to the community B. Study starts after a period of stabilization in the community C. Data from both phases of the study D. Mixed patient groups E. Not specified F. Not applicable
4. *Duration of Study:*	A. $\leqslant$6 months B. $\geqslant$6 months to 1 year C. $\geqslant$1 to 2 years D. $\geqslant$2 years E. Not specified
5. *Type of Medication:*	A. Oral B. Long-acting phenothiazines (LAPs)

6. *Social Support Provided:* Minimal social support refers to the situation in which the patient–provider interaction is confined to relatively brief (e.g., 20 minutes), possibly regular (e.g., once a month) visits that permit the provider to assess the patient's medical, psychiatric and functional status. Assessment of drug-taking behavior may occur, but the visits are not associated with the drug

administration. Thus, patients receive social support incidental to what is essentially a patient-monitoring visit. In contrast, in programmed social support the patient visits have a specific therapeutic objective: providing either social therapies and/or psychotherapy (B) or drug therapy (C), as well as a patient-monitoring function. We have also included studies in which the family has provided systematic support for the patient as an example of programmed social support (B).

A. Minimal Patient Monitoring
B. Programmed Psychotherapy, Social Therapies, and/or Systematic Family Support
C. Programmed Clinic Support

7. *Calculation of Noncompliance Rate*: The denominator was determined by subtracting from the total sample patients who were removed from the study because of:

A. side effects (a physician's decision)
B. relapse/rehospitalization
C. lack of drug effectiveness
D. suicide and/or death
E. a physician who refused to allow the patient to participate in the study, or
F. miscellaneous reasons (see paper).

The numerator was calculated by including patients who refused to:

G. participate in the study
H. comply with all aspects of the drug regimen
I. keep appointments for drug or psychotherapy, or who transfered to another treatment facility, or
K. sought treatment elsewhere but remained in the area.

If, on the other hand, the information provided was not specific enough to accurately calculate the noncompliance rate, then the rate provided was based on the:

L. available data (attrition data). In some studies measurement of noncompliance starts as soon as a patient becomes an outpatient, and in some only after it has been shown that the patient can comply with his or her medication regimen in the community. Measurement of noncompliance included both the initial and stabilized outpatient behavior where possible (see Criteria #3 and Table II).

8. *Calculation of the Relapse/Rehospitalization Rate*: Where possible the re lapse/rehospitalization rate was based on maintenance or chronic-treatment-

phase data only. If data for both relapse and rehospitalization were available, then the rehospitalization rates were presented. The denominator included noncompliant patients, but patients who were noncompliant during the chronic phase of the study only. Excluded were:

A. patients with whom contact was lost (i.e., they moved), or who
B. died or committed suicide, or for
C. miscellaneous reasons (see paper).

The numerator included all patients who relapsed or were hospitalized. It was assumed that admissions required a physician's acquiescence, independent of who initiated the hospitalization procedure—the patient, the patient's family, the police or a physician.

D. Characteristics of the sample were not specified.
E. Data on relapse/rehospitalization rate not available.

9. *Noncompliance Measures*: A wide variety of measures were used to determine if patients were noncompliant in these studies. Included were physician, patient or family reports, pill counts, and urine tests and broken appointments (such as for the patients receiving long-acting phenothiazines).

Part II: *References and Study Characteristics*

1. Engelhardt, D. M., Freedman, B. S. N., Glick, L. D., Hankoff, D. Mann, and Margolis, R. Prevention of psychiatric hospitalization with use of psychopharmacological agents. *Journal of American Medical Association* 173: 147-149 (1960).

   A. Chlorpromazine; Experimental Study; Diagnostic Status = A; Data Source = E; Duration = 1 to 2 years; Oral; Support = Minimal; Noncompliance Rate = 40.3%(L); N = 62; Relapse Rate = 4.8%(D); N = 62.

   B. Promazine; Experimental Study; Diagnostic Status = A; Data Source = E; Duration = 1 to 2 years; Oral; Support = Minimal; Noncompliance Rate = 34.5%(L); N = 55; Relapse Rate = 18.2%(D); N = 55.

2. Michaux, W. W. Side-effects, resistance and dosage deviations in psychiatric outpatients treated with tranquilizers. *Journal of Nervous and Mental Diseases* 133: 203-212 (1961).

   Chlorpromazine; Experimental Study; Diagnostic Status = D; Data Source = C; Duration = <6 months; Oral; Support = Programmed B; Noncompliance Rate = 47.0%(L); N = 32; Relapse Rate = E.

3. Renton, C. A., Affleck, J. W., Carstairs, G. M., and Forrest, A. D. A follow-up of schizophrenic patients in Edinburgh. *Acta Psychiatrica Scandinavica* 39: 548-581 (1963).

86% of sample on Phenothiazines; Follow-up; Diagnostic Status = C; Data Source = F; Duration = >1 to 2 years; Oral; Support = Minimal; Noncompliance Rate = 52.1% (B,D,F); N = 121; Relapse Rate = 16.2% (B); N = 130.

4. Willcox, D. R. C., Gillian, R., and Hare, E. H. Do psychiatric outpatients take their drugs? *British Medical Journal* 1: 790-792 (1965).

Chlorpromazine; Follow-up; Diagnostic Status = D; Data Source = F; Duration = <6 months; Oral; Support = Minimal; Noncompliance Rate = 32.0%(L), N = 22; Relapse Rate = E.

5. Winkelman, Jr., N. W. A clinical and socio-cultural study of 200 psychiatric patients started on chlorpromazines 10½ years ago. *American Journal of Psychiatry* 120: 861-869 (1964).

Chlorpromazine; Follow-up; Diagnostic Status = D; Data Source = F; Duration = >2 years; Oral; Support = Programmed C; Noncompliance Rate = 61.2%(B); N = 49; Relapse Rate = 21.0%(D); N = 62.

6. Hippius, H. Long-term pharmacotherapy of schizophrenia in *Biological Treatment in Mental Illness*, Rinkel, M., ed. New York, 1966, 497-505.

Perazine; Follow-up: Diagnostic Status = C; Data Source = F; Duration = > 2 years; Oral; Support = Minimal; Noncompliance Rate = 54.1% (L); N = 255; Relapse Rate = 47.0%(D); N-117.

7. Keskiner, A., Holden, J. M. C., and Itil, T. M. Maintenance treatment of schizophrenic outpatients with a depot phenothiazine. *Psychosomatics* 9: 166-171 (1968).

Fluphenazine; Experimental Study; Diagnostic Status = B; Data Source = B; Duration = ≤6 months; LAP: Support = Programmed C; Noncompliance Rate = 0.0%, (L); N = 12; Relapse Rate = 7.7%(D); N = 13.

8. Bucci, L., Fuchs, M., Simon, J., and Fink, M. Depot fluphenazine in the treatment of psychosis in a community mental health clinic. *Diseases of the Nervous System* 31: 28-31 (1970).

Fluphenazine; Experimental Study: Diagnostic Status = B; Data Source = B; Duration = ≤6 months; LAP; Support = Programmed C; Noncompliance Rate = 37.1%, (L); N = 62; Relapse Rate = E.

9. Denham, J., and Adamson, L. The contribution of fluphenazine enanthate and decanoate in the prevention of readmission of schizophrenic patients. *Acta Psychiatrica Scandinavica* 47: 420-430 (1971).

Fluphenazine; Mirror-Image Study; Diagnostic Status = C; Data Source = F; Duration = ≥1 to 2 years; LAP; Support = Programmed C; Noncompliance Rate = 10.1% (A, B, C,); N = 69; Relapse Rate = 33.0%(D); N = 103.

10. Case, W. G., Ryder, B. L., Dhopheshwarkar, V. P., Pereira-Ogan, J. A., and Rickels, K. Clomacran and chlorpromazine in psychotic outpatients: A controlled study. *Current Therapeutic Research* 13: 337-343 (1971).

Chlorpromazine; Experimental Study; Diagnostic Status = C; Data Source = C; Duration = <6 months; Oral; Support = Minimal; Noncompliance Rate = 50% (A,B); N = 20%; Relapse Rate = 12.5 (D); N = 24.

11. Irwin, D. S., Weitzel, W. D., and Morgan, D. W. Phenothiazine intake and staff attitudes. *American Journal of Psychiatry* 127: 1631-1635 (1971).

Chlorpromazine or Thioridazine; Follow-up; Diagnostic Status = D; Data Source = F; Duration = E; Oral; Support = Minimal; Noncompliance Rate = 35.0%(L); N = 40; Relapse Rate = E.

12. Leff, J. P., and Wing, J. K. Trial of maintenance therapy in schizophrenia. *British Medical Journal* 1: 599-604 (1971).

Chlorpromazine or Trifluoperazine; Experimental Study; Diagnostic Status = B; Data Source = B; Duration = ≥1 to 2 years; Oral; Support = Minimal; Noncompliance Rate = 71.4% (B,F); N = 42, Relapse Rate = 35.0%(A,B); N = 20.

13. Johnson, D. A. W., and Freeman, H. Drug defaulting by patients on long-acting phenothiazines. *Psychological Medicine* 3: 115-119 (1973).

Fluphenazine; Follow-up; Diagnostic Status = D; Data Source = F; Duration = ≥1 to 2 years; LAP; Support = Programmed C; Noncompliance Rate = 23.6% (A,D,E); N - 123; Relapse Rate = E.

14. Hirsch, S. R., Gaind, R., Rohde, P. D., Stevens, B. C., and Wing, J. K. Outpatient maintenance of chronic schizophrenic patients with long-acting phenothiazines: Double blind placebo trials. *British Medical Journal* 1: 633-637 (1973).

Fluphenazine; Experimental Study; Diagnostic Status = B; Data Source = C; Duration = ≥1 year to 2 years; LAP; Support = Programmed C; Noncompliance = 23.3%(B); N = 43; Relapse Rate = 12.5%; N = 40.

15. Carder, S. L. and Snibbe, J. Outpatient management of chronic schizophrenics with fluphenazine enanthate (Prolixin Enanthate): A clinical evaluation. *Current Therapeutic Research* 14: 589-598 (1973).

Fluphenazine; Follow-up; Diagnostic Status = C; Data Source = A; Duration = ≥6 months to 1 year; LAP; Support = Programmed C; Noncompliance Rate = 53.6%(F); N = 28; Relapse Rate = 10.3%(C); N = 29.

16. Routsonis, K. G. and Photiadis, H. The use of fluphenazine enanthate in psychotic patients. *Current Therapeutic Research* 15: 92-96 (1973).

Fluphenazine; Follow-up; Diagnostic Status = D; Data Source = F; Duration = ≥6 months to 1 year; LAP; Support = Programmed C; Noncompliance Rate = 2.5%(L); N = 40; Relapse Rate = E.

17. Crawford, R. and Forrest, A. Controlled trial of depot fluphenazine in outpatient schizophrenics. *British Journal of Psychiatry* 124: 385-391 (1974).

A. Trifluoperazine; Experimental Study; Diagnostic Status = B; Data Source = B; Duration = ≥6 months to 1 year; Oral; Support = Programmed C; Noncompliance Rate = 52.9%(L); N = 17; Relapse Rate = 26.7%(D); N = 15.

B. Fluphenazine; Experimental Study; Diagnostic Status = B; Data Source = B; Duration = ≥6 months to 1 year; LAP; Support = Programmed C; Noncompliance Rate = 35.7%(L); N = 14; Relapse Rate = 0.0%(D); N = 14.

18. Claghorn, J., Johnstone, E. E., Cook, T. H., and Itschner, L. Group therapy and maintenance treatment of schizophrenics. *Archives of General Psychiatry* 31: 361-365 (1974).

A. Phenothiazines; Experimental Study; Diagnostic Status = B; Data Source = E; Duration = ≥6 months to 1 year; Oral; Support = Minimal; Noncompliance Rate = 54.5%(L); N = 22; Relapse Rate = E.

B. Phenothiazines; Experimental Study; Diagnostic Status = B; Data Source = E; Duration = ≥6 months to 1 year; Oral; Support = Programmed B; Noncompliance Rate = 59.6%(L); N = 27; Relapse Rate = E.

19. Kolivakis, T., Azim, H., and Kingstone, E. A double-blind comparison of pimozide and chlorpromazine in the maintenance care of chronic schizophrenic outpatients. *Current Therapeutic Research* 16: 998-1004 (1974).

Chlorpromazine; Experimental Study; Diagnostic Status = B; Data Source = B; Duration = $\geq$6 months to 1 year; Oral; Support = Minimal; Noncompliance Rate = 20%(A,D); N = 20; Relapse Rate = E.

20. Gottfries, C. G. and Green, L. Flupenthixol decanoate in treatment of outpatients. *Acta Psychiatrica Scandinavica* Supp. 255: 15-24 (1974).

    Flupenthixol; Mirror-Image; Diagnostic Status = C; Data Source = F; Duration = $\geq$6 months to 1 year (minimum); LAP; Support = Programmed C; Noncompliance Rate = 44.7% (A,B,C,D,E); N = 47; Relapse Rate = 34.0% (A,B); N = 94.

21. Chien, C. Drugs and rehabilitation in schizophrenia, in *Drugs in Combination With Other Therapies*, M. Greenblatt, ed. New York: Grune and Stratton, 1975, pp. 13-34.

    Fluphenazine; Experimental Study (Group 2 only); Diagnostic Status = B; Data Source = B; Duration = $\geq$1 to 2 years; LAP; Support = Programmed C; Noncompliance Rate = 33.3%(E); N = 15; Relapse Rate = 33.3%(C); N = 15 ("Failure rate" was assumed to be equivalent to a relapse).

22. Nelson, A. A., Gold, B. H., Hutchinson, R. A., and Benezra, E. Drug default among schizophrenic patients. *American Journal Hospital Pharmacy* 32: 1237-1242 (1975).

    Chlorpromazine or Thioridazine; Experimental Study; Diagnostic Status = B; Data Source = A; Duration = $\leq$6 months; Oral; Support = Minimal; Noncompliance Rate = 46.2%(A,E); N = 40; Relapse Rate = E.

23. Del Giudice, J., Clark, W. G., and Gocka, E. F. Prevention of recidivism of schizophrenics treated with fluphenazine enanthate. *Psychosomatics* 16: 32-36 (1975).

    A. Fluphenazine; Experimental Study; Diagnostic Status = B; Data Source = B; Duration = $\geq$1 to 2 years; Oral; Support = Minimal; Noncompliance Rate = 21.4%(L); N = 28; Relapse Rate = E.

    B. Fluphenazine; Experimental Study; Diagnostic Status B; Data Source = B; Duration = $\geq$1 to 2 years; Oral; Support = Programmed C; Noncompliance Rate = 37.9%(L); N = 29; Relapse Rate = E.

    C. Fluphenazine; Experimental Study; Diagnostic Status = B; Data Source = B; Duration = $\geq$1 to 2 years; LAP; Support = Programmed C; Noncompliance Rate = 32.0%(L); N = 25; Relapse Rate = E.

24. Carney, M. W. P. and Sheffield, B. F. Comparison of anti-psychotic depot injections in the maintenance treatment of schizophrenia. *British Journal of Psychiatry* 129: 476-481 (1976).

Phenothiazines; Follow-up; Diagnostic Status = D; Data Source = F; Duration = ⩾1.5 years; LAP; Support = Programmed C; Noncompliance Rate = 12.1% (A,B,D,F); N = 338; Relapse Rate = E.

25. Polonowita, A., and Mc I. James, N. Fluphenazine decanoate maintenance in schizophrenia: A retrospective study. *New Zealand Medical Journal* 83: 316-318 (1976).

Fluphenazine; Mirror-Image Study; Diagnostic Status = C; Data Source = F; Duration = ⩾1 to 2 years; LAP; Support = Programmed C; Noncompliance Rate = 36.4% (Includes an unknown number of patients who had side effects. It was not possible to separate these patients from those who were noncompliant. Thus, rate is an overestimate.); N = 65; Relapse Rate = E.

26. Hiep, A., and Marriott, P. Long-acting neuroleptics—a fairy story? *Nursing Times*, 863-866 (1976).

Fluphenazine; Mirror-Image Study; Diagnostic Status = C; Data Source = F; Duration = ⩾1 to 2 years; LAP; Support = Programmed C; Noncompliance Rate = 12.9%(A,B,C,D,E,F); N = 364; Relapse Rate = E.

27. Rifkin, A., Quitkin, F., Rabiner, C. J., and Klein, D. F. Fluphenazine decanoate, fluphenazine hydrochloride given orally, and placebo in remitted schizophrenics. I. Relapse rates after one year. *Archives of General Psychiatry* 34: 43-47 (1977).

A. Fluphenazine; Experimental Study; Diagnostic Status = C; Data Source = B; Duration = ⩾1 to 2 years; Oral; Support = Programmed B; Noncompliance Rate = 4.8%(A,B); N = 21; Relapse Rate = 4.3%(B); N = 23.

B. Fluphenazine; Experimental Study; Diagnostic Status = C; Data Source = B; Duration = ⩾1 to 2 years; LAP; Support = Programmed B; Noncompliance rate = 23.0%(A,B); N = 13; Relapse Rate = 5.3%(D); N = 19.

28. Donlon, P. T., Swaback, D. O., and Osborne, M. L. Pimozide versus Fluphenazine in ambulatory schizophrenics. A 12-month comparison study. *Diseases of the Nervous System* 38: 119-123 (1977).

Fluphenazine; Experiment Study; Diagnostic Status = B; Data Source = A; Duration = ≥6 months to 1 year; Oral; Support = Minimal; Noncompliance Rate = 11.8% (A,C,F,G,J); N = 19; Relapse Rate = E.

29. Fallon, W., Watt, D. C., and Shepherd, M. A comparative controlled trial of pimozide and fluphenazine decanoate in the continuation therapy of schizophrenia. *Psychological Medicine* 8: 59-70 (1978).

Fluphenazine; Experimental Study; Diagnostic Status = B; Data Source = B; Duration = ≥ 1 to 2 years; LAP; Support = Programmed C; Noncompliance Rate = 46.2%(B); N = 13; Relapse Rate = 35.0%(D); N = 20.

30. Goldstein, J. J., Rodnick, E. H., Evans, J. R., May, P. R. A., and Steinberg, M. R. Drug and family therapy in the aftercare of acute schizophrenia. *Archives of General Psychiatry* 34: 1169-1177 (1978).

Fluphenazine; Experimental Study; Diagnostic Status = A; Data Source = A; Duration = ≥6 months to 1 year; LAP; Support = Programmed C; Noncompliance Rate = 8.4%(B); N = 95; Relapse Rate = 9.4%(D); N = 96.

31. Pinto, R., Baunerjee, A., and Ghosh, N. A double-blind comparison of flupenthixol decanoate and fluphenazine decanoate in the treatment of chronic schizophrenia. *Acta Psychiatrica Scandinavica* 60: 313-322 (1979).

A. Flupenthixol; Experimental Study; Diagnostic Status = B; Data Source = B; Duration = ≥1 to 2 years; LAP; Support = Programmed C; Noncompliance Rate = 0.0%; N = 31; Relapse Rate = E.

B. Fluphenazine; Experimental Study; Diagnostic Status = B; Data Source = B; Duration = ≥1 to 2 years; LAP; Support Programmed C; Noncompliance Rate = 21.9%(D); N = 32; Relapse Rate = E.

32. Knights, A., Okasha, M. S., Allsalih, M., and Hirsch, S. R. Depressive and extra pyramidal symptoms and clinical effects: A trial of fluphenazine versus flupenthixol in maintenance of schizophrenic out-patients. *British Journal of Psychiatry* 135: 516-523 (1979).

A. Flupenthixol; Experimental Study; Diagnostic Status = B; Data Source = A; Duration = ≥6 months to 1 year; LAP; Support = Programmed C; Noncompliance Rate = 30%(B); N = 20; Relapse Rate = 28.6%(D); N = 28.

B. Fluphenazine; Experimental Study; Diagnostic Status = B; Data Source = A; Duration = ≥6 months to 1 year; LAP; Support = Programmed C; Noncompliance Rate = 47.8%(B); N = 23; Relapse Rate = 21.0%(D); N = 29.

33. Hogarty, G. E., Schooler, N. R., Ulrich, R., Mussare, F., Ferro, P., and Herron, E. Fluphenazine and social therapy in the aftercare of schizophrenic patients. *Archives of General Psychiatry* 36: 1283-1294 (1979).

Fluphenazine; Experimental Study; Diagnostic Status = B; Data Source = A; Duration = ≥1 to 2 years; Oral and LAP; Support = Programmed B and C; Noncompliance Rate = 13%(A); N = 100; Relapse Rate = 49.5 (L; Oral); N = 50; Relapse Rate = 54.9; (L; LAP); N = 55 (Although this was a Drug x Social Therapy study, noncompliance rate was not broken out into specific treatment groups).

34. Chowdhury, M. E. H., and Chacon, C. Depot fluphenazine and flupenthixol in the treatment of stabilized schizophrenics. A double blind comparative trial. *Comprehensive Psychiatry* 21: 135-139 (1980).

Phenothiazines; Experimental Study; Diagnostic Status = B; Data Source = B; Duration = 6 months; LAP; Support = Programmed C; Noncompliance Rate = 21.4%(B); N = 28; Relapse Rate = 4.0%(C); N = 25.

35. Schooler, N. R., Levine, J., Severe, J. B., Brauzer, B., Di Mascio, A., Klerman, G. L., and Tuason, V. B. Prevention of relapse in schizophrenia: An evaluation of fluphenazine decanoate. *Archives of General Psychiatry* 37: 16-24 (1980).

A. Fluphenazine; Experimental Study; Diagnostic Status = B; Data Source = B; Duration = ≥1 to 2 years; Oral; Support = Programmed C; Noncompliance Rate = 39.7%(A,B); N = 68; Relapse Rate = 35.7%(B); N = 98.

B. Fluphenazine; Experimental Study; Diagnostic Status = B; Data Source = B; Duration = ≥1 to 2 years; LAP; Support = Programmed C; Noncompliance Rate = 35.5%(A,B); N = 76; Relapse Rate = 27.1%(B); N = 96.

36. Dencker, S. J., Lepp, M., and Malm, W. Clopenthixol and flupenthixol depot preparations in outpatient schizophrenics. I. A one-year double blind study of clopenthixol decanoate and flupenthixol palmitate. *Acta Psychiatrica Scandinavica.* Supp. 279 61: 10-28 (1980).

A. Clopenthixol; Experimental Study; Diagnostic Status = B; Data Source = C; Duration = ≥6 months to 1 year; LAP; Support = Programmed C; Noncompliance Rate = 0.0%(C); N = 27; Relapse Rate = E.

B. Flupenthixol; Experimental Study; Diagnostic Status = B; Data Source = C; Duration = ≥6 months to 1 year; LAP; Support = Programmed C; Noncompliance Rate = 8.0%(C,D); N = 25; Relapse Rate = E.

PART II

PSYCHOSOCIAL TREATMENT PRINCIPLES

EDITOR'S COMMENTARY: PART II

This section addresses the individual in the psychosocial context of his family, his work, his living situation and his social environment. The vulnerable patient when skillfully approached with insight and sensitivity within a meaningful social setting can often respond with health and strength. Good community care, as represented in these pages, is usually delivered by a comprehensive and multifaceted program. A prototypical patient—his family situation having been assessed as unsatisfactory as a result of a crisis intervention in an acute psychiatric service—may well be referred to a community residential program which will serve as an alternative living arrangement. Additionally, this same patient could conceivably be considered for vocational assessment while at a partial hospital program or social club during the day, as well as for individual therapy to help him understand his unique dynamics. Ideally, the various players upon this stage—all of the various clinicians—will meet together both initially for assessment and planning and periodically thereafter to assure a coordinated, knowledgeable treatment. This section describes the background and practice of the various components of this psychosocial program. All of these are practiced in the context of deinstitutionalization—the preservation of the "patient's assets for self-care" and social networks, as described in the previous section. The partial program is the component which would likely assess, prescribe and monitor the pharmacologic needs of the patient, as is described in the next section. Discussion of the problems in delivering all of these services in different environments (suburban and rural) and exploration of issues common to all programs (fiscal, legal and advocacy) follow in subsequent sections of the text.

In the first chapter, Stanton writes a thoughtful introduction to the role of the psychosocial therapies. He highlights man's social need to interact with his fellow man. He then distinguishes the essential differences between psychotherapy and other beneficial human interactions. He also relates psychotherapy to the importance of group living for the patient. He carefully reviews, in addition, the history of the development of psychotherapy. He emphasizes the therapist's expectation of change, and the importance of this in the therapeutic interaction with the chronic patient. He reviews the four types of psychotherapy used with chronic patients as well as the elements common to all of these. Stanton demonstrates how psychotherapy alone or psychotherapy only with medication "is clearly inadequate for many of the more seriously disturbed patients." He believes that the addition of an experience in a therapeutic community as a simultaneous part of the patient's program can give major aid in working toward recovery. He reviews six different therapeutic community models and then interrelates the practice of psychotherapy with that of the therapeutic milieu. He importantly points out how more benefits are gained when the therapeutic milieu can be explored in the course of a simultaneous, ongoing individual psychotherapy. Conversely, individual psychotherapy is enriched through the ongoing reality confrontation the patient experiences in the therapeutic milieu. Ultimately, Stanton suggests that the therapeutic community itself may be a necessary condition for the successful individual psychotherapy of the chronic patient.

Leff highlights in his chapter the increased burden carried by the families of psychiatric patients who have been discharged into the community. He recognizes the unique day-in and day-out strain on the family which has a chronically ill member living with it. He suggests that professionals who only spend a few hours a week with these patients may not be sensitive to the problems of patients' families. Leff makes a clear distinction between the two major diagnostic categories—manic-depressive illness and schizophrenia. He then divides his chapter between problems common to all patients and those specific to these two major illnesses. He discusses the problem of providing families with adequate information and education; the social problems encountered due to difficulties in employability and housing; and the problems encountered by the family members who are likely to experience greater social isolation due to either their own shame or to the aversion of friends and neighbors. Methods of decreasing the burden on relatives are considered. He reviews the significance of the family's influence on the course of schizophrenic disorders and on subsequently developed policies for managing these families. The issue of high-expressed emotion or emotional over-involvement in relatives of schizophrenics as directly associated with relapse of schizophrenia is explored. Protection of the patient is first obtained by prescribing regular antipsychotic medication and then by reducing the amount of time spent with the relatives. The latter is accomplished by the use of either supervised lodgings or a day hospital, two methods of removing the patient from a noxious environment. It is important to note that in an effort to decrease the overintense contact with the family, Leff advocates the use of a variety of different modalities described in this volume, including residential care, day center care and sheltered occupations.

Aguilera describes crisis intervention as an inexpensive, short-term therapy that focuses on solving the immediate problem. First, she reviews the historical background of urbanization leading to a greater likelihood of crisis development. Then she describes the history of the development of the technique of crisis intervention. She reviews the psychoanalytic contributions of Freud, Hartmann, Rado, Erikson, Lindemann and Caplan. Following this, the technique of crisis intervention is described in relation to the family's adjustment to the return of the patient to the home. This clearly relates directly to the previous chapter by Leff. Also, her comment that the social isolate in particular is more vulnerable to crisis recalls to the reader the issues explored by Hammer in an earlier chapter. Her focus on urban life relates to the Lamb chapter that follows in a later section.

Hursh and Anthony emphasize how work is not only a normalizing activity but also a provider of therapeutic benefits. In particular, work contributes to "shedding one's patienthood" and improving one's self-concept. These authors focus on the psychiatrically disabled client's skills instead of on his symptoms. They approach this subject through what they describe as client-skill development in community support. In contrast to Leff, and in accordance with their focus on the patient's potential for productivity, the notion of the traditional psychiatric diagnosis is entirely repudiated, and instead a "rehabilitation diagnosis" is used. They distinguish work/environment behaviors as being either physical, emotional or intellectual. Interviewing techniques are specifically described as "attending, observing, listening and responding," and these are used in order to acquire an assessment of "where the client is" in relation to his/her goal. The authors review work-sample techniques that help to assess the client's different work skills, as well as situational-assessment techniques, on-the-job evaluation techniques and psychometric testing techniques. The authors then take up some of the practical interferences with the setting-up of an effective program. In particular, they address the problem that results too often when vocational assessment is done in a separate geographical site, which leads to poor communication among the entire rehabilitative team. They also feel that the common view of the vocational evaluator as a specialist with unique knowledge that is different from that of other rehabilitation practitioners contributes to poor interdisciplinary communication, and they propose a number of corrective measures to ameliorate this problem. The authors then explore rehabilitation programming strategies including work adjustment, career counseling, occupational skill training and career placement. Several unique training situations are described, including workshop without walls, transitional employment programs and projects with industry. This chapter is overall a very technical one; it addresses specific techniques in assessment and programming for rehabilitation counseling. It focuses more on the importance of recognizing the special value of a proper vocational assessment than on collaboration with other mental health professionals. Nevertheless, it is important that other mental health professionals begin to recognize that symptomatology and the capacity to work are two very different variables. It appears that the human personality is too complex to allow us to make a prediction regarding the capacity to work from one set of pathologic symptomatology. Rather, one would have a more accurate predictive measure using Hursh and Anthony's assessment techniques.

Washburn reviews the early development of the day hospital as a replacement to a great extent for the inpatient service. He describes the criteria used to determine eligibility for his programs as well as the issue of staffing. Then he reviews outpatient vs. inpatient placement. He explores extensively a variety of followup research studies comparing the day hospital to inpatient care. He makes the general point that most patients can be handled in a day hospital, especially after a short hospital stay, and can thereby avoid the use of long-term hospitalization altogether.

Grob sets the historical development of psychosocial rehabilitation centers in the context of the two major presidential commissions on mental health in 1961 and 1978. Following this, he reviews the historical antecedents to the social approach. With stunning accuracy, Harry Stack Sullivan predicted in the 1930s that patients would be helped through social psychiatry, and that there would be an increase in relapse rate if there were no intermediate facilities such as "convalescent camps and communities for those on the way to mental health." Further, it is remarkable how other authors of the same era, such as Marsh, working at Worcester State Hospital in Massachusetts, advocated expatient organizations on a national basis. The influence of the study and development of group psychotherapy is discussed, as well as the influence of Adler. Grob reviews how the experience of World War II and the rapid funding of mental health services thereafter promoted the development of psychosocial rehabilitation centers. Grob's chapter clearly relates to Hammer's in its focus on socialization. He concludes with a list of what he calls the model elements required in a quality program. He warns that these could too easily be lost in the bureaucratic mechanics and fiscal intricacies of expanded programs.

Finally, Budson describes the evolution of community care deriving from pharmacologic, social and legal developments in the 1950s, 60s and 70s. He then reviews ten different types of sheltered housing used for the chronically mentally ill. He explores problems in appraising the effectiveness of these community residential alternatives, including the problem of "client/milieu matching." Following this, he discusses some issues in starting a new program and covers some pithy clinical topics. He concludes with an exploration of some controversial administrative issues facing community residential care—regulatory, financial, building codes, staffing and community opposition.

These chapters described the elements of psychosocial treatment. In the following section, we describe the other major treatment modality: pharmacotherapy.

CHAPTER 5

THE INDIVIDUAL PSYCHOTHERAPIES AND THEIR RELATIONSHIP TO THE THERAPEUTIC COMMUNITY

ALFRED H. STANTON, M.D.

The needs and activities of human beings reflect the fact that they are members of a species of social animals. Humans need each other and interact with each other almost continually, except when asleep, and sometimes then also. In many patients with psychiatric disorders, withdrawal from the group or society becomes conspicuous and is the object of much attention and therapeutic effort by the patients' therapists. Even here, however, it is only very occasionally that withdrawal is complete and lasts for a long period of time. Human beings want groups, they live in groups of their own making and they eat, sleep, play, work and dream with each other with few exceptions, sick or well. To a considerable extent, human beings are not aware of the degree of their dependence upon interaction with other humans, and it is only in exceptional circumstances—in prison, in seclusion, as hermits, or in preferential solitude in the wilderness for recreation—that they recognize the degree to which their lives are built around their relations and prospects of relations with other human beings.

If human function is analyzed scientifically, this central fact becomes apparent in a different way. Developmental psychology starts from the obvious total dependence of the newborn infant on others and describes changes in his relations to his "objects" at different stages in his development, together with the increasing complexity and discrimination which characterizes his dealings with others—his family and the broader society. Psychodynamic and psychoanalytic theories have also come increasingly to focus upon "object relations," the nature of the drives which can be satisfied only in interaction with others, and of the drive controls whose necessity and whose form arise from the larger social group to whom the patient or person gives his allegiance. Behavioral therapy, although apparently dealing with the details of drive, behavior and reward, tends to obscure the overriding fact that reward is expected or gained almost entirely from other people. It is necessary to emphasize the degree of social commitment of the human organism because an awareness of it is needed to distinguish psychotherapy from other human interaction.

The need for other people, and for experience with them, are reflected in the fact that talking and dealing with other people in a friendly or in a hostile way (or more commonly in some complex mixture of the two) meet the needs of the person who is reacting, and are consequently beneficial and satisfying. Those peppery, shy or shattered people who claim not to want to have anything to do with others are rarely able to make good on their claim; they benefit from telling others how they feel, albeit irritably, and often from the fact that the other person does not accept their statement and obey the injunction. In general, people are good for people, whether patients or not, and regardless of one's superficial preferences. This fact is a source of confusion in trying to analyze psychotherapy, since so many things people can do with others are recognized as beneficial. The benefits of everyday social intercourse are often intimately comingled with benefits that might be sought as a result of individual psychotherapy. Indeed, the practice of some types of psychotherapy implies that the mechanism of benefit is little more than meeting this need arising from the human condition.

INDIVIDUAL PSYCHOTHERAPY

Individual psychotherapy can be discriminated from friendly discourse by the fact that it is to some degree (1) planned, (2) systematic, (3) deliberate, and (4) self-conscious. It is (5) asymmetric in that its aim is for the benefit, indeed the treatment of, one of the two parties, and it is conducted (6) upon the basis of a theory of what is wrong with the other person and how the therapy is expected to ameliorate it. The theory may be only an elementary, primitive—even unrecognized—theory, but it is used nevertheless. Individual psychotherapy, of course, will include many of the more generalized features of helpful, friendly, human interaction—warmth, giving, stimulation, instruction, recognition of the other, reliability, sympathy and searching for the needs of the other. All these and many other characteristics of human beneficence may, and often are, included in the practice of psychotherapy, but they are not identical with it. They do not supplant the deliberate, aimed, systematic effort to bring the patient more specifically designed benefits than these more general ones. Psychotherapy, in this sense, began to be discriminated in the nineteenth century from the much more generalized ancient doctor-patient or therapist-patient relationship whose history has been described in an illuminating way by Entralgo (1969).

Psychotherapy quickly became an experimental discipline of varying sorts. The French dominated this development of psychotherapy, at first with the Nancy School of Bernheim (1889) in which hypnosis was studied and from which Charcot developed many of his ideas of the nature of the major neuroses. Dubois (1909), Janet (1924) and Dejerine (1913) all published highly influential books on psychotherapy in the short period around the turn of the century. The influence spread to Switzerland where Forel (1907) and later Adolph Meyer (1913) described their own differing techniques. It was, of course, in Vienna that the recognition of psychotherapy received its greatest development at the hands of Sigmund Freud and, following him, psychoanalysts in Vienna, Germany, England, Canada and the United States. The deepening influence of the psychoanalytic formulations of the personality, psychoneurosis and treatment should not blind us to Freud's early experimentation with techniques; many other psychotherapists also were experimenting with various technical innovations. The dynamism of the psychoanalytic movement and of its theory were such as to dominate the first half of the century in psychotherapy. Most new variations and innovations in psychotherapy were originally presented as alterations in psychoanalysis. Although Meyer's distributive analysis and Sullivan's study of interpersonal relations each sought to establish a separate and distinct identity, both finally came to be regarded as variants of psychoanalysis.

The end of World War II brought notable changes. These arose *first* from the increasing recognition of the importance to individual psychotherapy of the group living of the patient being treated—a topic we will consider further below—and *second* from a great though gradual increase in interest in the empirical characteristics of psychotherapy, at the hands primarily of clinical psychologists, particularly Carl Rogers and his group of scholars. In a somewhat different way, Kurt Lewin and his group, had a major focus upon group practices. Rogers developed and greatly emphasized the empirical evaluation of therapy, as well as its analysis, and the use of tape recording to gain a more accurate and manageable record of what happened in the therapeutic sessions. The interest in objective and empirical evaluation spread slowly but broadly throughout the western world. Evaluation has proved to be difficult in view of the complexity of the treatment modality, the complexity of the original complaints of patients, the length of time that many treatments require, and the complexity of improvement of patients (particularly where chronic patients are treated). A considerable amount of effort has left appreciable areas of uncertainty about how to interpret the studies. Bergin and Garfield (1971), Glass (1976), and Smith and Glass (1977) have summarized these findings.

The difficulties in interpreting the results of studies evaluating the effects of psychotherapy arise not only from the intrinsic difficulties of the subject matter, but also from reluctance on the part of many psychotherapists to engage in systematic, quantified and controlled research. There is evidence that over half of the institutions engaging in intensive psychotherapy with schizophrenia as a prominent part of their program are so convinced of the value of intensive psychotherapy that they do not find it ethically permissible to randomize patients into a control group. Beyond this type of resistance toward setting up systematic controls, the very nature of quantified, objective, testing research is somewhat alien to the humanistic, individualistic attitude which dominates much of psychotherapeutic clinical experience. In this connection, however, it should be emphasized that systematic evaluation of psychotherapy has not only had the effect of developing information bearing upon how effective the therapy is, but has also had a further reflex effect of strengthening and clarifying the theoretical conceptions of the psychotherapists. The development of an objective and testable hypothesis requires a degree of analytic clarity which in some cases has proved highly beneficial to the development of psychotherapy in recent decades.

Efforts at evaluation point up still one more difference between psychotherapy and the humane care of patients—psychotherapy is expected to bring about change and is undertaken with this aim in view. It is at its best when this aim is completely and unreservedly shared by *both* participants, but it should always be an expectation of the therapist. Psychotherapy of a particular patient may move slowly, glacially, but it should move. In certain therapeutic prescriptions, so much emphasis has been placed upon acceptance of the patient, upon avoiding moralistic demands and upon recognizing the facts of the patient's mind rather than trying to change them, that the opposite has been a danger—the development of a systematic effort to create a holding environment that is completely static, as if the patient were expected to go out where he comes in. On the contrary, it is the usual belief that static patients, particularly chronic patients, leave worse, not the same as they came in. The expectation of change, and collaboration in working to bring it about, are not at all incompatible with fully accepting the patient as a person.

Since often the distinction between humane relations and psychotherapy is not clearly made, one general development in the 60s and 70s of this century has been the creation, sometimes by unsupported imagination, of a bewildering array of types of psychotherapeutic intervention—such that Klerman (1980) recently spoke of 140 different types of psychotherapy that are now "on the market." The array is, of course, bewildering in a completely literal sense. Such a wide variety of expectation, theory and technique has been developed, often quite uncritically, that even a specialist gets lost. This has meant, of course, that not only have the boundaries between different types of psychotherapy been blurred, but the boundaries between psychotherapy on the one hand, and education, religious exhortation, esthetic and artistic experience on the other have also been lost. Indeed, the boundary between psychotherapy and sheer quackery has also become blurred.

Nevertheless, with regard to the chronic patient, at least, recent years have seen the development of a widely shared set of general assumptions about psychotherapy, making it possible to divide the psychotherapies used with chronic patients into four different types—(1) the instructive/prescriptive, (2) the behavioral, (3) the interpersonal, and (4) the psychoanalytic.

Before describing them, however, it will be well to review the degree to which therapists of all four groups generally share certain assumptions and practices. *First*, they share a considerable reliance upon theory; whether elementary or elaborated, some degree of allegiance to theory beyond that held idiosyncratically by the therapist himself is characteristic of psychotherapists of all these schools of thought. *Second*, there is a general tendency to insist upon adequate time; this entails a degree of continuity of therapeutic effort with the same therapist; "adequate" time is not always seen as the same amount, but it is more than a few minutes every now and then. *Third*, the widespread practice is to ask for a reasonably regular frequency of meetings; the most common is probably one hour per week, although there are many variations. *Fourth*, all share a considerable sensitive attention to the clarity and completeness of communication between patient and therapist, with a corollary emphasis upon privacy and confidentiality of the communications—whose purpose, aside from the ethical protection of the patient, is to induce the patient to recognize that he is in fact free, as he must be, to express aspects of his experience unwise to express in any other situation. *Fifth*, there is a general tendency to minimize educational and directive comments, except as they are focused on symptoms and the disturbance the patient has, or on advising and instructing the patient how to cooperate in the treatment. *Sixth*, most emphasize the importance of the management of unusual and/or strong emotional responses of the patient to the therapist and to the treatment situation itself. There is a widespread recognition of the vulnerability of the patient to exploitation because of these emotional responses, and of the opposite effect—that the patient may interrupt treatment unwisely because of them. In any case, and with widely different ways of management, all note the importance of these emotional responses.

The *instructive/prescriptive* type of psychotherapy descends directly from the narrowly defined doctor/patient relationship—in which the role of the physician as expert in the knowledge of what is the matter with the patient and of how to treat it, and his advice, explanation, education and directions to the patient are all a prominent part of the treatment. This approach differs from simple medical care, however, by the therapist's recognition that his way of acting itself has therapeutic effects upon the patient; thus it is being used, in addition to medications and prescribed activities, as a way of treating the patient. The definiteness, clarity, and indeed the therapist's position—since his technical and theoretical authority are not open to debate—are often highly reassuring to patients. A need for direction and some sense of certainty about the disturbing experience of mental illness predisposes patients to welcome a degree of comfort, confidence and faith in this type of treatment; the faith indeed, like faith elsewhere, is not only reassuring, but may contribute in more serious ways to facilitating the patient's competence in dealing with his disturbance. Goldstein and Stein (1976) have given a description of this type of therapy; it is otherwise hard to find except in conjunction with other aspects of the treatment situation. The latter situation is outlined well for the reader who wishes to follow the subject further in Strauss (1964). The use of medication is nearly always a prominent part of this treatment regimen.

Practitioners of the *behavioral group* of psychotherapies expect to achieve benefit to the patient by developing a proper emotional climate in which he may take action, and then, consistently and promptly, rewarding the most appropriate actions of the patient. Such a course may require, in some techniques, an initial period of "desensitization," by which the patient's resistance and fears of the procedure are allayed. Since rewarding patients can only consist heavily of interpersonal rewards, there is the possibility that the desensitization period during which the therapist is trying to gain the confidence, faith and trust of the patient may prove to be, or seem to the patient to be, excessively seductive, and may lead to the patient's termination. The behavioral therapist depends considerably upon common sense instruction about conduct vis-a-vis symptoms and how to control them. Patients may be encouraged to talk to themselves, or to teach themselves, and are usually urged in the direction of confronting a situation which is frightening. Third, many behavioral therapists tend to discourage "too much" self-observation, with the belief that patients may become self-absorbed and lost in their symptoms and preoccupations. Fourth, there is considerable attention to the management of low self-esteem by the patient's achievements; indeed, this is almost a primary area of reliance for therapeutic effect. The patients must act. Fifth, in some cases there is considerable interest in analysis and management of interpersonal relations by the thoughtful planning of scenarios which the patient can discuss in advance, analyze, practice, and in the case of psychodramatic programs, act out in a preliminary and experimental way. Whatever else such practices do, they cannot help but reinforce the common sense perception of circumstances which the patient had perceived with fright and anxiety. Sixth, in many cases programs of this sort tend to avoid or deny the role of "patient" and "illness," although usually "therapy" is permitted to remain. The reason for this is not clear, although it may be derivative from a simplistic "labeling theory" of mental illness, which implies that illness is heavily influenced by, and to some extent caused by, the fact that the patients are labeled as mentally ill. There has been considerable work done in the behavioral type of therapy; see Beck (1979); Paul and Lenz (1977).

The *Interpersonal cluster* of therapies stem from a number of sources, including Otto Rank and his relationship therapy and Harry Stack Sullivan and interpersonal psychiatry (1956) and, to a considerable extent, from various sources known loosely as existentialist; they share certain general approaches and theories of benefit to the patient: (1) Attention is carefully given to the growth in the patient's awareness of his interpersonal relations, especially with his intimates.

The complexity, anxiety and false types of relationships which occur become a central area of interest. (2) There is a self-conscious search for insight, that is, for a new self-understanding and a new self-knowledge into the ways of dealing with others. (3) There is a search for the relationship between symptoms and identified interpersonal experiences. (4) The enhancement of self-esteem is sought by a progressive growth in understanding of the experience of the self as reflected in the appraisal of others; how the appraisals of others are internalized by the patient and his responses to them are all part of a central interest in self-esteem. (5) There is a recognition of, even an emphasis on, the relations to the therapist as a source of information about the self, as a source of deepening self-acceptance, as may occur in communion with the other person. To a variable extent, the source of actual therapy is sought in the "relationship," or a "good relationship," or "authentic relationship," which is self-consciously sought by some therapists in collaboration with the patient. (6) There is usually a lack of emphasis upon the illness, without denying it. There is considerable interest in patient actions, but without attributing to them the degree of therapeutic importance mentioned in the behavioral groups.

Psychoanalytic psychotherapy is a group of psychotherapies derived by modifying, or selecting relevant aspects of, psychoanalytic theory, and applying them, often in the treatment of patients who are sicker than those originally treated by psychoanalysis. Frequently the therapy is comparatively short term, but in some cases, unfortunately, the distinction from psychoanalysis itself has been blurred, at the expense of clarity.

Psychoanalytic psychotherapy is characterized by the following:

One. There is an emphasis upon expressiveness and the permissiveness of verbal expression and the absence of conscious reserve in communication between patient and therapist; the asymmetry of the relationship is highlighted by the fact that there is a variable degree of emphasis upon an incognito for the therapist, which is used to clarify transference misapprehensions. In contrast to psychoanalysis, free association, the use of the couch and minimal stimulation, and other devices facilitating regression in the service of the ego are less often used.

Two. There is a recognition of the complexity of the relations to the therapist—especially conflicting, dependent wishes and defenses against them, coexisting transference and nontransference relations, and the aim of the patient to recognize all of this as fully as possible.

Therapists have less confidence in such phrases as a "good relationship," or full communion, or a constructive versus a destructive relationship; they prefer instead to encourage or insist upon the patient's awareness of the coexistence of many conflicting wishes and the ways in which these conflicts are managed helpfully or unhelpfully.

Three. There is considerable attention to the illness, to symptoms and to their structure, with the patient.

Four. With considerable variation, there is often a trend toward "open" unstructured exploration, in some analogy to the free association and basic rule of psychoanalysis itself.

Five. There is a high priority about the patient's developing insight through his own work at self-exploration. Although variable from therapist to therapist, there is great emphasis in general upon the patient's developing insight, not just upon the therapist's doing so.

Six. There is a heavy emphasis upon a developmental point of view —upon illness as either immaturity or regression and upon progressive maturation as improving health. It is upon maturation that the therapists rely primarily for the therapeutic effects of their therapy.

Seven. There are often ambitious aims compared to those of others. Although limited insight is recognized, there is often a hope for "structural change" in the patient's personality, and even in some cases that a patient who has been psychotic may at the end of treatment be in better health than he was prior to his first breakdown—that is, that he may be less likely to break down again than he was before his first break.

Although its practice and theory have been seminal for many of the psychotherapies, *psychoanalysis* itself is a relatively uncommonly practiced treatment for chronically ill patients of the sort often thought of as in partial hospital institutions. Psychoanalysis has always treated "chronic" patients, but it has not been adapted to those patients with more ego disturbance or ego regression than characterizes the severe neuroses. There is an area of semantic confusion here, since some therapists speak of "psychoanalysis" without requiring that its elementary technique be the basic rule—that the patient put every thought and feeling into words as they occur to him without censorship—and that free association be the technique which leads to analysis of the transference, from which a deeper and more ambitious therapy may be achieved than is usual in any of the other therapies. The expense of psychoanalysis in time, money and discipline has led to a consistent and repeated search for other techniques of therapy which do not require as long a training for the therapist and perhaps do not attempt such ambitious goals. At any rate, psychoanalysis remains an actively practiced and continuing fertile source of stimulation for students of personality and psychiatric illness.

For the chronic psychiatric patient in the community, individual psychotherapy of one sort or another ought to be the cornerstone of treatment. Certainly, the free and discriminating use of medication has equally come into prominence in recent years, and in the hands of most practitioners is united with at least the instructive/directive type of psychotherapy to compose a program for the care of patients.

Unfortunately, there are many persons counseling or advising chronic patients who are inadequately educated, if at all, for the more specific, useful practice of psychotherapy. Much of this counseling is administered under the label of psychotherapy. Such a diffusion is all the easier because there is no widely agreed-upon, clear and sharp distinction between psychotherapy and other interpersonal helping efforts. To some extent, these are the unavoidable casualties of the widespread, uninforned acceptance of the importance of individual psychotherapy among the therapies available today. However, the combination of medication and individual psychotherapy is clearly inadequate for many of the more seriously disturbed patients, who can, however, be given major aid in working toward recovery by the combination of individual psychotherapy, judicious medication and an experience in the therapeutic community, overlapping and at the same time. The interaction among these different types of therapy is complex and may be controversial depending upon where primary values are placed, but this does not alter the fact that the combination of the three approaches often proves a great deal better than any two, or any one alone.

THE THERAPEUTIC COMMUNITY

The small community institutions for the care and treatment of the mentally ill springing up in recent years are examples and important representatives of an effective treatment for illness which is entirely new in the twentieth century—the therapeutic community. While groups (temples, hospitals, hostels and group religious ceremonies) have been used in one form or another by mankind throughout its urban and tribal existence, it is only in this century that the self-conscious, planned use of a community designed for the treatment of sick patients has been instituted. Treatment is to be contrasted to containment, custody, care and protection of patients, functions carried out by other institutions from hotels to the family.

Not only is the treatment new in the sense of its explicit and planned character, but it has been instituted on the basis of information from new basic sciences of medicine—sociology and social psychology. Beginning, perhaps, with the small group retreats instituted by Trigant Burrow in the twenties, the concept of the therapeutic community crept almost surreptitiously into the practice of psychiatry up until World War II. Following the war, it became the center of much psychiatric attention in England following the Northfield experiment. A short time later Maxwell Jones (1953) conducted his well-know study of the therapeutic community. This was followed by similar developments in the United States. Wilmer (1958) in the Navy and Artiss in the Army, the study *The Mental Hospital* by Stanton and Schwartz (1954), and further analysis of therapeutic implications by John and Elaine Cumming (1962) established a trend of interest which continues until the present. The Cumming study first brought direct attention to the relation between community phenomena and the psychopathology which brought their patients to the hospital.

A direct effect of these studies was the growing recognition of the ineptitude of the usual psychiatric hospital for the conducting of therapy, particularly therapy on a community basis and, indeed, the unwarranted reawakening of an ancient prejudice which indicated that hospitals only made patients worse, at least, if patients stayed for more than a few days or weeks. Evidence that this, indeed, could happen was taken as grounds for eliminating the psychiatric hospital, or at least the government psychiatric hospital. What resulted was an impersonal, at times almost frantic, emptying out of the hospitals "into the community," on the basis of a mathematical formula for the number of patients who should be out. The full consequences of this pressure to discharge were only belatedly appreciated. The discharge of patients from a mental hospital "into the community" meant the substitution of a different subcommunity for that of the mental hospital. The differing relationships of the two subcommunities to the overarching community were uncritically accepted as a universal sign of benefit to patients who otherwise would be "destroyed" in a state hospital. The cost of such inadequate social planning is now being widely recognized. As it turned out, the new community institutions could be extremely good, or terrible.

Just as in the case of psychotherapy, where we noted that the association of one person with another is likely to have a beneficial effect for the nonspecific reason that people are good for each other, the same is true regarding small groups. The same distinction needs to be made between a therapeutic community and a small, good care-taking institution, where people eat, sleep, work or play. While any lasting collection of people are likely to create at least some degree of community organization and awareness, the degree varies. In a community, members become a self-conscious group with which each member to some extent identifies himself, even if in opposition. A community, as opposed to a simple collection of people, must share a certain underlying consensus of how things should be done, and to some extent a consensus of values. Its members should share and develop a sense of identity, both of the person and of the group or the community. What the individual members of a community do is to some extent colored at all times by some recognition of their identity in the community, their sense of belonging to a collective, or perhaps more actively, of being a member of a group.

There is no secret as to the nature of the consensus in a therapeutic community—the purpose of the community is not only the maintenance but also the therapy of the members of the community. True, the nature of the therapy and the nature of the illness to be treated may be vague, or controversial, but the consensus survives, and the nature of treatment and illness is analyzed in the light of this consensus.

The characteristics of a therapeutic community vary, but within the context of a general overall agreement. The operations of such a community have been described by Paul and Lentz (1977). They emphasize the law of expectancy in which a certain level of behavior and certain aims of behavior are quietly expected by, and from, all members of the group. To expect something is, of course, an ambiguous concept—it may mean to demand something, or it may mean to predict something. Whichever it means, the expectancy that surrounds each patient in the therapeutic community has its effect. The expectancy must be communicated to the patient so that he knows of it, and therefore it is common that standards of behavior are publicly posted, and, if the community is alive, altered from time to time.

Besides the expectancy that characterizes a therapeutic community, there is also an understanding of involvement. Members of the community are expected in some sense to "do it themselves"—to act upon challenges, to show the way in which they are community members along with their fellows, and in fact, to continuously construct and reconstruct the community itself.

There is also a vaguely defined but often fairly strong sense of group cohesiveness, even rising to the point of loyalty which surmounts the sense of belonging and the sense of identity with the group. All of these combine to create a therapeutic community, but this does not imply that everybody agrees with the consensus that the community expresses. The consensus exists, and everybody responds to some extent to it by incorporating it, by living in terms of it, but a certain number of people will always—or should always—express their membership in the community by an oppositional standpoint. There should be challenges to the community, alternatives, insistences upon privacy, and other humanly inconvenient but unavoidable opinions and actions. In the words of Sapir, "the way in which a rebel objects to church membership in a culture is itself laid down and prescribed by that culture."

Therapeutic environments or therapeutic communities have begun to differentiate into various types, although the movement is little more than thirty years old. The various types have not been combined into one organization planned to remedy several different identified types of patient disability. There are several reasons for this. First, for practical reasons, most therapeutic communities have had as their function the treatment and care of patients of many different types of illness at the same time; and if the needs of the individual types are different from each other, the same community may have difficulty in being equally responsive to all of the needs. This is made more prominent because of the fact that the structure and nature of the continuing processes known as emotional illness in individual patients have not been customarily analyzed in terms of group function. Increasing interest in family therapy and the family as the etiological background for developmental disorders, interest in group psychotherapy, and the development of a more sophisticated, and to some extent clinically oriented, group psychology as a science have all contributed some knowledge, but the understanding of psychiatric disorder in terms of group function is still rudimentary and patchy.

The development of therapeutic community types has also been heavily influenced by the fact that in many cases therapeutic communities have been created within preexisting institutions with their own community characteristics. Even when a new institution has been designed, the people doing the planning have themselves very often been products of prior institutional experience which they have brought to bear in designing the therapeutic milieu. The third factor is, of course, a product of the expense of creating any community; this makes the development of the community a political process in which a very large number of people of diverse interests are engaged; thus forthright, nonconservative planning is often not reached under these circumstances. It is instructive to think of a modern surgical operating room and the degree to which its various characteristics are derived directly from the needs of surgery, asepsis, resuscitation, anesthesia and the like. If we did not understand the nature of surgery, an operating room would seem to be a nightmarish boondoggle, indeed. In contrast, the theoretical background for the structure of the therapeutic community is much weaker and provides much less guidance in its continuation. The operating room can perhaps serve as a reminder of the power and effectiveness of consistent, scientifically based planning, given time for its application.

In spite of these difficulties, there is a considerable common ground among therapeutic communities. Canter and Canter (1979) have given an excellent general summary of their types.

They speak first of the *custodial model*, an institution specializing in the care and usually the relative isolation of particular groups of people over a considerable time, protecting both the patients and the outside community from each other and usually emphasizing the boundary between them. The apparent economy and efficiency, and the possibility of unusual sympathy based upon special understanding of the particular characters of the patients, are all significant advantages. Tolerance for deviant behavior and eccentricity is easier to achieve, even if at times tolerance of patients' deviant behavior may prejudice the expectancies for nondeviant behavior which the therapeutic community must require.

The static characteristics of the custodial model have been difficult to accept, and together with the ease with which patients can be "warehoused," has given custodial institutions a reputation, partly deserved, which has led to a flight from them, with an unwitting substitution of other custodial institutions.

The *medical model* is a direct descendant of the practices of hospital medicine in which the activity of the community is primarily based on delivering certain identified and particular treatments—medications, operations, exercises and the like, prescribed by a central authority (nearly always a physician) for each individual patient, in the light of the illness that the patient is conceived to be suffering from. The treatments are generally administered specifically by nursing personnel whose duties also include evaluative observation of the course of patients, usually primarily oriented around observing the effects of the medication or the specific treatments that are prescribed for the patient. The familiarity and high degree of coherent organization that often characterize communities of this sort are sources of immediate and lasting security for new patients, and also for personnel. The medical hospital is a part of western culture as a whole—familiar, generally trusted and generally effective. If the difficulties of psychiatric disorder can be handled in this way, it is a source of reassurance and optimism.

The model does, however, have certain serious shortcomings. The focus upon the patient's illness and his symptoms leaves outside of the central field of vision those aspects of his personality and general social functioning which, in the case of psychiatric disorders, are usually major parts of the psychiatric disorder itself. If the patient shows primarily behavioral disorders such as impulsivity, kleptomania, sexual deviation or other types of unusual behavior, the medical model seems inappropriate and unable to grapple with the manifestations of illness. Further than this, the focus upon illness has the effect of encouraging those impersonal ways of treating patients which may occur. To the extent that the patient's personality finds its central expression in a symptom, that patient is likely to be worse than otherwise. The impersonality is exaggerated by the fact that there are usually few physicians who can see the patients for whom they prescribe only once every week or two, after a brief passing interview.

The behavioral treatment is best manifested by the type of therapeutic community based upon "*normalization*," in which great effort is made to keep the institution as normal as it is possible to make it. Unusual practices are avoided and normal behavior is expected from patients. What is normal behavior and what is a normal institution? The model most often used is that of the nuclear family. Usual domestic arrangements, for instance, require that food be prepared and served in family style, dishes washed in a similar way, housekeeping done by each person for himself and the general problems of housekeeping shared in some equable manner. If the family is considered to be one of those small institutions where a member is sought if he does not come "home" when expected, where each person is known closely, not to say intimately, by each other on a fully personal basis, it conforms to the model sought by those considering the family as a model. Provisions for the growth and development of its members, and ultimately for their leaving when "grown up," is usually intrinsic to the model. Budson (1978) has emphasized this model for the halfway house and has shown, by means of a sophisticated analysis of function within the family, the similarities in the way the family and the halfway house function or should function. Extended families may continue for many years to adapt to the family member's state of development, with support of various types of creativity and maturation. The halfway house can and should try to do this also.

In contrast, scepticism has been expressed over the wisdom of using the family as a model, Bettelheim specifically mentions the harm he attributes to welcoming patients to a hospital with the analogy to a family. Generally, the use of the family as a model should focus upon the characteristics that distinguish it from other small institutions, rather than solely upon its functional analysis; if members arrange a division of labor in the family, they also do so in a scout troop, in a vacation group, in school, in church, and finally in business. The important point here is that the arrangements for division of labor are made on the assumption that the members are responsible, grown-up members, competent or close to it; the therapeutic community can and should do this. In much of family experience, people are either parents or children, with severely asymmetric duties and responsibilities and privileges; there is the ever-present opportunity for members of the community to slip into either one of these authoritative or regressive roles. Aside from these limitations, the normalization model rests as heavily as it can upon overt and describable behavior and thus tends to settle for the mediocre and the conventional—characteristics about which the staff can agree. Further, the failure of a patient to meet the requirements of the normal must be handled, since patients cannot always meet them immediately and completely. The way in which failure is handled gives a tone to the whole community which can be seriously stultifying for both patients and staff.

The *prosthetic model* is one of an institution in which the essential activity is to compensate for deficits in either the behavior or experience of a patient. This of course includes spectacles, wheelchairs and the like, but also social difficulties, intellectual limitations, undue self-centeredness and the like. The provision of prosthetics, while essentially human and universal (it should be characteristic, of course, of all therapeutic institutions), can result in a community's becoming another static one, differentiated only quantitatively from a custodial institution.

The prosthetic model is close to what Canter and Canter called *the enhancement model.* This type of institution is built upon the determined provision of a better environment than usual, in the expectation first that patients will need it, and secondly that it is a characteristic of the institution which leads to the actual improvement of patients, much more easily than does the simple expectation of a normal behavior pattern. Many people in the enhancement type of institutions believe that the behavioristic normal model is unnecessarily demanding for many people.

When carried further, the enhancement model merges into the *individual growth model.* This is an institution in which one of the understood functions is to seek out and find those special tendencies, abilities and potentials which each individual is assumed to possess, and having identified them, to try to help the patient develop them as much as possible. This is an activity which is expected, to some extent, from every member of the community for every other member of the community. While the enhancement of the staff's ability is hardly the purpose of such an institution, nevertheless, if it happens, everyone is pleased and there is no great loss of face in recognizing the fact that it has. This model would require the development of schools, practice sessions, group activities, but always focused upon individuals and their development. Clearly, such an individual growth model also contains within it expectancies that the patients will improve, and in many cases leave to go on to better and fuller living elsewhere. The focus is so highly personal that the degree of personal interest is often overlooked. Nevertheless, the development of those aspects of a patient's personality which are characteristic of psychiatric disorders become easily the focus of attention.

In trying to describe the characteristics of therapeutic institutions in general by describing several types of them, it is necessary to remind ourselves of some of the general characteristics—the most important being the continued and quiet expectation of benefit to the patients, and the recognition that this is the purpose of the therapeutic community. While the custodial type of institution does not fit this characteristic, precisely for that reason it occupies a somewhat marginal position in the classification. The expectancies that the staff and other patients maintain need not be always directly and overtly expressed in institutions where people are living together all of the time. They will be revealed and they will be recognized and understood, but it is true that in some forms of therapeutic community, the explicit defined listing of expectations is helpful.

Most therapeutic communities contain a very active group life in which the involvement of all patients is expected. Regular scheduled meetings, long enough to permit detailed discussion of personal and personality issues which appear before the group, perhaps individual discussions after periods of disturbance, manipulation of the patient's participation in group, or temporary restriction to his own private area—these are the agencies through which the therapeutic milieu expresses itself, through which it is perceived and built. The withdrawal characterizing many psychiatric states and particularly chronic ones, or the spurious participation which masks a withdrawal, is grist for the mill in the therapeutic community. Both are dealt with by everyone else, not just by the patient or by the patient and one other person; they become problems for everyone, and the efficacy is enormously augmented by this fact. For although it is hard to parcel out just what it does, there is repeated evidence that the therapeutic community is not only an effective therapeutic agent, but an enormously effective one. The best way in which one can gain some grasp of the importance of it is by moving from an institution which has no therapeutic community of substance into a therapeutic community that treats the same kind of patients. The first assumption will always be the same—that they could not possibly be the same kind of patients and how did they get picked for what they were doing? And, indeed, they are no longer the same kind of patients precisely because they have been a part of a therapeutic community.

INDIVIDUAL PSYCHOTHERAPY WITHIN THE THERAPEUTIC COMMUNITY

While there have been many studies of individual psychotherapy and a number of descriptions of the therapeutic community as a way of treatment, the interaction between individual psychotherapy and the therapeutic community has been considered in the clinical literature only marginally. The early development of individual psychotherapy focused upon difficulties "within the patient," and there was a strong, if not very articulate, pressure against considering the environment as contributing either to illness or to recovery. "Interpretation of reality" was widely discouraged in psychoanalytic practice except for patients suffering from severe ego disturbance, who were often not seen in psychoanalysis precisely because of their limitations. Freud's early case in which he attributed the cause of a psychoneurosis to the patient's being seduced was followed by his reevaluation and his emphasis that seduction was a memory, probably a fantasy, and that patients in general suffer from memories and from fantasies, rather than from events. While Freud never made this statement in this definite a way, the tenor of early practice reflected this reevaluation made by Freud in obscuring any environmental contributions to illness. Indeed, it was only many years later that Erikson reviewed Freud's Dora case and indicated the importance of the agreement between Dora's father and Freud in influencing the conduct of psychoanalytic treatment, and presumably, in Dora's prematurely breaking off the treatment. But it was to be many years before the recognition of the family as the matrix within which illness grew and developed was given the attention it merited, and the influence of the environment upon the therapy itself has not yet been carefully explored.

While the Menninger Clinic was among the first hospitals to plan systematically for programs for patients on the basis of their psychopathology, it is noteworthy that the separation of the milieu from psychotherapy is maintained quite consistently throughout the Menninger Clinic's descriptions. If patients were to be handled with firm kindness, for instance, there is no observation of the effect that this milieu handling could be expected to have upon the psychotherapy which the patients were receiving, and conversely, the extensive and detailed study of the psychotherapy of thirty patients at the Menninger Clinic is totally silent on the relation of psychotherapy to the Clinic, to discharge and to the environment to which the patients were discharged. The early effort at activation in mental hospitals, which was named "total push," also had no reference to its effect on psychotherapy, in spite of the fact that patients were engaged in psychotherapy at McLean and other hospitals where the total push method was explored. On the contrary, without focusing upon it, Stanton and Schwartz (1954) did treat the therapist and the milieu as two components of the patient's environment and noted a frequent complimentary relationship between them, so that the therapist tended to deal with ward issues as the patient brought them up, a procedure which was replete with the possibility of considerable gain and the possibility of grave disturbance. In particular, therapists were as likely as anyone else to engage in covert disagreements with other members of the staff, with often devastating effects on the patient and on his treatment. In situations of serious differences between patient and ward staff, therapists found it extraordinarily difficult to open up inquiry into the inner sources of the patient's experience without at the same time seeming to cast blame upon the patient as the cause of controversy. At the other end of the spectrum, when rapid improvement of patients occurred in a ward which was highly organized and in general harmony with what the patient needed, the therapist was usually unable to identify the sources of the patient's improvement in his interactions on the ward.

Clinical accounts of the relations between psychotherapy and milieu therapy tend to focus upon difficulties, as difficulties are more conspicuous and easily identified; they always represent a problem to the staff which must be dealt with. Nevertheless, even if less easily noted, psychotherapy generally contributes important supportive ingredients to the patient's experience in a therapeutic community. The most widespread, relatively unrecognized value of individual psychotherapy is its reinforcing of a patient's discrimination of his own individual identity. There are many different levels of participation in a community or in any group, some of which tend to support the merging of the patient's identity into that of the group in a regressive and often gravely pathogenic way. The heightening of one's own individual identity may occur as a particular way of participating in a group, but the ideology of therapeutic milieu is often subtly biased in favor of the loss of the patient's sense of his separate and individual identity. Individual psychotherapy—however much difficulty may arise from its practice—strongly and continuously, if subtly, keeps the patient's own self and his career, past and future, identified and to some extent discriminated from that of the group of which he is a part (Christ 1968). While it is possible for the psychotherapist in individual psychotherapy to treat the patient impersonally, and thus to rob him to some extent of his experience of being fully human, it is hard to do, and therapists rarely do treat patients consistently in an impersonal way.

There are more specific advantages. The experience in the therapeutic milieu can be subjected in individual therapy, to detailed and concrete observation which is beyond the reach of even the most successful group psychotherapy efforts. The necessary time is available to put a patient's experience in the group in the context of his own biography, with a growth in his recognition of the kind of person he is and the kind of disturbance that he shows, based upon the much greater amount of detailed information which can become available in the course of successful individual psychotherapy.

In its turn, individual psychotherapy can benefit from the effects of the group, particularly with chronic patients. Ingrained and established patterns of disturbance or of inadequate interpersonal relations may frequently be so familiar to a patient that he adapts to them and to their effects rather quietly, without noticing enough to provide grounds for exploration in individual psychotherapy. In the well functioning therapeutic milieu, the requirements of community participation and the likelihood of some kind of friendly but novel confrontation from peers bring to the patient the opportunity and the material to grow in his grasp of himself and his illness, which will often have escaped his work and treatment for many years. The therapeutic community may be, for many issues, a necessary condition for the best improvement that the chronic patient can make in individual psychotherapy.

REFERENCES

Artiss, K. L. *Milieu Therapy in Schizophrenia.* New York: Grune & Stratton, 1962.

Beck, A. T., Rush, A. J., Shaw, B. F., and Emery, G. *Cognitive Therapy of Depression.* New York: Guilford Press, 1979.

Bergin, A. E. and Garfield, S. L. *Handbook of Psychotherapy and Behavior Change.* New York: Wiley, 1971.

Bernheim, H. *Suggestive Therapeutics: A Treatise on the Nature and Uses of Hypnotism.* Translated from second French edition by Christian Herter. New York: Putnam, 1889.

Budson, R. D. *The Psychiatric Halfway House: A Handbook of Theory and Practice.* Pittsburgh: University of Pittsburgh Press, 1978.

Burrow, T. *Structure of Insanity. A Study in Phylopathology.* London: Paul, 1932.

Canter, D., and Canter, S., eds. *Designing for Therapeutic Environments.* New York: Wiley, Chichester, 1979.

Christ, J. Psychoanalytical treatment of a dissociative state with hallucinations, in *Psychotherapy in the Designed Therapeutic Milieu*, S. Eldred and M. Vanderpol, eds. Boston: Little Brown, 1968, pp. 33-44.

Cumming, J., and Cumming, E. *Ego and Milieu: Theory and Practice of Environmental Therapy.* New York: Atherton Press, 1962.

Dejerine, J. J. *The Psychoneuroses and their Treatment by Psychotherapy.* Trans. by Smith Ely Jelliffe. Phila.: Lippincott, 1913.

Dubois, P. *The Psychic Treatment of Nervous Disorders.* New York: Funk & Wagnalls, 1909.

Entralgo, P. L. *Doctor and Patient.* New York & Toronto: World University Library, McGraw-Hill, 1969.

Forel, A. *Hygiene of Nerves and Mind in Health and Disease.* New York: Putnam, 1907.

Garfield, S. L., and Bergin, A. E., eds. *Handbook of Psychotherapy and Behavior Change: An Empirical Analysis.* New York: Wiley, 1978.

Glass, G. V. Primary, Secondary, and Meta-Analysis of Research. Presidential Address, 1976 Annual Meeting, American Education Association. San Francisco, April 21, 1976.

Goldstein, A., and Stein, N., eds. Prescriptive Psychotherapies. New York: Pergamon Press, 1976.

Hogarty, G. E., Goldberg, S. C., and the Collaborative Study Group. Drug and sociotherapy in the Aftercare of schizophrenic patients: One Year Relapse Rates. *Arch. Gen. Psychiat.* 28: 54-64 (1973).

Hogarty, G. E., Goldberg, S. C., Schooler, N. R., Ulrich, R. F., and the Collaborative Study Group. Drug and sociotherapy in the aftercare of schizophrenic patients: III. Adjustment of non-relapsed patients. *Arch. Gen. Psychiat.* 31: 609-618 (1974).

Janet, P. *Principles of Psychotherapy.* Trans. by H. M. and E. R. Guthrie. New York (1924).

Jones, M. *The Therapeutic Community: A New Treatment Method in Psychiatry.* New York: Basic Books, 1953.

Klerman, G. Quoted in B. S. Herrington: Klerman weighs role in therapy efficacy study. *Psychiatric News*, 15, p. 10, May 2, 1980. Washington, American Psychiatric Assoc.

Malan, D. *Individual Psychotherapy and the Science of Psychodynamics.* London, Boston: Butterworths, 1979.

Meyer, A. Treatment of Paranoic and Paranoid States, in *Modern Treatment of Nervous and Mental Disease*, W. A. White and Smith Ely Jelliffe. Philadelphia: Lea, 1913, pp. 614-661.

Paul, G. L., and Lentz, R. J. *Psychosocial Treatment of Chronic Mental Patients: Milieu vs. Social Learning Programs.* Cambridge, Mass.: Harvard U. Press, 1977.

Rank, O., in Fay B. Karpf. *The Psychology and Psychotherapy of Otto Rank.* New York: Philosoph Library, 1953.

Rogers, C., and Dymond, R. F., eds. *Psychotherapy and Personality Change; Coordinated Research Studies in the Client Centered Approach.* Chicago: U. of Chicago Press, 1954.

Smith, M. L., and Glass, G. V. Meta-Analysis of Psychotherapy Outcome Studies. *Amer. Psychologist.* 752-760 (1977).

Stanton, A. H., and Schwartz, M. S. *The Mental Hospital.* New York: Basic Books, 1954.

Strauss, A. L. *Psychiatric Ideologies and Institutions.* Free Press of Glencoe, 1964.

Sullivan, H. S. *Clinical Studies in Psychiatry.* New York: Norton, 1956.

Wilmer, H. A. *Social Psychiatry in Action.* Springfield, Ill.: Thomas, 1958.

CHAPTER 6

THE MANAGEMENT OF THE FAMILY OF THE CHRONIC PSYCHIATRIC PATIENT

JULIAN P. LEFF, B.Sc., M.D., F.R.C.Psych., M.R.C.P.

INTRODUCTION

Unfortunately, psychiatry appears to have more than its fair share of chronic conditions. This throws a considerable burden on the psychiatric services and professional personnel. With the advent of community care, there has been a substantial increase in the burden carried by the families of psychiatric patients. As the number of psychiatric beds falls progressively, and the length of hospital stay decreases, the relatives are asked to contribute more and more of their own resources, both material and emotional, to the care of the patients. In addition to ethical considerations, the shift of the focus of psychiatric care to the community was seen by many politicians as a way of saving money. Community care appeared to be a cheap alternative to hospital beds, which are extremely expensive to maintain. The truth is that only *poor* community care is cheap. If adequate professional support is provided for the families of psychiatric patients, and if the necessary facilities are built up in the community, the cost is probably no less than for hospital care. The fact that this has not been appreciated by the relevant authorities has meant that inadequate support has been given to relatives, some of whom have refused to have patients back to live with them, while others have developed psychiatric illnesses themselves as a result of the excessive strain placed on them.

Few professionals realize what a strain it is to cope with chronic psychiatric patients day in and day out, and often at night as well, for years without any respite. This is because their experience of patients is confined to a few hours a week, or at most to a daily shift, and because they rarely see the patients in their home setting. Many of the problems that arise in the home are never seen in the hospital, so that professional staff have not built up the necessary experience of dealing with them on which to base advice to the relatives. Only when research workers ask relatives directly about their experience of dealing with patients at home, as Creer and Wing (1975) did, do the majority of these problems emerge.

DIAGNOSIS

In considering the details of management of families, it is necessary to pay regard to the diagnosis of the patients. Although there are problems common to all chronic psychiatric patients, there are also features that are specific to each diagnostic category. Thus, manic-depressive patients are likely to suffer from recurrent episodes of florid symptoms, but to be symptom free between episodes and to show little social impairment. On the other hand, although schizophrenic patients may also show discrete episodes, they are likely to suffer from a multiplicity of neurotic symptoms between episodes and to exhibit a progressive decline in social functioning. Furthermore they may also develop the so-called negative symptoms, which are particularly difficult for relatives to deal with. Because of the way problems vary with the patient's condition, we will divide this chapter into two parts. In the first part we will deal with the management of problems that are common to all chronic psychiatric patients. In the second part we will discuss problems specific to particular psychiatric conditions.

COMMON PROBLEMS

Information and Education

One of the most pressing concerns relatives have is uncertainty about the future. This is particularly so if the patient suffers from recurrent episodes. Relatives are justifiably apprehensive about the possible return of symptoms and may seize on minor abnormalities of behavior as evidence of impending relapse. They often claim to be unaware of the patient's diagnosis and have unrealistically optimistic or pessimistic views of the prognosis. Relatives interviewed a few weeks after patients' admission to hospital deny being told the diagnosis by the psychiatrist responsible for the patient's care, and claim they have been given no indication of what to expect in the future. When checks are made in these cases, it is found that they have indeed been told both the diagnosis and the prognosis. It is evident that one brief session with the psychiatrist, the usual allocation of time, is insufficient. The reasons for this are partly the complex nature of the information to be imparted, and partly emotional reactions in the relatives which prevent the absorption of information at the time. For example, one relative reported that as soon as the psychiatrist told her that her son was suffering from schizophrenia, her mind went numb with the shock and she heard nothing more of what was said in the interview. Other relatives have complained that they cannot think of the questions they want to ask at the time, and later, when appropriate questions occur to them, it is too late.

It is clearly necessary for the psychiatric team to spend a lot more time on informing and educating the relatives about the nature of the patient's illness than is customary at present. The relatives need to be told the diagnosis, if the team is certain about it, and what to expect in the future. This is a difficult task for the psychiatric team because it deals in probabilities, which are often not specific enough for the individual case. However, this is not different in principle from prognostication in other branches of medicine, so that relatives can be expected to be familiar with this form of information. They can usually understand and deal with a statement of the form that "if the patient takes regular medication there is a one in three chance that he will relapse in the next year, while if he doesn't take regular medication the chance of relapse is doubled."

The team needs to make a distinction between what is preventable in the way of illness and what is remediable, or what cannot be expected to alter. For example, the relatives can be told the chances of preventing relapses if the patient follows a particular course of treatment. They can be informed that the patient's poor social skills are likely to be improved by the appropriate therapy; and it can be made clear that the patient's excessive jealousy, which was present long before the illness appeared, is unlikely to abate much. This involves quite subtle judgments as to what constitute episodes of illness, what are secondary handicaps accruing as a consequence of protracted illness and what may be identified as premorbid personality characteristics. Despite the difficulty of the task, it is important to convey these distinctions to the relatives so that they may have as realistic a view of outcome as is possible.

It is vital for all members of the psychiatric team to agree on what is to be told to the relatives in any particular case. There is nothing more confusing for relatives than to be given different information by different professionals. It also provides an opportunity for manipulative relatives to pit one member of the team against another, leading to internecine tension which impairs the efficiency of the team. Therefore it is advisable for the team to meet in conference on each case and decide on a unanimous view of the condition, which is to be imparted to the relatives. If it is impossible to reach a unanimous view, then the dissenting minority must agree not to sabotage the efforts of the majority to inform the relatives with their version. In this respect it is important to admit to relatives that there are still large areas of ignorance in our understanding of psychiatric illness. Once the psychiatric professional steps down from a Godlike stance, it is easier for relatives to bring into play their own observations of patients, which are potentially of great value both in management and in furthering our understanding of these conditions.

Social Services

Patients suffering from chronic psychiatric conditions are either unemployable or else only able to work at a reduced capacity or in a less skilled job than they occupied before the onset of symptoms. The financial burden this represents rests heavily on the patient's family. This situation appears to be no different from that arising from any chronic handicapping condition, for instance, rheumatoid arthritis, but there is one major difference: the very nature of psychiatric illnesses impairs the patients' ability to seek out the resources provided by official agencies for their relief. It is in the history and nature of social welfare agencies that a client has to be determined, equipped with more than ordinary social skills, and well informed to extract from them what is due to him by law. Most chronic psychiatric patients are severely deficient in these qualities, so that it falls to their relatives to act on their behalf. To do this effectively they need advice, support and active help from mental health professionals. Sadly, this is rarely forthcoming.

The scale of the problem is indicated by a study carried out by Leff and Vaughn (1972). They selected two groups of patients suffering from functional psychoses, that is, schizophrenia and manic-depressive illnesses. An In Contact group consisted of persons who contacted local psychiatric services in South-East London during the year prior to being sampled. An Out of Contact group was limited to persons out of contact with services for one year, but in contact during the year before that. In each case the patient was interviewed, and also a relative if available. Ninety percent of the In Contact group and 88 percent of the Out of Contact group were living with relatives. Structured interviews were used to assess the patient's current mental state, the adequacy of the patient's social functioning in the community, and attitudes to contact and the services. The latter two areas were also covered in independent interviews with the relatives.

One of the principal aims of this study was to determine whether the existing psychiatric and social services were meeting the needs of patients. In terms of the patients' clinical status the services were functioning effectively. Few patients in any group had active symptoms, and those out of contact with the services were clinically better than those in contact. However, the services were much less adequate in coping with social needs. Of the In Contact group 16 patients (32%) were in need of help from the housing department and other social agencies, irrespective of whether they were being seen by social workers. In the Out of Contact group 20 patients (50%) were in need of similar help.

Patients' and relatives' complaints reflected the disproportionately greater social than medical nature of the needs. Only one patient and four relatives in the In Contact group and one patient and three relatives in the Out of Contact group complained of inadequate in-patient or out-patient care, whereas in the case of all the patients with social needs, complaints were made by the patient, the relatives or both. Taking the two groups as a whole, housing was found to be a particular problem, reflecting both the housing shortage in the general population and the shortage of halfway houses for psychiatric patients. Nineteen patients (21%) urgently needed alternative accommodation, four of them requiring a halfway house or convalescent home. Most of them were on local authority housing lists but had been waiting many years for rehousing, meanwhile living in appalling circumstances. In some instances overcrowding was the main problem, with as many as five persons sleeping in one room. Conditions of cold and damp, collapsing ceilings and floorboards, and inadequate or absent plumbing were also common. Repeated requests for repairs had been ignored or put off by the local authority or private landlords, especially if rehousing was believed to be "imminent."

In addition to their housing problems, four In Contact patients (10%) and six Out of Contact patients (15%) had other needs as well, for example, a day nursery, visits from a social worker, financial assistance, a Home Help or a social club. A further eight In Contact patients (16%) and nine Out of Contact patients (23%) were adequately housed but could have benefited from other services such as the above.

It is evident from the above findings that despite the Welfare State set up in the United Kingdom, a large proportion of the social needs of patients and their relatives are not being met. It is reasonable to suppose that the situation is at least as bad as this in the United States.

Emotional Support

In addition to their needs for social services, relatives often have emotional needs which are unmet. Because the patients suffer from psychiatric conditions, relatives feel they cannot unburden themselves to them. Furthermore, the relatives often lack other intimate relationships in their social circle that they could use as an emotional outlet. There are a number of reasons for this: relatives often feel that the patient's condition carries a stigma and deal with their sense of shame by withdrawing from company. On the other hand, the patient's behavior may actually cause friends and neighbors to cease visiting the household. A further problem affects the blood relatives of schizophrenic patients, who tend to have schizoid personalities. This is particularly true of female blood relatives (Stephens et al. 1975) and contributes to their lack of intimate relationships. Whatever the reasons, relatives are often attempting to cope with the emotional strains of living with a psychiatric patient without any support from other people. What this may lead to is illustrated by the study of Leff and Vaughn (1972) described above. In two of the cases in their sample the relatives felt they had reached breaking point and questioned how much longer they could provide twenty-four-hour supervision and care without severe damage to their own mental and physical health. Both relatives were being treated for depression by their family doctors, and one relative (the patient's brother) found the situation so unbearable he regularly contemplated suicide as an escape.

It is advisable for the professional team responsible for the patient to keep a close eye on the relatives with whom the patient is living, from the point of view of their mental health. If the team decides that a relative has developed a psychiatric illness and needs treatment, it is preferable for this to be given by someone other than the individual dealing with the patient. This is to avoid problems of confidentiality and the possibility of the patient becoming paranoid about what might be going on between his relative and his therapist.

Ways of alleviating the burden relatives carry, either long- or short-term, should be considered. For instance, it may be advisable to admit patients to hospital or to sheltered accommodation for brief periods from time to time to allow relatives to take a holiday on their own. Admission of patients for "social" rather than medical reasons may not be popular with the authorities, but it can be argued that in the long run it contributes to a reduction in psychiatric morbidity in the community. Long-term measures include regular visits by a social worker or community nurse to allow relatives to unburden themselves about current problems, and the encouragement of relatives to join social clubs or other groups which enable them to spend some of their leisure time independently of the patients.

A growing source of emotional support is the formation of relatives' groups. These usually result from the initiative of individuals who have relatives suffering from a particular illness. A good example in the psychiatric field is the National Schizophrenia Fellowship (Creer and Wing 1974), which organizes groups of relatives in each area of the United Kingdom. The groups bring together relatives, who are able to give each other emotional support to combat the sense of isolation, and to bring pressure to bear on the relevant authorities to improve services for the patients. Such groups tend to attract articulate middle class people, but they are of course open to all, and less verbal, lower class relatives should be encouraged to join them.

PROBLEMS SPECIFIC TO DIAGNOSTIC GROUPS

In this section we will deal with the functional psychiatric disorders as divided into the psychoses and neuroses, but will not attempt to cover the management of the demented patient.

Schizophrenia

The majority of chronic psychiatric patients suffering from functional disorders are diagnosed as schizophrenic. Roughly two thirds of these can be expected to be living with relatives. In the preceding section we have indicated ways in which the burden of caring for chronic psychiatric patients can be alleviated, and all of these apply to the relatives of schizophrenics. However, there is another major consideration, and that is the role family members play in perpetuating the chronicity of the illness.

There is considerable controversy about the possible etiological contribution of family attitudes to the origin of schizophrenia. The major methodological problem is the retrospective nature of the enquiry (Hirsch and Leff 1975). The handful of studies that have employed strategies to overcome this problem have pinpointed two characteristics of the families of people who later develop schizophrenia: the mothers tend to be overprotective during the patients' childhood, and there tends to be excessive conflict between the parents. These two findings are echoed in the work that has been carried out in the Medical Research Council Social Psychiatry Unit on the influence of families on the *course* of schizophrenic disorders. This work, which has been recently summarized (Leff 1976), employs a prospective design, assigning relatives to different groups at the time the patients present with a schizophrenic episode, and then following up the patients after their return home to live with their relatives. It is necessary to present a summary of this work in order to justify the policies for managing the families.

The key measure in this series of studies is of Expressed Emotion (EE). This consists of four components: critical comments, hostility, warmth and emotional overinvolvement (Brown and Rutter 1966; Rutter and Brown 1966). These ratings are made from interviews with relatives in which a standard list of questions are asked about the patient's behavior and symptoms and the quality of interpersonal relationships. The interviews are conducted shortly after the patient's admission to hospital with a first attack or relapse of schizophrenia. Trained raters achieve a high inter-rater reliability on the above measures both in live interviews and from tape recordings. Ratings are made on content and on vocal aspects of speech including tone, volume and speed. In the initial studies the interviews took an average of over four hours to administer. However, it was found that the key measures could be made from a greatly shortened interview lasting no more than an hour and a half (Vaughn and Leff 1976a), and this has become the standard procedure. A series of three studies conducted over 15 years has employed these measures (Brown et al. 1962, 1972; Vaughn and Leff 1976b) all studies have shown a strong association between high Expressed Emotion in relatives and relapse of schizophrenia. The crucial components of EE have proved to be critical comments and emotional overinvolvement. Critical comments are made as commonly by spouses as by parents, whereas overinvolvement is seen much more often in parents, particularly mothers, than in spouses. On the basis of their scores on these two scales, relatives are assigned to High EE or Low EE groups. Patients returning to live with High EE relatives have a relapse rate (not necessarily rehospitalization) of 48% in nine months, compared with only 6% for those returning to Low EE homes, a highly significant difference (Vaughn and Leff 1976b).

It appears from these findings that living with High EE relatives is dangerous for patients who have suffered from schizophrenia. However, they can protect themselves in two ways: by taking regular phenothiazine medication, and by reducing the amount of time they spend with their relatives. The latter factor was studied by constructing a time budget of the patient's typical week. Ideally, one would like to know how much time is spent in social interaction between patient and relative, but this is impossible to estimate. Instead, questions are asked which enable one to determine how much of the day the relative and patient spend in the same room together (periods of sleep are excluded). The number of hours per week spent in what is termed face-to-face contact is assumed to reflect the amount of social interaction. An arbitrary cutting point of 35 hours per week was used to differentiate high from low face-to-face contact. It was found that patients who were in high face-to-face contact with High EE relatives had a higher relapse rate (69%) than those in low face-to-face contact (28%). Even if they were maintained on regular phenothiazine treatment, their relapse rate was still alarmingly high, reaching 53% in nine months after discharge.

These results indicate that phenothiazine medication alone is insufficient to protect schizophrenics living in high contact with High EE relatives. It is also necessary to do something about the emotional climate in the home. There are a variety of strategies that can be adopted, which are presented diagrammatically in Figure 1.

The most effective measure would appear to be removal of the patient from the High Emotion home and placement in a more neutral environment, such as a halfway house or supervised lodgings. This would not usually be considered in the case of a married couple, since proposing to break up a marriage is ethically dubious. Even when the patient is living with parents, this obvious course of action proves difficult to implement for a number of reasons. In practice, sheltered accommodation of the type suitable for schizophrenic

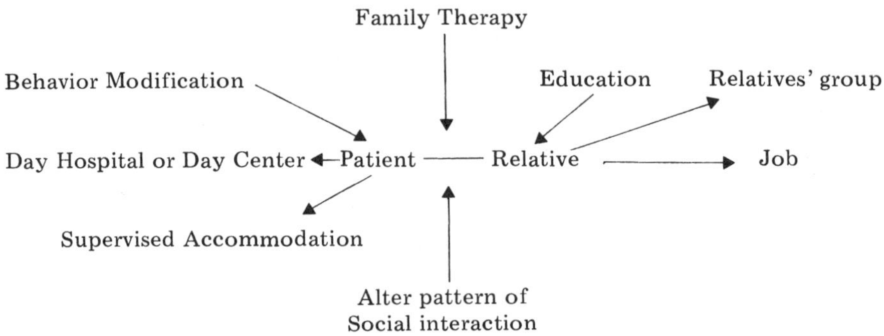

Figure 1. Social Intervention Strategies in High EE Homes

patients is rarely available. Too few facilities have been built, and the turnover of occupants in existing accommodation is low. Furthermore, it is usually very difficult to persuade parents and patients that they would be better off living apart. When the Expressed Emotion concerned is overinvolvement, the resistance to letting the patient leave home stems naturally from this. However, even parents who are purely critical without any hint of overinvolvement are also reluctant to part from the patient because of their sense of guilt and responsibility. It is necessary to explore these feelings before the patient can be extricated from such homes. Unfortunately opposition is not confined to the parents, but is often expressed by the patients as well. Schizophrenic patients are often lacking in elementary social skills and have no friends outside of the family. They are understandably nervous about moving to a new environment where they will have to form relationships with strangers and will probably be expected to do more in the way of looking after themselves than they have been accustomed to at home.

If removal from the home is impractical, the next best strategy is to attempt to reduce the time relatives and the patient spend together. Frequently the patient is unemployed and unable to compete with healthy people in open employment. The unemployed patient spends a great deal of time at home and is usually in high face-to-face contact with a relative. Arranging for the patient to attend a day hospital or day center ensures that he will be out of the house for a large part of the day, and this effectively reduces face-to-face contact with the relative. Another strategy, which is appropriate if the patient is an unemployable man married to a healthy woman, is to persuade the wife to go out to a job. This not only reduces the time they spend together, but enables her to socialize with healthy people, often a welcome relief. Even patients who are in full employment can be in high face-to-face contact with their relatives. For these reasons it can be useful to attempt to alter the way patients and relatives spend their leisure time. They can be encouraged to attend day or evening classes provided by the local authority, or even to spend less time in the same room when they are at home together. Some relatives develop their own strategies to achieve the same result; for example, one mother would tell her schizophrenic son to take the dog out for a walk whenever the atmosphere between them became tense.

So far we have considered methods of separating patients and relatives in space and time without tackling the root of the problem, namely, the emotional attitudes of the relatives. We have accumulated evidence that they can be altered, mainly from their own accounts of the patient's illness. Every now and then we encounter relatives whose current attitudes place them firmly in the Low EE group, but who describe their emotional responses at an earlier period in the history of the illness in a way that would undoubtedly characterize them as High EE. We have not come across a spontaneous change of this kind in the reverse direction. In an attempt to understand the development of critical attitudes in relatives, we examined the detailed content of critical comments (Leff and Vaughn 1976). It was somewhat surprising to discover that only one third of the criticisms related to behavior stemming from the florid symptoms of schizophrenia, namely, delusions and hallucinations. Two thirds of the critical comments were aimed at long-standing behavior which did not appear to the relatives to be part of the illness. In particular they were upset by the patients' lack of communication, inertia, apathy and failure to show warmth and affection. These findings are supported by a study of relatives of schizophrenics, the majority of whom were contacted through the National Schizophrenia Fellowship, while the remainder were randomly sampled from families living in South-East London (Creer and Wing 1974, 1975). On being asked about management problems, they complained most commonly of social withdrawal (74%), underactivity (56%), lack of conversation (54%) and few leisure interests (50%). By contrast only 34% complained of odd ideas and odd behavior.

The professional view of schizophrenia is that the so-called negative symptoms—apathy, inertia, emotional blunting and social withdrawal—are as much a part of the illness process as delusions and hallucinations. It is not surprising, though, that relatives do not recognize the negative symptoms as products of an illness, viewing them instead as personality characteristics which are under the patients' control. Hence they criticize the patients for being lazy, stubborn, cold and selfish. It is reasonable to suppose that if the relatives were educated to see the negative symptoms as an integral part of schizophrenia, their attitudes might become much less critical. We have already stressed the importance of informing and educating relatives about psychiatric illnesses, but with these high-risk schizophrenic patients, this endeavor takes on a special significance.

Unfortunately, the negative symptoms of schizophrenia are not amenable to drug treatment, but it is claimed that they respond to behavioral modification techniques (Liberman et al. 1974). The early enthusiasm for this approach has cooled somewhat with disappointing reports of short-lived effects (Falloon et al. 1978), but there is hope that changes in technique will overcome these problems.

We have emphasized earlier that approximately half of the relatives living with schizophrenic patients fall into the Low EE group and are coping very adequately with the problems of daily management of this condition. One might imagine that in contrast to the High EE relatives, these others are cool and remote and uninvolved with the patients. Recent work on psychophysiological responses of patients to their relatives suggests that this is far from the case, and that Low EE relatives play an active role in helping the patients to adjust to environmental stress (Tarrier et al. 1979). It was therefore considered possible that Low EE relatives could teach their own coping skills to High EE relatives. A relatives' group was set up two years ago composed of both types of relatives, who were unaware of their categorizations. The group meets once every two weeks for an hour and a half, has a maximum of eight members at any one time and a flexible policy on attendance. The therapists act as catalysts to draw out the relatives on the problems they face and how they tackle them. The group undoubtedly counters the sense of isolation felt by many relatives and referred to earlier. In addition, it does appear to have led to changes in attitude and behavior of the kind we were hoping for. However, it is too soon to pronounce on this, as the relatives' group is part of a scientifically evaluated program which has yet to run its course before any analysis can be done. Nevertheless, we consider it worthwhile to present a number of major themes that have emerged from the groups, as they throw light on the emotional attitudes of relatives towards schizophrenic patients.

Themes From the Relatives' Group

Intolerance of illness

Some relatives are totally unable to come to terms with the patient's illness. They may relate well to the patient while he or she is healthy, but find it extremely difficult to maintain that relationship during periods of illness. Their reaction is to want to escape from the situation at all costs. They seem to be people who find mental illness frightening, perhaps because it represents a threat to their own, rather precarious, stability.

Intolerance of handicap

Others can accept the idea that their relative is ill, but never come to terms with the chronic incapacity that is so common with schizophrenia. They find it very difficult to modify their preillness expectations of the patient. Commonly these are parents who wanted their children to do better than they did, so that the patient is under pressure to make up for the parents' lack of fulfillment. It is particularly hard for such parents to accept that their child may actually achieve *less* than they did. Spouses may also show this kind of intolerance, particularly if they have rigid views of family roles. Thus, the wife who can only see her husband as the breadwinner and herself as the homemaker finds it hard to accept that she may have to contribute the major portion of the family income, while her handicapped husband takes over some of the household chores.

Displaced aggression

Relatives may be very resentful of the patients' behavior but find it hard to confront him directly for fear of making him worse. Their aggression then becomes displaced onto other members of the household. Thus, the wife of a patient may become very irritable with their children. The group acts as a useful forum for discharge of relatives' aggressive feelings, but we are careful to put a limit on this use of the group to allow more positive ways of coping to be discussed.

Inability to separate

Some relatives realize that both they and the patient would be better off living apart, but are quite unable to achieve the separation. In some cases, usually parents, this is because of a great emotional investment in the patient. We have encountered a particular family pattern of relationships in which the healthy parents have a poor relationship of long standing. One of them, almost always the mother, turns to the child, either son or daughter, for emotional satisfaction, and then cannot bear to let the child leave home because of having to face the problems in the marital relationship. This is a particularly difficult situation for the schizophrenic patient, who often has to cope not only with the mother's emotional overinvolvement but also with the father's criticism, because he disapproves of the mother-child bond.

Spouses may also find it difficult to contemplate separation because they feel very responsible for the patient. They worry about the patient's ability to cope on his own, and get trapped into remaining in a mutually antagonistic relationship by their sense of guilt.

Power of madness

Some of the above themes come together in a feeling expressed by many relatives that patients wield power over them by virtue of their illness. Relatives are afraid to criticize patients directly or be firm with them about unacceptable behavior in case this will upset them and make them worse. There is no doubt that some patients use their illness to manipulate relatives into doing much more for them than is necessary. In addition to these understandable aspects of patients' and relatives' behavior, there is a less rational element of fear of the unknown, stemming from the incomprehensible. Sensational presentations of the mass media undoubtedly play a part here.

In addition to these specific themes, we have been able to identify different coping patterns in the two types of relatives. The High EE relatives are intolerant of the patients' behavior at home and deny the validity of the patients' experiences, leading to angry confrontations. The Low EE relatives show a tolerant, even collusive, attitude towards the patients' symptoms and retain a remarkable ability to defuse the most explosive situations. They show no hint of blaming or criticizing the patients.

It should be apparent from this brief account that the relatives' group cannot be confined to a simple exchange of coping skills. There is a great deal of emotion to be discharged, giving the members an opportunity to explore the nature and formation of emotional attitudes to the patients, and possibly to modify them. In forming the group we deliberately excluded patients, partly to shield them from the intense emotions we anticipated would be discharged, and partly to allow relatives to discharge the emotions, uninhibited by the presence of the patients. However, there is a long tradition of family therapy that includes the patient, which is strongest in the U.S.A. and is beginning to gain adherents in the U.K. There seems to have been some disillusionment with family therapy for schizophrenia in the twenty years since its inception (Leff 1979), and there are less than a handful of scientific studies of its effectiveness. However, a recent scientific trial of crisis-oriented family therapy for acute schizophrenia showed encouraging results (Goldstein et al. 1978) and should stimulate more enthusiasm for this form of treatment.

Manic-Depressive Psychosis

There is very little work on the effects of this group of conditions on relatives, but we can refer again to the study of Leff and Vaughn (1972) quoted above. In this study of functional psychoses 20% manic-depressives were included in the In Contact group and 33% in the Out of Contact group. In almost every respect the schizophrenic patients showed more severe social impairment than the manic patients. It would be anticipated that with the increasing use of prophylactic lithium treatment, manic episodes would be better controlled, allowing the patients to maintain a more stable job record. However, there remains a small group of uncontrollable manics who lose their jobs whenever they fall ill and who eventually may become unemployable. The problems faced by their relatives are similar to those encountered by the relatives of unemployable schizophrenic patients, dealt with above.

There is one aspect of lithium prophylaxis that may affect patients and their relatives, and that is the possibility that controlling manic episodes may result in lowered productivity and creativity in creative workers (Schou 1979). Creativity may be shown by artists, scientists, business-men, politicians, etc., but only a small proportion of manics controlled by lithium experience this effect, so that the problem is not likely to be widespread, and lithium remains the treatment of choice in these cases.

Apart from occupational problems, the relatives of manic-depressive patients also suffer as a result of the symptoms in acute episodes. In our study (Leff and Vaughn 1972), we were surprised to discover that these relatives actually reported greater and more persistent distress than the relatives of schizophrenic patients. This appeared to be due to the high proportion of manic patients who developed paranoid delusions centered on their relatives. These findings suggest that the relatives of manic patients could benefit from emotional support given by professionals, at least during episodes of florid symptoms.

Neuroses: Phobic Neurosis

Until recently phobias were considered to be chronic intractable conditions, but the introduction of behavioral methods of treatment has brought the possibility of rapid cure in many cases. One of the commonest phobias in the general population is agoraphobia, which presents much more often in women than in men (Marks 1969). Although very handicapped by their symptoms, many women do not seek help from the medical services, the reason being that their families rearrange their lives to compensate for the handicap. For instance, a woman who is unable to go out by herself may keep a child out of school to accompany her on shopping expeditions. Sometimes if there are several children, the oldest acts as a companion for a while until pressure from the school authorities becomes too insistent. He then starts to attend school regularly, and his place is taken by the next eldest child. The agoraphobic mother may work her way down the whole line of children until she gets to the youngest, for whom there is no substitute, and hence there is no escape. Alternatively, the husband makes up for the wife's restrictions, doing the shopping for her, accompanying her on all her outings and even coming home for lunch during the working day to keep her company.

It is evident that the rapid removal of a phobic patient's symptoms in a compensating family of this kind will have a profound effect on the healthy members of the family. Indeed, the change in role required, particularly for a healthy husband, may be actively resisted, thus tending to perpetuate the patient's symptoms. Evidence for this has been presented by Hafner (1977a) in a study of agoraphobic women and their husbands. He found that the husbands were far less dissatisfied with their wives' symptoms than the patients themselves. Furthermore, husbands and wives showed strongly complementary hostility patterns; extrapunitive women with very high total hostility scores were married to relatively intrapunitive men with normal hostility scores; while intrapunitive women with low total hostility scores were married to extrapunitive men with high hostility scores. This suggests that assortative mating had taken place, leading to the sort of relationship in which a psychological change in one partner necessitates a complementary change in the other. In fact, when the agoraphobic women were treated with behavior therapy, there was a fall in the total hostility of the most hostile group of patients, and a *rise* in their spouses' total hostility score (Hafner 1977b). The most hostile patients showed an overall symptomatic improvement at a three-month followup, whereas their husbands showed an increase in scores on a symptom questionnaire. One husband attempted suicide about four months after the treatment. He said that he had done so because he had felt useless and inadequate since his wife's recovery, as she was no longer almost totally dependent on him. It follows from these findings, as Hafner suggests, that husbands should be included in the treatment of their wives' agoraphobic symptoms to facilitate any complementary changes required of them and to avoid any resistance to their wives' improvement.

Depressive Neurosis

Evidence has been accumulating that the spouses of depressed patients play an important part in perpetuating or curtailing the illness. In a series of studies Brown and his colleagues have identified life events as important precipitants of depression in women, but only in the presence of vulnerability factors (Brown and Harris 1978). One of these is the availability of an intimate, that is, another person with whom the depressed woman can share her concerns in an uninhibited manner. An intimate is frequently, but not invariably, the woman's sexual partner. Brown's findings come from studies carried out on samples of the general population, but have been confirmed for depressed women treated as out-patients and in-patients by Roy (1978). In his study he rated marriages as either "good" or "poor" in addition to determining whether a confiding relationship was present. He found that several depressed women had a "poor" marriage yet were able to confide in their husbands, whereas only one subject with a "good" marriage claimed she was unable to confide in her husband. Thus, there is a considerable degree of overlap between "poor" marriages as assessed in this study and lack of a confiding relationship. This leads us into the study by Vaughn and Leff (1976b), the findings of which for schizophrenic patients and their relatives were discussed above. In addition to studying schizophrenics, we also included a comparison group of depressed neurotic patients. We measured Expressed Emotion in the relatives of both groups of patients in the same way, although all but two of the 30 depressives were living with spouses, compared with only 13 of the 37 schizophrenics. We found a strong association between critical remarks made by spouses and subsequent relapse of depressed patients. Critical attitudes in the spouses of depressives were linked with a generally poor relationship between patient and relative which antedated the illness. In a later analysis of the interaction of life events and Expressed Emotion (Leff and Vaughn 1980), we found that a high proportion of patients living with critical spouses had experienced a life event in the three months before the onset of depression. It should be noted that whereas Brown and his colleagues and Roy studied depressed women exclusively, one third of our depressed patients were men.

We have presented the experimental work on this topic in some detail because the findings have potentially far-reaching implications for treatment of depressive neurosis, one of the commonest psychiatric conditions. The various studies reviewed all point to the relationship between the depressed patient and his or her spouse as being of great importance in determining whether the patient will respond to a life event with a recurrence of depression. At present the findings are of strong associations, which suggest but do not prove that the relationship with the spouse plays a causal role in the maintenance of depressive states. Further experimental work is required, but in the current state of knowledge it is certainly worth assessing the marital relationship in any case of depressive neurosis in a married patient. If found to be unsatisfactory in any way, it is justifiable to intervene therapeutically in an attempt to improve the relationship. If successful, this might not only benefit the marriage but could play an important part in curtailing the chronicity of the depressive condition.

SUMMARY AND CONCLUSIONS

We have seen that relatives play crucial roles in respect to chronic psychiatric patients in the community. On the one hand they are often carrying the major burden of community care with little or no support from the medical and social services. On the other hand they are implicated in the perpetuation of symptoms in a number of psychiatric conditions as diverse as schizophrenia and agoraphobia. In order to alleviate the burden on the relatives it is necessary to provide them with as much information about the illness with which they are coping as is available, to mobilize the social services to provide the maximum statutory care, and to give them emotional support *ad libitum*. The latter function is very demanding of professional resources, but the value of self-help groups in this respect is being increasingly recognized (Katz and Bender 1976).

From the point of view of relatives' etiological role in various psychiatric conditions, a great deal more research needs to be done. However, work already completed is suggesting increasingly specific links between emotional attitudes in relatives and recurrence of episodes of psychiatric illness (Leff et al. 1982). If these links do indeed prove to be causal, then the therapeutic focus will need to shift to the relatives, and new techniques will be required to modify their attitudes.

It is evident that for both these major functions to be carried out by the psychiatric team demands a wide range of skills and abilities that need to be complementary and well integrated. It is of the first importance that members of the team share the same aims and work towards the same ends. This ideal may prove hard to attain but needs to be sought after if community care for the chronic psychiatric patient and his family is to become preferable to a lifetime in a psychiatric institution.

REFERENCES

Brown, G. W., Birley, J. L. T., and Wing, J. K. Influence of family life on the course of schizophrenic disorders: A replication. *Brit. J. Psychiat.* 121: 241-258 (1972).

Brown, G. W., and Harris, T. *Social Origins of Depression.* London: Tavistock Publications, 1978.

Brown, G. W., Monck, E. M., Carstairs, G. M., and Wing, J. K. Influence of family life on the course of schizophrenic illness. *Brit. J. Prev. Soc. Med.* 16: 55-68 (1962).

Brown, G. W., and Rutter, M. The measurement of family activities and relationships: A methodological study. *Human Rel.* 19: 241-263 (1966).

Creer, C., and Wing, J. K. *Schizophrenia at Home.* Surbiton, Surrey: National Schizophrenia Fellowship, 1974.

Creer, C., and Wing, J. K. Living with a schizophrenic patient. *Brit. J. Hosp. Med.* 73-82 (1975).

Falloon, I. R. H., Lindley, P., McDonald, R., and Marks, I. M. Social skills training of out-patient groups: A controlled study of rehearsal and homework. *Brit. J. Psychiat.* 131: 599-609 (1977).

Goldstein, M. J., Rodnick, E. H., Evans, J. R., May, P. R. A., and Steinberg, M. R. Drug and family therapy in the aftercare of acute schizophrenics. *Arch. Gen. Psychiat.* 35: 1169-1177 (1978).

Hafner, R. J. The husbands of agoraphobic women: assortative mating or pathogenic interaction? *Brit. J. Psychiat.* 130: 233-239 (1977a).

Hafner, R. J. The husbands of agoraphobic women and their influence on treatment outcome. *Brit. J. Psychiat.* 131: 289-294 (1977b).

Hirsch, S. R., and Leff, J. P. *Abnormalities in Parents of Schizophrenics.* Maudsley Monograph No. 22. Oxford University Press, London (1975).

Katz, A., and Bender, E. I., eds. *The Strength in Us: Self-Help Groups in the Modern World.* New York: Franklin Watts, 1976.

Leff, J. P. Schizophrenia and sensitivity to the family environment. *Schiz. Bull.* 2: 566-574 (1976).

Leff, J. P. Developments in family treatment of schizophrenia. *Psychiat. Quart.* 51: (1979).

Leff, J. P., Kuipers, L., Berkowitz, R., Eberlein-Vries, R., and Sturgeon, D. A controlled trial of social intervention in the families of schizophrenic patients, *Brit. J. Psychiat.* 141: 121-134 (1982).

Leff, J. P., and Vaughn, C. E. Psychiatric patients in contact and out of contact with services, in *Evaluating a Community Psychiatric Service*, J. K. Wing and A. M. Hailey, eds. London: Oxford University Press, 1972.

Leff, J. P., and Vaughn, C. E. Schizophrenia and family life. *Psychol. Today* 2: 13-18 (1976).

Leff, J. P. and Vaughn, C. E. The interaction of life events and relative's expressed emotion in schizophrenia and depressive neurosis. *Brit. J. Psychiat.* 136: 146-153 (1980).

Liberman, R. P., Wallace, C., Teigen, S., and David, J. Interventions with psychotic behaviors, in *Innovative Treatment Methods in Psychopathology*, H. D. Adams, and K. M. Mitchell, eds. New York: John Wiley & Sons, Inc., 1974.

Marks, I. M. *Fears and Phobias.* London: Heinemann, 1969.

Roy, A. Vulnerability factors and depression in women. *Brit. J. Psychiat.* 133: 106-110 (1978).

Rutter, M., and Brown, G. W. The reliability and validity of measures of family life and relationships in families containing a psychiatric patient. *Soc. Psychiat.* 1: 38-53 (1966).

Schou, M. Artistic productivity and lithium prophylaxis in manic-depressive illness. *Brit. J. Psychiat.* 135: 97–103 (1979).

Stephens, D. A., Atkinson, M. W., Kay, D. W. K., Roth, M., and Garside, R. F. Psychiatric morbidity in parents and sibs of schizophrenics and nonschizophrenics, *Brit. J. Psychiat.* 127: 97–108 (1975).

Tarrier, N., Vaughn, C., Lader, M. H., and Leff, J. P. Bodily reactions to people and events in schizophrenics. *Arch. Gen. Psychiat.* 36: 311–315 (1979).

Vaughn, C. E., and Leff, J. P. The measurement of expressed emotion in the families of psychiatric patients. *Brit. J. Soc. Clin. Psychol.* 15: 157–165 (1976a).

Vaughn, C. E., and Leff, J. P. The influence of family and social factors on the course of psychiatric illness: A comparison of schizophrenic and depressed neurotic patients. *Brit. J. Psychiat.* 129: 125–137 (1976b).

CHAPTER 7

THE ROLE OF CRISIS INTERVENTION IN THE MANAGEMENT OF THE CHRONIC PSYCHIATRIC PATIENT

DONNA CONANT AGUILERA, Ph.D., F.A.A.N.

HISTORICAL DEVELOPMENT OF CRISIS INTERVENTION METHODOLOGY

A person in crisis is at a turning point. He faces a problem that he cannot readily solve by using the coping mechanisms that have worked for him before. As a result, his tension and anxiety increase, and he becomes less able to find a solution. A person in this situation feels helpless—he is caught in a state of great emotional upset and feels unable to take action on his own to solve his problem.

Crisis intervention can offer the immediate help that a person in crisis needs in order to reestablish equilibrium. This is an inexpensive, short-term therapy that focuses on solving the immediate problem. Increasing awareness of sociocultural factors that could precipitate crisis situations has led to the rapid evolution of crisis intervention methodology. Therefore, these factors will be discussed first in order to create a better understanding of their social and cultural implications.

Everywhere today we hear talk of the changes in our lives that have been made by "urbanization" and "technology." A closer study of these changes will add to our understanding of what they have meant to families and to individuals.

Before the revolution in technology and industrialization, most people lived on farms or in small rural communities. They were chiefly self-employed, either on their farms or in small, associated businesses. When sons and daughters married, they were likely to remain near their parents, working in the same occupations, and in this way, trades and occupations were a link between generations. Families therefore tended to be large, and because family members lived and worked together and relied chiefly upon each other for social interaction, they developed strong loyalties and a sense of responsibility for one another.

Contemporary urban life, however, does not encourage or allow this kind of sheltered, close-knit family relationship. People who live in cities are likely to be employed by a company and paid a wage. They work with business associates and live with neighbors rather than with their immediate family. Because of housing conditions and the necessity of living on a wage, families in cities usually consist of parents and unmarried children.

These differences between rural and urban life have important repercussions with regard to individual security and stability. The large, extended rural family offered a large and relatively constant group of associates. Family size and the varying strength of blood ties meant that there was always someone to talk to, even about a problem involving two family members. But urban life is highly mobile. There is often a rapid turnover in business associates and neighbors, and there is no certainty that these relative strangers will share the same values, beliefs and interests. All these factors make it difficult for people to develop real trust and interdependence outside the small immediate family. In addition, urban life requires that people meet each other only superficially, in specific roles and in limited relationships rather than as total personalities.

All of these factors taken together mean that people in cities are more isolated than ever before from the emotional support provided by the family and close and familiar peers. As a result, there are no role models to follow—the demands of urban life are constantly changing, and coping behavior that was appropriate and successful several years before may be hopelessly ineffective today.

This creates a favorable environment for the development of crises. As defined by Caplan (1961:18) crisis may occur when the individual faces a problem that he cannot solve. There is a rise in inner tension and signs of anxiety and inability to function in extended periods of emotional upset.

HISTORICAL DEVELOPMENT

The crisis approach to therapeutic intervention has been developed only within the past few decades and is based upon a broad range of theories of human behavior, including those of Freud, Hartmann, Rado, Erickson, Lindemann and Caplan. Its current acceptance as a recognized form of treatment cannot be directly related to any single theory of behavior; all have contributed to some degree.

The intent in presenting an overview of historical development is to create awareness of the broad base of knowledge incorporated into present practice. Although not all theories of human behavior are necessarily dependent on Freudian concepts, and only a selected few are presented here, we chose to begin with the psychoanalytic theories of Freud because these are a major basis for further investigation of normal and abnormal human behavior. The fundamental procedures of brief psychotherapy are derived from hypotheses based upon studies of the reasons for normal as well as abnormal human behavior.

Sigmund Freud was the first to demonstrate and apply the principle of causality as it relates to psychic determinism (Bellak, Small 1965:6). Simply put, this principle states that every act of human behavior has its cause, or source, in the history and experience of the individual. It follows that causality is operative whether or not the individual is aware of the reason for his behavior. Psychic determinism is the theoretical foundation of psychotherapy and psychoanalysis. The technique of free association, dream interpretation and the assignment of meaning to symbols are all based upon the assumption that causal connections operate unconsciously.

A particularly important outcome of Freud's deterministic position was his construction of a development or "genetic" psychology (Ford, Urban 1963:117). Present behavior is understandable in terms of the life history or experience of the individual, and the crucial foundations for all future behavior are laid down in infancy and early childhood. The most significant determinants of present behavior are the "residues" of past experiences (learned responses), particularly those developed during the earliest years to reduce biological tensions.

Freud assumed that a reservoir of energy that exists in the individual initiates all behavior. Events function as guiding influences, but they do not initiate behavior; they only serve to help mold it in certain directions (Ford, Urban 1963:178).

Since the end of the nineteenth century, the concept of determinism, as well as the scientific bases from which Freud formulated his ideas, have undergone many changes.

Although the ego-analytic theorists have tended to subscribe to much in the Freudian position, there are several respects in which they differ. These seem to be extensions of Freudian theory rather than direct contradictions. As a group, they conclude that Freud has neglected the direct study of normal or healthy behavior.

Heinz Hartmann was an early ego analyst who was profoundly versed in Freud's theoretical contributions (Loewenstein 1966:475). He postulated that the psychoanalytic theories of Freud could prove valid for normal as well as pathological behavior. Hartmann began with the study of ego functions and distinguished between two groups: those that develop from conflict, and those that were "conflict free," such as memory, thinking and language, which he labeled "primary autonomous functions of the ego." He considered these important in the adaptation of the individual to his environment. Hartmann emphasized that man's adaptation in early childhood as well as his ability to maintain his adaptation to his environment in later life had to be considered. His conception of the ego as an organ of adaptation required further study of the concept of reality. He also described man searching for an environment as another form of adaptation—the fitting together of the individual and his society. He believed that although the behavior of the individual is strongly influenced by his culture, a part of the personality remains relatively free of this influence.

Sandor Rado developed the concept of adaptational psychodynamics, providing a new approach to the unconscious as well as new goals and techniques of therapy. Rado saw human behavior as based upon the dynamic principle of motivation and adaptation. An organism achieves adaptation through interaction with its culture. Behavior is viewed in terms of its effect upon the welfare of the individual, not just in terms of cause and effect. The organism's patterns of interaction improve through adaptation, with the goal being the increase of possibilities for survival. Freud's classical psychoanalytic technique emphasized the developmental past and the uncovering of unconscious memories, and little if any importance was attached to the reality of the present. Rado's adaptational psychotherapy, however, emphasizes the immediate present without neglecting the influence of the developmental past. Primary concern is with failures in adaptation "today," what caused them and what the patient must do to learn to overcome them. Interpretations always begin and end with the present; preoccupation with the past is discouraged. As quickly as insight is achieved, it is used as a beginning to encourage the patient to enter into his present, real-life situation repeatedly. Through practice the patient automatizes new patterns of healthy behavior. According to Rado, it is this automization factor that is ultimately the curative process, not insight. He does not believe that it takes place passively in the doctor's office but actively in the reality of daily living.

Erik H. Erikson further developed the theories of ego psychology, which complement those of Freud, Hartmann and Rado by focusing on the epigenesis of the ego and on the theory of reality relationships (Rappaport 1952:14). Epigenetic development is characterized by an orderly sequence of development at particular stages, each depending upon the other for successful completion. Erikson perceived eight stages of psychosocial development, spanning the entire life cycle of man and involving specific developmental tasks that must be solved in each phase. The solution that is achieved in each previous phase is applied in subsequent phases. Erikson's theory is important in that it offers an explanation of the individual's social development as a result of his encounters with his social environment. Another significant feature is his elaboration on the normal rather than the pathological development of man's social interactions. He dealt in particular with the problems of adolescence and saw this period in life as a "normative crisis," that is, a normal maturational phase of increased conflicts, with apparent fluctuations in ego strength. Erikson integrated the biological, cultural and self-deterministic points of view in his eight stages of man's development and broadened the scope of traditional psychotherapy with his theoretical formulations concerning identity and identity crises. His theories have provided a basis for the work of others who further developed the concept of maturational crises and began serious consideration of situational crises and man's adaptation to his current environmental dilemma.

Lindemann's initial concern was in developing approaches that might contribute to the maintenance of good mental health and the prevention of emotional disorganization on a community-wide level. He chose to study bereavement reactions in his search for social events or situations that predictably would be followed by emotional disturbances in a considerable portion of the population. In his study of bereavement reactions among the survivors of those killed in the Coconut Grove nightclub fire, he described both brief and abnormally prolonged reactions occurring in different individuals as a result of the loss of a significant person in their lives (Lindemann 1956:310).

In his experiences in working with grief reactions, Lindemann concluded that it might be profitable for investigation and useful for the development of preventive efforts if a conceptual frame of reference were to be constructed around the concept of an emotional crisis, as exemplified by bereavement reactions. Certain inevitable events in the course of the life cycle of every individual can be described as hazardous situations, for example, bereavement, the birth of a child, marriage and so forth. He postulated that in each of these situations emotional strain would be generated, stress would be experienced and a series of adaptive mechanisms would occur that could lead either to mastery of the new situation or to failure with more or less lasting impairment to function. Although such situations create stress for all people who are exposed to them, they become crises for those individuals who by personality, previous experience or other factors are in the present situation especially vulnerable to this stress, and whose emotional resources are taxed beyond their usual adaptive capacities.

Lindemann's theoretical frame of reference led to the development of crisis intervention techniques, and in 1946 he and Caplan established a community-wide program of mental health in the Harvard area, called the Wellesley Project.

According to Caplan (1961:35), the most important aspects of mental health are the state of the ego, the stage of its maturity and the quality of its structure. Assessment of its state is based upon three main areas: (1) the capacity of the person to withstand stress and anxiety and to maintain ego equilibrium, (2) the degree of reality recognized and faced in solving problems and (3) the repertoire of effective coping mechanisms employable by the person in maintaining a balance in his psychobiosocial field.

Caplan believes that all the elements that compose the total emotional milieu of the person must be assessed in an approach to preventive mental health. The material, physical and social demands of reality, as well as the needs, instincts and impulses of the individual, must all be considered as important behavioral determinants.

As a result of his work in Israel and his later experiences in Massachusetts with Lindemann and with the Community Mental Health Program at Harvard University, he evolved the concept of the importance of crisis periods in individual and group development (Caplan 1951:235).

Crisis is defined as occurring when a person faces an obstacle to important life goals that is, for a time, insurmountable through the utilization of customary methods of problem solving. A period of disorganization ensues, a period of upset, during which many abortive attempts at solution are made.

In essence, the individual is viewed as living in a state of emotional equilibrium, with his goal always to return to or to maintain that state. When customary problem-solving techniques cannot be used to meet the daily problems of living, the balance or equilibrium is upset. The individual must either solve the problem or adapt to nonsolution. In either case, a new state of equilibrium will develop, sometimes worse insofar as positive mental health is concerned. There is a rise in inner tension, there are signs of anxiety and there is disorganization of function, resulting in a protracted period of emotional upset. This he refers to as "crisis." The outcome is governed by the kind of interaction that takes place during that period between the individual and the key figures in his emotional milieu.

The Emergence of Crisis Intervention in the Evolution of Community Psychiatry

Community psychiatry is, even now, emerging as a new field. New concepts and new psychobiosocial problems arise continually in rapidly changing cultures, so that it is a broad, fluid field. A difference is now perceived between long-term, psychoanalytic therapy of the individual and short-term, reality-oriented psychotherapy practiced in community psychiatry.

In the middle 1960s the term crisis intervention was not yet included in psychiatric dictionaries. In 1970 the fourth edition of *Hinsie and Campbell's Psychiatric Dictionary* listed crisis intervention as one of several modes of community psychiatry: "In the crisis-intervention model, the focus is on transitional-situational demands for novel adaptational responses. Because minimal intervention at such times tends to achieve maximal and optimal effects, such a model is more readily applicable to population groups than the medical model."

According to Bellak (1964:190), community psychiatry evolved from multiple disciplines and is intrinsically bound to the development of psychoanalytic theory. The social and behavioral sciences that advanced during the first half of this century were predicted on psychodynamic hypotheses. At the same time, concepts of public health and epidemiology were advancing in community health programs.

After World War II the general public's increasing awareness and acceptance of the high incidence of psychiatric problems created changes in attitudes and demands for community action.

The discovery and utilization of psychotropic drugs was an important step forward. This resulted in opportunities for open wards and rehabilitation of the hospitalized patient in his home milieu.

It would be incorrect to assume that all of these factors merged spontaneously, creating a successful, structured cure for psychiatric illness. Rather, this was a slow process of trial and error. Widely different programs, each striving to meet problems involving different cultures, interests, knowledge and skills, communicated with and related to other programs similarly initiated. Disciplines once separated in goals became cognizant of their interdependence in attaining mutually recognized goals. New allied disciplines developed; roles changed and expanded. There was a diffusion of tasks, and lines between disciplines became more flexible.

The origin of day hospitals for the care of psychiatric patients grew out of a shortage of hospital beds (which forced premature discharge of patients to their homes) rather than as a treatment innovation. The first reported day hospital was associated with the First Psychiatric Hospital in Moscow in 1933. As Dzhagarov (1937:147) states: "The need to continue treatment and for special observation in a setting similar to that of a hospital suggested a practical solution in the form of admission to the preventive section of the hospital. In a short time a transformation took place, the day hospital was created, proving to be adequately prepared to meet the new needs." In referring to this day hospital in Moscow, Ross (1964:190) states: "While this day center is little known and probably had little effect on later developments in the Western world, it is accurate to say that this was the first organized Day Hospital for individuals with severe mental illness."

In the late 1930s Bierer began the Marlborough Experiment in England. Patients, as members of a "therapeutic social club," lived outside the hospital and were treated at day hospitals or part-time facilities. According to Bierer, the primary goal of the program was to change the patient's concept of his role from that of a passive object of treatment to one of an active participant-collaborator. At the same time, the psychiatrist and his staff had to reconceptualize the patient as a human being accessible to reason, emphasizing his assets rather than concentrating on his psychopathology and conflicts. The reality of here and now was the focus of attention.

These innovations in attitude gave rise to the concept of "therapeutic community." The patient became a partner and collaborator with the staff and was granted equal rights, opportunities and facilities. The medical staff and their assistants functioned as advisors.

The patient group assumed responsibility for the behavior of its members, as well as planning of activities, planning of their futures and the offering of support to each other. Group and social methods that encouraged the constant interaction of the members were used.

Other complementary projects developed in the Marlborough Program were the Day Hospital, the Night Hospital, the Aftercare Rehabilitation Center, the Self-Governed Community Hostel, Neurotics Nomine and the Weekend Hospital. With this frame of reference it was only natural that the general hospital should add to the various roles in which it served the community—that of becoming a focal point of preventive medicine and public health functions in psychiatry.

In 1958 a "Trouble Shooting Clinic" was initiated by Bellak (1960:174) as part of City Hospital of Elmhurst, New York, a general hospital with 1,000 beds. The clinic was designed to offer first aid to emotional problems and was not limited to urgent crises. It combined two aspects of service: major emergencies, and minor problems involving guidance, legal problems and marital relations, on a walk-in basis around the clock.

After the passage of the California Community Mental Health Act (1958), the California Department of Mental Hygiene established the first state agency in the country (1961) to undertake the training of specialists in community psychiatry.

It was recognized that clinics were needed to accommodate those individuals in the community who were unfamiliar with established forms of psychiatric treatment. A cause for these individuals' exclusion from treatment conceivably could have been due to divergences in social-cultural background, lack of communication and lack of recognition of the need for services by both the population and the existing agencies.

In January 1962 the Benjamin Rush Center for Problems of Living, a division of the Los Angeles Psychiatric Service, was opened as a no-waiting, unrestricted-intake, walk-in crisis intervention center.

In 1967 crisis intervention replaced emergency detention at the San Francisco General Hospital. On each of the psychiatric units interdisciplinary teams were established whose primary goals were to reestablish independent functioning of the clients as soon as possible. A followup study by Decker and Stubblebine (1972:103) concluded that the crisis-intervention program achieved the anticipated reduction in psychiatric inpatient treatment.

In the early 1970s the Bronx Mental Health Center (Centro de Hygiene Mental del Bronx) was created for crisis intervention for low socioeconomic Spanish-speaking people and was staffed by Spanish-speaking psychiatrists.

At about the same time, brief crisis intervention services were being offered by suburban churches in Montreal, Canada, on an experimental basis. The goal of the program was to reach families undergoing a variety of stress through a roving walk-in clinic. The clinics served to facilitate delivery of these services to a latent population at risk, not reached by other means and at a point early in the evolution of a life crisis.

The first hotline was started at Children's Hospital in Los Angeles in 1968. Hotlines and youth crisis centers have been created in recognition of the failure of traditional approaches to make contact with adolescents. Twenty-four-hour crisis telephones, free counseling with a minimum of red tape, walk-in contacts and crash pads, with young people serving as volunteer staff in such services, are becoming increasingly attractive to those youth who are emerging as the locus in a counterculture.

Trends such as these are being repeated around the country as community mental health programs recognize the value of providing service in primary and secondary prevention that is unique to the needs of their particular clients. Increasing recognition is also being given to the need to provide more services for those clients who require continuing support in rehabilitation after resolution of the immediate crisis.

Crisis Intervention as Practiced Today

Crisis intervention has gained recognition as a viable therapy modality to assist individuals through acute traumatic life situations. As large psychiatric facilities are beginning to shorten the length of hospitalization, slowly or rapidly according to individual state laws, the chronic psychiatric patient is returning to his community where continuity of care must be maintained. The questions to be asked and answered are: (1) Does crisis intervention work successfully with chronic psychiatric patients, and (2) if not, what other methods must be employed to keep this patient functioning in his community?

With a chronic psychiatric patient, as with any patient, identification of the precipitating event, the symptoms the patient is exhibiting, his perception of the event, his available situational supports and his usual coping mechanisms are crucial factors in resolving his crisis. Situational supports are those persons in the environment whom the therapist can find to lend support to the individual. A patient may be living with his family or friends; are they concerned enough—and do they care enough—to give him help? The patients situational supports can serve as "assistants" to the therapist and the patient. They are with him daily and are encouraged to have frequent communication with the therapist. Usually situational supports are included in some part of the therapy sessions. This provides them with the knowledge and information they need to help the identified patient.

If the patient is living in a board-and-care facility, one must determine if any of its members are concerned and willing to work with the therapist to help the individual through the stressful period. This involves visits to the facility and the conducting of collateral or group therapy with the patient and other members to get and keep them involved in helping to resolve the crisis.

Occasionally the patient has no situational supports. He may be a social isolate; he may have no family, and may have acquaintances but no real friends with whom he can talk about his problems. Usually an individual such as this has many difficulties in interpersonal relationships, at work, in school and socially. It is then the therapists's role to provide situational support while the patient is in therapy.

Our experiences have verified for us that crisis intervention can be an effective therapy modality with chronic psychiatric patients. If a psychiatric patient with a history of repeated hospitalizations returns to the community and his family, his reentry creates many stresses. While much has been accomplished to remove the stigma of mental illness, people are still wary and hypervigilant when they learn that a "former mental patient" has returned home to his community.

In his absence the family and community have, consciously or unconsciously, eliminated him from their usual life patterns and realities. They then have to readjust to his presence and include him in activities and decision making. If for any reason he does not conform to their expectations, they want him removed so that they can continue their lives without his possible disruptive behavior.

The first area to explore is to determine who is in crisis: the patient or his family. In many cases the family is overreacting because of its anxiety and is seeking some means of getting the "identified" patient back into the hospital. The patient is usually brought to the center by a family member because his original maladaptive symptoms have begun to reemerge. Questioning the patient or his family about medication he received from the hospital and determining if he is taking it as prescribed are essential. If the patient is unable to communicate with the therapist about what has happened or what has changed in his life, the family is questioned as to what might have precipitated his return to his former psychotic behavior.

There is usually a cause-and-effect relationship between a change, or anticipated change, in the routine patterns of life style or family constellation and the beginnings of abnormal overt behavior in the identified patient. Often families forget or neglect to tell a former psychiatric patient when they are contemplating a change because "he wouldn't understand." Such changes could include moving or changing jobs. This is perceived by the patient as exclusion or rejection by the family and creates stress that he is unable to cope with; thus he retreats to his previous psychotic behavior. Such cases are frequent and can be dealt with through the theoretical framework of crisis intervention methodology.

Rubinstein (1972) stated that family-focused crisis intervention usually brings about the resolution of the patient's crisis without resorting to hospitalization. In a later article in 1974, he advocated that family crisis intervention is also a viable alternative to rehospitalization. Here the emphasis is placed on the period immediately after the patient's release from the hospital. He suggested that conjoint family therapy begin in the hospital before the patient's release and then continue in an outpatient clinic after his release. His approach has also served to develop the concept that a family can and should share responsibility for the patient's treatment.

In Decker's 1972 study, two groups of young adults were followed for 2½ years after their first psychiatric hospitalization. The first group was immediately hospitalized and received traditional modes of treatment, and the second group was hospitalized after the institution of a crisis intervention program. The results of the study indicated that crisis intervention reduced long-term hospital dependency without producing alternate forms of psychological or social dependency and also reduced the number of rehospitalizations.

The following brief case studies illustrate how one can work with chronic psychiatric patients in a community mental health center using the crisis model; one was successful and the other was not.

CASE STUDY: JIM

Assessment of the Individual and His Problem

Jim, a man in his late thirties, was brought to a crisis center by his sister because, as she stated, "he was beginning to act crazy again."

Jim had many prior hospitalizations, with a diagnosis of paranoid schizophrenia. The only thing Jim would say was, "I don't want to go back to the hospital." He was told that our role was to help him stay out of the hospital if we possible could. A medical consultation was arranged to determine if he needed to have his medication increased or possibly changed.

Information was then obtained from his sister to determine what had happened (the precipitating event) when his symptoms had started, and specifically, what she meant by his "acting crazy again." His sister stated that he was "talking to the television set . . . muttering things that made no sense . . . staring into space . . . prowling around the apartment at night," and that "this behavior started about 3 days ago." When questioned about anything that was different in their lives before the start of his disruptive behavior, she denied any change. When asked about any changes that were contemplated in the near future, she replied that she was planning to be married in 2 months but that Jim did not know about it because she had not told him yet. When asked why she had not told him, she reluctantly answered that she wanted to wait until all of the arrangements had been made. She was asked if there was any way Jim could have found out about her plans. She remembered that she had discussed them on the telephone with a girl friend the week before.

She was asked what her plans for Jim were after she married. She said that her boyfriend had agreed, rather reluctantly, to let Jim live with them.

Since her boyfriend was reluctant about having Jim live with them, other alternatives were explored. She said that they had cousins living in a nearby suburb but that she did not know if they would want Jim to live with them.

Planning the Intervention

It was suggested that Jim's sister call her cousins, tell them of her plans to get married and her concerns about Jim, and in general find out their feelings about him living with them. The call was placed, and she told them her plans and concerns. Fortunately their response was a positive one. They had recently bought a fairly large apartment building and were having difficulty getting reliable help for the yard work and minor repairs. They felt that Jim would be able to manage this, and they would let him live in a small apartment above the garage.

Intervention

Jim was asked to come back into the office so that his sister could tell him of her plans to marry and the arrangements she had made for him with their cousins. He listened but had difficulty comprehending the information. He just kept saying, "I don't want to go back to the hospital."

He was asked if he had heard his sister talking about her wedding plans. He admitted that he had and that he knew her boyfriend would not want him around—"they would probably put him back in the hospital." As the session ended he still had not internalized the information he had heard. He was asked to continue in therapy for 5 more weeks and to take his medication as prescribed. He agreed to do so.

By the end of the sixth week he had visited his cousins, seen the apartment where he would be living and had discussed his new "job." His disruptive behavior had ceased, and he was again functioning at his precrisis level.

Anticipatory Planning

Since Jim had had many previous hospitalizations and did not want to be rehospitalized, time was spent in discussing how this could be avoided in the future. He was given the name, address and telephone number of a crisis center in his new community and told to visit them when he moved. He was assured that the center could supervise his medication and be available if he needed someone to talk to if he felt he again needed help.

Summation of Paradigm

Jim's sister neglected to tell him about her impending marriage, which he perceived as rejection. Because of his numerous hospitalizations, he feared that his sister would have him rehospitalized "to get rid of him." He was unable to verbalize his fears, retreated from reality and experienced an exacerbation of his psychotic symptoms.

The therapist adhered to the crisis model by focusing the therapy sessions on the patient's immediate problems, not on his chronic psychopathology.

The next case study illustrates how the crisis intervention model was ineffective with a chronic psychiatric patient.

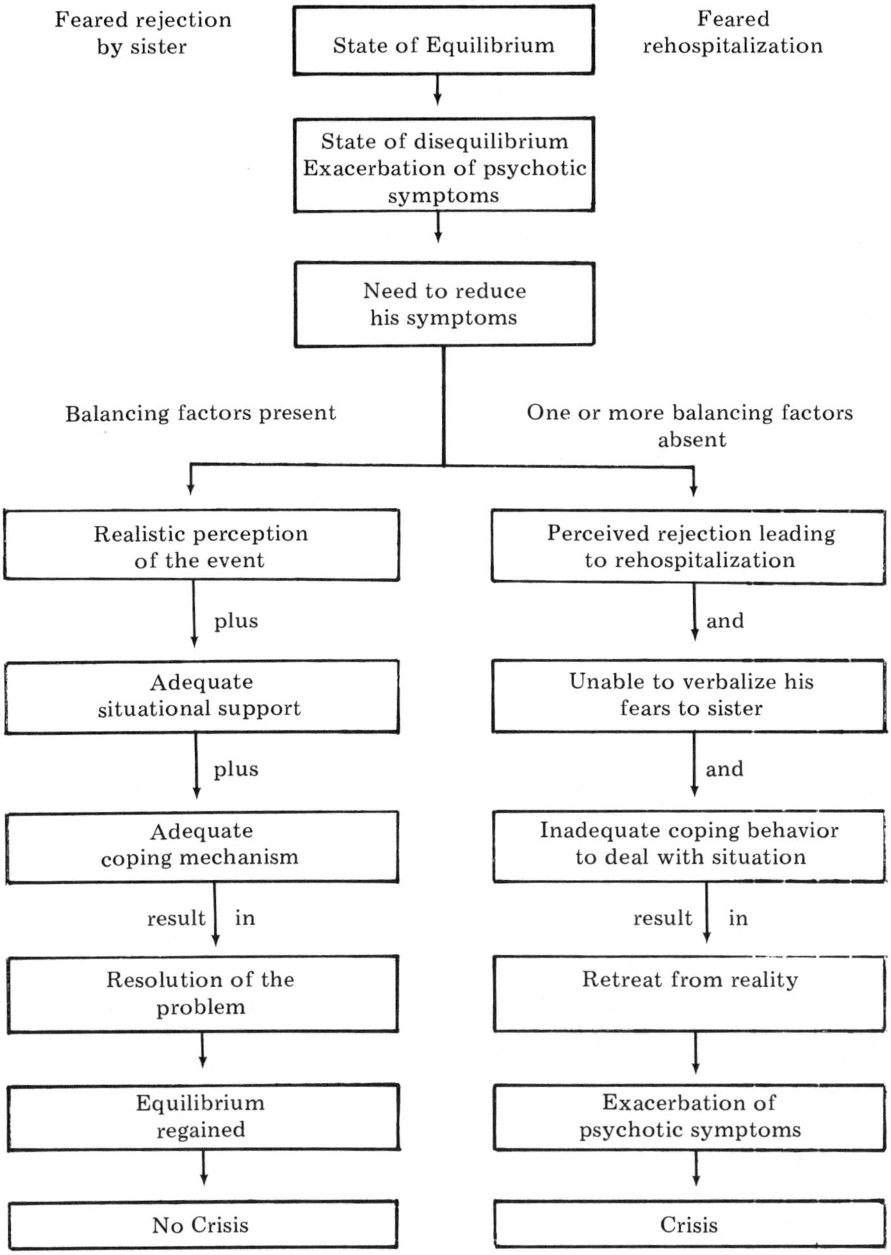

Figure 1. Case study: Jim

CASE STUDY: MATTIE

Assessment of the Individual and the Problem

Mattie was a twenty-four-year-old female who had had three prior hospitalizations with a "nebulous" diagnosis of schizophrenia, affective disorder. Mattie was a fairly attractive, but poorly groomed, young lady who was brought to a crisis center by her mother, Mrs. S. Mattie was quite willing to discuss her prior hospitalizations and the medications she was taking; she then stated with a smile, "I really don't have a problem—*she* does" (pointing to her mother). During this brief interchange, Mrs. S. (who was impeccably groomed) would try to interrupt Mattie by saying very firmly, "Mattie, *I* will explain everything!" Mrs. S. was told by the therapist, just as firmly, that she wanted to hear what Mattie had to say, since she was the "identified patient"—which made Mrs. S. compress her lips even tighter and sit up rigidly.

Mattie stated that she had been out of the "last hospital" for two months and that she had thought that she was doing alright—but that her mother did not; she laughed and said sarcastically, "I am not perfect—but she is." When asked what had precipitated her first hospitalization, she looked down at her clenched hands and then replied softly, "I did a dumb thing—I was smoking 'pot' (marijuana) and *she* caught me. I am dumb—but I am *not* crazy."

When questioned about her subsequent hospitalizations, Mattie said, "You don't understand—I have never lived up to *her* expectations and I never will. The easy way out for her is to stick me in a fancy hospital and forget I am there." (These statements were made with tears, anger and inappropriate laughter.)

The therapist looked at Mrs. S. and said, "How do you feel about what your daughter has said?" While shrugging her shoulders, Mrs. S. stated very calmly, "What can I say. I have been told by the finest psychiatrists that she is a nonconformist, incorrigible and incapable of taking care of herself, and that she should be cared for in a hospital."

Mrs. S. was then questioned about the reason for this visit to the crisis center. Her response was immediate and vehement. In essence, she told what had happened that day. She said that this was her "day" to have the luncheon and "bridge party" for the "ladies." While they were having the luncheon, Mattie came downstairs dressed in a "bathrobe," into the dining room, and flippantly said, "Hi!" She then went into the kitchen to get something to eat. Mrs. S.

said, "She *knows* that she should never come downstairs in a robe—and she could have had the housekeeper bring a tray to her room." She knew I had guests—she just wanted to embarrass me, she always does things like that!"

Again the therapist asked, "How do you feel about what your daughter said and did?" Mrs. S. smiled slightly, paused and stated, "I don't *feel* anything—I just want her out of the house." The therapist asked, "Is that why you brought her to the center, so that we would hospitalize Mattie?" Mrs. S. replied, "Yes, of course!" She was informed that our role was to *prevent* hospitalization, and that while Mattie's appearance in a robe while she was entertaining guests might be considered inappropriate, it was not that bizarre.

Mattie sat quietly during the interchange between her mother and the therapist; only the expression on her face betrayed her feelings of increasing anxiety. The therapist then asked Mattie how she felt about the statement her mother made regarding rehospitalization. She said, "I don't want to go to a hospital, I want to stay home." She looked at her mother and said in a pleading voice, "Don't send me away again—I'll stay upstairs in my room—I'll never come down!" Mrs. S. did not reply, she just looked casually out the window.

The therapist, hoping a compromise could be reached, asked Mrs. S. to let Mattie come to the center one day a week for therapy and to have her medications monitored. Mrs. S. replied, "You don't understand—she will still be there every day and will disrupt the entire household." The therapist explained that the center also had a day treatment center where Mattie could spend every day and become involved in individual therapy, group therapy, occupational therapy, recreational therapy and psychodrama. Mattie enthusiastically said, "Mother, I could do that—and then stay in my room at night, you would never even know I was there!" Mrs. S. sighed and said, "Well, I guess we could try that."

Mattie and Mrs. S. were taken to the day treatment center and introduced to the director, and the situation was explained to him. He thought that Mattie would do well there and asked her to return the following day at 9:00 A.M.

The therapist received a telephone call from the director the next day, who stated that Mattie had not come to the day treatment center as arranged, and that no one had answered the telephone at Mrs. S.'s home. The therapist said she would continue to try to reach Mrs. S. and Mattie.

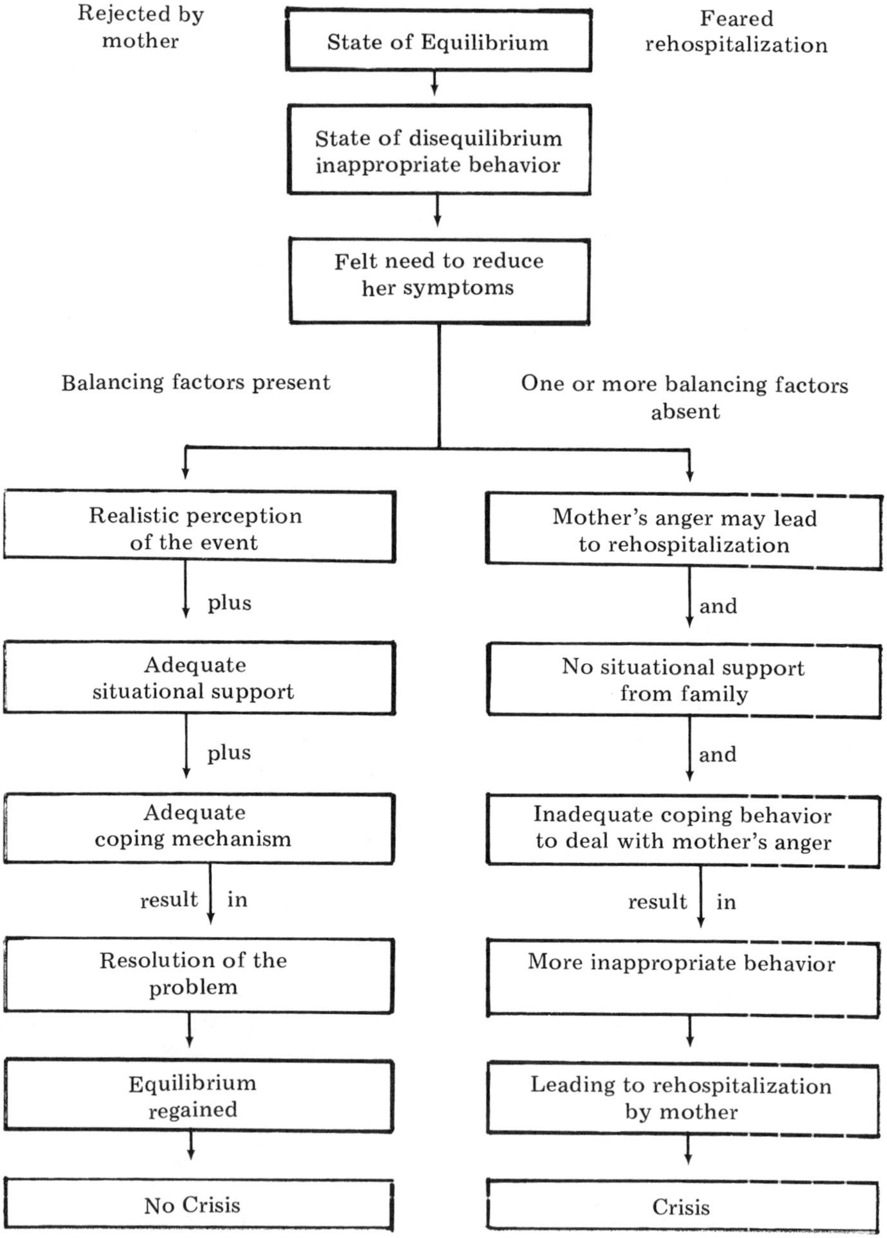

Figure 2. Cast study: Mattie

At approximately 9:30 P.M. that evening, the housekeeper answered the telephone; the therapist gave her name and asked to speak to Mrs. S. Mrs. S. came to the telephone and said "Yes?" The therapist explained why she was calling. Mrs. S. replied, "It won't be necessary for Mattie to attend the center, I managed to contact a marvelous psychiatrist and Mattie is in a lovely hospital."

As stated earlier, if the family is uncaring or unwilling to assist in the care of the identified patient, then no solution to the problem can be reached within the home setting. This was the case with Mattie; her mother just wanted her out of the way, so she had her rehospitalized.

An alternative approach of the therapist could have been the recommendation that Mattie and her mother work toward an alternative home for Mattie—other than a hospital—for instance, a community residence.

Programmatic Issues

Since community mental health centers have a well-known philosophy of prevention, maintenance of the patient in his community and hospitalization only as a last resort, more chronic psychiatric patients and their families are seeking help from crisis centers. Increasing demand from the community calls for an expansion of services, and this is not always easy.

Community mental health centers have established various techniques to accommodate the influx of new patients. Some have established day treatment centers, where the patients may spend the day in a structured environment and return home in the evenings. Others have established small emergency inpatient units that are staffed around the clock to care for patients for a maximum of 48 hours while the patients are being assessed for possible hospitalization, or are medicated and hopefully stabilized. Many maintain a 24-hour, 7-days-a-week medication station where medications can be obtained as needed for the patients. Many also have instituted an emergency hotline to handle calls from patients or their families. Some have ongoing, long-term group therapy sessions for the chronic psychiatric patient.

Smitson (1972) states that an effective mental health delivery system must include three levels of intervention: a crisis intervention unit, a maintenance walk-in service, and a time-limited individual and group therapy program. Such a system, he feels, can maintain individuals outside the hospital and can in many cases minimize the need for rehospitalization.

De Smit (1972) writes that interest in crisis theory and intervention is intense among the public in the Netherlands, indicating dissatisfaction with the present structure of mental health care. Long waiting lists and complicated and prolonged admission procedures of institutionalized care are contrasted with easy accessibility, low threshold and absence of waiting lists in crisis intervention centers. Another aspect is the absence of a psychiatric label. De Smit states that a well-functioning mental health center can greatly reduce hospitalization and rehospitalization of the chronic psychiatric patient.

Wales (1972) stated that placement of trainees in clinical psychology in crisis intervention centers has produced many positive results for the trainees. Some of these are: (1) the development of a sense of responsibility for patients, (2) the development of self-confidence on the part of the trainee, and (3) the more rapid development of professional maturity than is possible at the slow pace that most clinical placements allow.

An interesting and unanswered question is the extent to which a hospital-based program sees patients with more serious pathological conditions than does the typical community-based crisis intervention program. The percentage of individuals with previous hospitalizations seen at the Benjamin Rush Center in Los Angeles was 12.2%. This percentage is almost identical with that reported for a hospital-based program, Kings County of New York, where it was 12.5%. At the same time the Rush Center diagnosed only 16.7% of the patients in the same series as being psychotic, whereas the Kings County program diagnosed 46% of their admissions as psychotic (Jacobson 1974).

What may appear to be a greater pathological condition in a hospital-based program may, at least in part, be due to different diagnostic conventions and a greater staff orientation toward seeing pathological conditions rather than life problems, with a reverse orientation in community-based crisis intervention programs.

Conclusion

In summary, crisis intervention can be used successfully with chronic psychiatric patients; however, the approach may have to be modified and the therapist should be flexible. An extension of emergency services should be maintained on a 24-hour basis to meet the needs of the patient and his family.

In essence, one must determine: Can the patient be helped using crisis intervention techniques only? Does he need longer-term outpatient care? Or does he in fact need to be rehospitalized?

If, as stated earlier, the family is concerned and caring, the task is one of reeducating the family and giving them support. If, on the other hand, the family members are uncaring and simply want the patient out of their lives and back into the hospital, then the task is more difficult. Unless great effort and skill are applied to effect another solution, the family will be likely to try to find a hospital to accept the patient, and the patient and family will never return to the center.

Thus, working in a community mental center with chronic psychiatric patients can be extremely rewarding or extremely frustrating. Crisis intervention is not a "bandaid" or a second-class citizen in the realm of therapy modalities. Rather, it is an important first line of defense in the community mental health center's armamentarium. It confronts the initial event precipitating psychosis in the social context where it has transpired. Its skillful application renders it an effective technique which is the treatment of choice in such situations.

REFERENCES

Aguilera, D. C. and Messick, J. J. *Crisis Intervention: Theory and Methodology.* 3rd edition, St. Louis: the C. V. Mosby Company, 1982.

Bellak, L. and Small, Leonard. *Emergency Psychotherapy and Brief Psychotherapy.* New York: Grune & Stratton, Inc., 1965.

Bellak, L. A general hospital as a focus of community psychiatry. *J.A.M.A.* 174: 2214 (1960).

Caplan, G. A public health approach to child psychiatry, *Mental Health* 35: 235-249 (1951).

Caplan, G. *An Approach to Community Mental Health.* New York: Grune & Stratton, Inc., 1961.

Decker, J. B., and Stubblebine, J. M. Crisis intervention and the prevention of psychiatric disability; a follow-up study. *Am. J. Psychiatry* 129(6): 725 (1972).

Decker, J. B., and Stubblebine, J. M. Crisis intervention and the prevention of psychiatric disability; a follow-up study. *Am. J. Psychiatry* 129: 101-105 (Dec. 1972).

De Smit, N. W. Crisis intervention and crisis centers; their possible relevance for community psychiatry and mental health care. *Psychiatria, Neurologia, Neurochirugia* 75(4): 299 (1972).

Dzhagarov, M. A. Experience in organizing a day hospital for mental patients. *Neuropatol. Psikhiatr.* 6: 147 (1937). (Translated for authors by G. Wachbrit.)

Ford, Donald, and Urban, Hugh. *Systems of Psychotherapy.* New York: John Wiley & Sons, Inc., 1963.
Hinsie, L. E., and Campbell, R. J. *Psychiatric Dictionary*, ed. 4. New York: Oxford University Press, Inc., 1970, p. 606.
Jacobson, G. F. Emergency services in community mental health; problems and promise. *Am. J. Public Health* 64(2): 124 (1974).
Lecker, S., et al. Brief intervention; a pilot walk-in clinic in suburban churches. *Can. Psychiatr. Assoc. J.* 16(2): 141–146 (1971).
Lindemann, Erich: The meaning of crisis in individual and family. *Teachers Coll. Rec.* 57: 310 (1956).
Loewenstein, Rudolph M. Psychology of the ego, in *Psychoanalytic Pioneers*, F. Alexander, S. Eisenstein, and M. Grotjahn. New York: Basic Books, Inc., 1966.
Morales, H. M. Bronx Mental Health Center, N.Y. State Division Bronx Bull. 13(8): 6 (1971).
Ovesy, Lionel, and Jameson, Joan. Adaptational techniques of psychodynamic therapy, in *Changing Concepts of Psychoanalytic Medicine*, S. Rado, and G. Daniels, eds. New York: Grune & Stratton, Inc., 1956.
Pumpian-Mindlin, Eugene. Contributions to the theory and practice of psychoanalysis and psychotherapy, in *Psychoanalytic Pioneers*, Alexander, Eisenstein, and Grotjahn, eds.
Rappaport, David: A historical survey of psychoanalytic ego psychology, in *Psychological Issues*, G. S. Klein, ed. New York: International Universities Press, 1959.
Ross, Matthew. Extramural treatment techniques, in *Handbook of Community Psychiatry and Community Mental Health*, L. Bellak, ed. New York: Grune & Stratton, Inc., 1964.
Rubenstein, D. Rehospitalization versus family crisis intervention. *Am. J. Psychiatry* 129(6): 715 (1972).
Rubenstein, D. Family crisis intervention as an alternative to rehospitalization. *Current Psychiatric Therapies* 14: 191 (1974).
Salzman, Leon. *Developments in Psychoanalysis.* New York: Grune & Stratton, Inc., 1962.
Smitson, W. Focus on service. *Men. Hyg.* 56(4): 22 (1972).
Wales, E. Crisis intervention in clinical training. *Professional Psychology* 3(4): 357 (1972).

ADDITIONAL READINGS

Arnhoff, F. M. Manpower needs, resources, and innovation, in *Progress in Community Mental Health*, vol. 2, H. H. Barten, and L. Bellak, ed. New York: Grune & Stratton, Inc., 1972, pp. 35-61.
Bard, M. The role of law enforcement in the helping system. *Community Ment. Health J.* 7(2): 151 (1971).
Barten, H. H. and Bellak, L., ed. *Progress in Community Mental Health*, vol. 2, New York: Grune & Stratton, Inc., 1972.
Barthal, H. S. Resistances to community psychiatry. *Psychiatr. Q.* 45(3): 333 (1971).

Board, M. The role of law enforcement in the helping systems. *Community Ment. Health J.* 7(2): 151 (1971).

Brandon, S. Crisis theory and possibilities of therapeutic intervention. *Br. J. Psychiatry* 117: 541 (Dec. 1970).

Bruder, E. E. The clergyman's contribution to community mental health. *Hosp. Commun. Psychiatry* 22: 207 (July 1971).

Cassell, W. A., and others. Comparing costs of hospital and community care. *Hosp. Commun. Psychiatry* 23: 197 (July 1972).

Chandler, H. M. Family crisis intervention, point and counterpoint in the psychosocial revolution. *J. Natl. Med. Assoc.* 64: 211 (May 1972).

Cobb, C. W. Community mental health services and the lower socioeconomic classes; a summary of research literature on outpatient treatment (1963–1969). *Am. J. Orthopsychiatry* 42: 404 (April 1972).

Daniels, R. S. Community psychiatry; a new profession, a developing subspecialty, or effective clinical psychiatry? *Community Ment. Health J.* 2: 47 (1966).

Decker, J. B., and Stubblebine, J. M. Crisis intervention and the prevention of disability; a followup study. *Am . J. Psychiatry* 129: 725 (Dec. 1972).

De Smit, N. W. The crisis center in community psychiatry; an Amsterdam experiment, in *Current Psychiatric Therapies*, vol. 2, J. H. Masserman, ed. New York: Grune & Stratton, Inc., 1971.

De Smit, N. W. Crisis intervention and crisis centers; their possible relevance for community psychiatry and mental health care. *Psychiatr. Neurol. Neurochir* 75: 299 (1973).

Donovan, James M., et al. Psychiatric crisis, a comparison of schizophrenic and non-schizophrenic patients. *J. Nervous and Mental Disease* 161: 172 (1975).

Edgerton, J. W. Evaluation in community mental health, in *Issues in Community Psychology and Preventive Mental Health*, G. Rosenblum, ed. Task Force on Community Mental Health, Division 27 of the American Psychological Association, New York: Behavioral Publications, Inc., 1971.

Ewalt, J. R., and Farnsworth, D. L. Psychiatry and religion, in *Textbook of Psychiatry*, J. R. Ewalt, and D. L. Farnsworth, eds. New York: ????????

Feirstein, A., Weisman, G., and Thomas, C. A crisis intervention model for inpatient hospitalization, in *Current Psychiatric Therapies*, vol. 11, J. H. Masserman, ed. New York: Grune & Stratton, Inc., 1971.

Flomenhaft, K., et al. After the crisis. *Ment. Hyg.* 55: 473 (Oct. 1971).

Huessy, H. R. Rural models, in *Progress in Community Mental Health*, vol. 2, H. H. Barten, and L. Bellak, eds. New York: Grune & Stratton, Inc., 1972.

Kretz, H. Structure and function of a psychiatric polyclinic; possibilities, limitations, and practical perspectives of work at the Polyclinic of the Heidelberg University Psychiatric Clinic, Nervenartz. 45(4): 215 (1974).

Mackenzie, M., et al. Family crisis unit. *Lancet* 1: 642 (March 1972).

McClennan, M. S. Crisis groups in special care areas. *Nurs. Clin. North Am.* 7: 363 (June 1972).

Morehead, M. A. Evaluating quality of care of the neighborhood health center program of O.E.O. *Med. Care* 8: 118 (1970).

Naylor, H. New trends in volunteer services for the mentally handicapped. *Hosp. Commun. Psychiatry* 22: 109 (April 1971).

Polak, P. Techniques of social system intervention. *Curr. Psychiatr. Ther.* 12: 185 (1972).

Polak, P., et al. Prevention in mental health; a controlled study. *Am. J. Psychiatry* 132(2): 146 (1975).

Raphael, B. Crisis intervention; theoretical and methodological considerations. *Aust. N.Z.J. Psychiatry* 5: 183 (1971).

Rosenbaum, C. P., and Beebe, J. E. *Psychiatric Treatment; Crisis/Clinic/Consultation.* New York: McGraw-Hill Book Co., 1975.

Schneider, B. Preparing general practitioners for community mental health work. *Hosp. Commun. Psychiatry* 22: 346 (Nov. 1971).

Schwartz, D. A. Community mental health in 1972; an assessment, in *Progress in Community Mental Health,* vol. 2, H. H. Barten, and L. Bellak, eds. New York: Grune & Stratton, Inc., 1972.

Schwartz, J. L. First national survey of free medical clinics, 1967-1969. *HSMHA Health Report* 86: 775 (Sept. 1971).

Schwartz, S. L. A review of crisis intervention programs. *Psychiatr. Q.* 45: 498 (1971).

Weinstein, R. M., and Brill, N. Q. Social class and patients' perceptions of mental illness. *Psychiatr. Q.* 45(1): 35 (1971).

Wellisch, D. K., and Gay, G. R. The walking wounded; emergency psychiatric intervention in a heroin addict population. *Drug Forum* 1: 137 (Jan. 1972).

Wilson, S. E., Courtney, C. G., Ota, K. Y., and Radauskas, B. Evaluating mental health associates. *Hosp. Commun. Psychiatry* 22: 371 (Dec. 1971).

Wolberg, L. R. Psychiatric technics in crisis therapy. *N.Y. State J. Med.* 72: 1266 (1972).

Zelbach, J. Z. Crisis in chronic problem families; psychiatric care of the underprivileged. *Int. Psychiatry Clin.* 8(2): 101 (1971).

CHAPTER 8

THE VOCATIONAL PREPARATION OF THE CHRONIC PSYCHIATRIC PATIENT IN THE COMMUNITY

NORMAN C. HURSH
WILLIAM A. ANTHONY

The psychiatrically disabled person's ability to assume the worker role in the community is viewed as a legitimate treatment goal for many persons with a psychiatric disability. Unfortunately, a review of outcome studies indicates that traditional methods of psychiatric treatment are not successful in providing the psychiatrically disabled client with the skills necessary to function on the job or in the community. This chapter discusses those assessment techniques and programming strategies which appear potentially effective in developing the client's vocational behaviors and skills necessary to function more successfully in various work environments. The chapter initially provides an overview of a comprehensive skills-based approach to psychiatric rehabilitation so that the vocational rehabilitation process can be understood within the context of the total psychiatric rehabilitation process. The chapter then focuses on the vocational assessment process and the various diagnostic assessment tools used in vocational rehabilitation. The following section discusses the most common vocational intervention programs. A separate section reviews some sample programs which illustrate how various assessment tools and training strategies have been utilized in the vocational preparation of the psychiatrically disabled client. The final section suggests some future directions for the field.

INTRODUCTION

Vocational choice and vocational training are becoming increasingly difficult tasks for any individual who is entering the world of work. Rapid changes in technology both displace persons from old jobs and require retraining for new jobs. While these tasks are difficult for most, the problems and barriers are greatly compounded for the chronic psychiatrically disabled client. Successful and extended employment for chronic psychiatric clients requires that they be prepared for a level of vocational functioning that reflects their work capacity, and this requires knowledgeable and skilled rehabilitation practitioners.

Mental health services have involved the psychiatrically disabled client in work as a "treatment" activity for over a century. Initially, work was viewed as "moral therapy," originating from the philosophy that idleness was consistent with evil and that physical and mental work were next to godliness (Bockoven 1963). With the advent of large state hospitals and institutions, patients were involved in work as an activity that served to maintain the large hospital system. The emphasis at that time was not on therapy but on activity useful to the hospital, such as "work" in the kitchen, laundry, farms and buildings and grounds. With the advent of pharmacological drugs after World War II, and subsequent symptom reduction for many patients, efforts were made to rehabilitate the psychiatrically disabled and return them to more effective levels of functioning. Today, with a strong emphasis on deinstitutionalization and community support programs, many chronic psychiatrically disabled clients are being returned to the community, albeit with varying degrees of success (Bachrach 1976). As a result of this community orientation, vocational training and involvement in work activities in the community are receiving increased emphasis as legitimate measures of rehabilitation outcome.

The rationale for this emphasis on work activities in the community is that work is a normalizing activity. Work activities take up approximately one third of a person's daily life, and approximately two thirds of an individual's life span. Those not involved in work are often stigmatized by a society which associates inability to work or to be self-supporting with deviance (Levine and Levine 1970). On the other hand, successful performance in the work environment is associated by society with value, worth, legitimacy and belonging.

While work is a normalizing activity, reinforced by societal expectations, it also provides therapeutic benefits. Olshansky (1969) observes that work provides structure and involvement in meaningful activity and a means of "shedding one's patienthood." He believes that by functioning in the adult worker role and becoming more self-supporting, the psychiatrically disabled person is able to improve his or her self-concept. Thus, work is viewed as a normalizing activity valued by society as well as a therapeutic activity for psychiatrically disabled clients. Perhaps more importantly, work performance is one easily discernible and direct reflection of the success or failure of the rehabilitation process. It is useful, then, to examine vocational outcome data as an index of overall rehabilitation outcome.

VOCATIONAL OUTCOME DATA

Unfortunately, traditional methods of treatment do not appear to have much impact on the community work activities of the psychiatrically disabled. In the first comprehensive review of psychiatric rehabilitation, Anthony et al. (1972) reported data indicating that only 20 to 30% of expatients were employed full-time—regardless of the follow-up period studied. Although there have been a paucity of studies reporting employment outcome measures, later surveys (Anthony et al. 1978) show that past results may in fact be a slight overestimation. A more accurate range may be only 10 to 30% of discharged patients employed at follow-up. Furthermore, specific inpatient work therapy programs do not improve posthospital employment outcome. Also, the type and amount of worklike activities in which a patient participates in the hospital do not correlate with the discharged patient's work activities in the community (Anthony 1979).

What, then, are the vocational assessment and treatment strategies with the most potential for improving these rather dismal community work outcome figures? In order to proceed toward an answer to this question, the vocational rehabilitation process must be understood within the context of the complete rehabilitation approach. The vocational component of treatment cannot occur in isolation. The failure of many psychiatric clients to obtain or retain a job is not just due to a deficit in their work-related skills. The clients' vocational failures may also occur because of their inability to function in their living environment, and/or their inability to cope in a learning or training setting. Thus, vocational interventions must be seen as part of a coordinated rehabilitation intervention.

In order to more accurately present the vocational assessment and treatment process, this chapter will first review the *rehabilitation* approach to treatment. Using this rehabilitation approach to treatment as the comprehensive intervention model, the chapter then will focus on various vocational assessment tools used in psychiatric rehabilitation. Next, the chapter will describe the most common vocational intervention programs. A separate section will demonstrate how various assessment tools and training strategies are utilized in specific community programs. The final section discusses some of the future directions for the field.

THE REHABILITATION APPROACH TO TREATMENT

Philosophically, the rehabilitation approach to treatment is analogous to the treatment approach used in physical medicine. In physical medicine the treatment focus is either on developing the physically disabled person's skill level or on modifying the environment in order to maximize the patient's present skill. For example, the techniques of physical therapy do not attempt to probe for or remove the cause of hemiplegia; rather, the physical therapist focuses on rebuilding the patient's damaged skills, teaching the patient new skills, or adapting the environment so as to better accommodate the patient's postmorbid skill level (Anthony 1977).

Similar to the approach used in physical rehabilitation, the rehabilitation approach with the psychiatrically disturbed client also focuses on diagnosing and building client skills. The research literature consistently indicates that it is the psychiatrically disabled client's skills, not symptoms, which relate to rehabilitation outcome (research summarized in Anthony 1979; Anthony, Cohen and Vitalo 1978). In addition, rehabilitation research has shown repeatedly that psychiatric clients can learn a variety of physical, emotional and intellectual skills regardless of their present symptomatology. Furthermore, these skills, when properly integrated into a comprehensive rehabilitation program that provides reinforcement and support for the use of these skills in the community, can have a significant impact on the client's rehabilitation outcome (Anthony and Margules 1974). In essence, the means of achieving the goal of rehabilitation is *client skill development and community support.*

Because of the fact that rehabilitation outcome is a function of the client's skills and his/her community supports, the rehabilitation diagnosis is strikingly different from the typical psychiatric diagnosis. In contrast to the latter type of diagnosis, the rehabilitation diagnosis neither attempts to label the psychiatrically disabled client nor to categorize the client's symptomatology. Rather, the rehabilitation diagnostic process yields information about the disabled client's level of skills and the skill demands of the community in which he or she wants or needs to function. Such information enables the rehabilitation practitioner to work with the client to develop a treatment plan designed to increase the client's strengths and assets, and/or to identify an environment more suitable to the client's functioning.

The vocational intervention approaches described in this chapter are only a part of a more comprehensive rehabilitation skill assessment and development process. For purposes of clarification, the vocational preparation of the psychiatrically disabled person is discussed separately in this chapter; in practice, however, vocational intervention specialists must be perceived as an integral part of the rehabilitation team. The vocational rehabilitation professional acts on the assumption that the psychiatrically disabled client's vocational functioning is clearly impacted by the client's successes and failures in the living and learning environments, and vice versa. The following descriptions of vocational assessment and vocational programming are based on this fundamental assumption of rehabilitation practice (Anthony, Pierce and Cohen 1980a).

VOCATIONAL ASSESSMENT STRATEGIES

The overall goal of the diagnostic assessment of vocational skills and behaviors is the presentation of an observable and measurable description of the client's strengths and deficits relevant to the working environment in which the client is or will be functioning. In assessing the psychiatrically disabled client's skills and deficits, the rehabilitation practitioner must go through three fundamental stages of the diagnostic assessment process. The stages are developmental in nature in that the initial stages must be completed before later stages can begin. Also, later stages use information from the earlier stages to both reinforce and add to the client's developing knowledge of self.

In the initial stage of vocational diagnostic assessment, the rehabilitation practitioner involves the psychiatrically disabled client in an *exploration* of his or her own unique strengths and deficits, and the feelings which the client experiences in relation to work and/or specific work environments. In the second phase the practitioner assists the client to focus on the client's own role in the process in order to *understand* his or her own unique strengths and deficits, and most importantly, how these strengths and deficits help or hinder the client's ability to function in specific work environments. The information concerning the client's vocational strengths and deficits

Exploration of client's unique problem and goal

1. Inform and encourage the client to become involved.
2. Attend to the client's presence.
3. Observe the client's nonverbal behavior and appearance.
4. Listen to the client's verbal expression.
5. Respond to the client's verbal, nonverbal, and behavioral expressions.
6. Involve the client in realistic concrete experiences.
7. Specify the client's situational problem and rehabilitation goals.

Understanding client's personal strengths and deficits

1. Involve the client in realistic concrete experiences (work samples, situational assessment).
2. Personalize the meaning of the client's exploration.
3. Categorize the client's strengths and deficits by skill areas.
4. Categorize the client's strengths and deficits by environmental areas.

Assessing client's personal strengths and deficits

1. Involve the client in realistic concrete experiences (work samples, situational assessments, job sites.
2. Operationalize each important strength and deficit.
3. Quantify present levels of function.
4. Quantify needed levels of function.

Figure 1. Stages and Skills of Diagnostic Planning Adapted from Anthony, W. A., Pierce, R. M., and Cohen, M. R. *The Skills of Diagnostic Planning. Psychiatric Rehabilitation Practice Series: Book 1.* Baltimore, MD: University Park Press, 1980.

gathered during the exploration phase must now be understood in relation to how they may or may not differ from the level of skill needed by the client to function on his or her present or potential job. In the third phase of vocational diagnostic planning, the rehabilitation practitioner *assesses* the client's previously identified strengths and deficits in observable, measurable terms. The diagnostic process is depicted in Figure 1.

To be compatible with the overall rehabilitation assessment approach, each vocational strength and deficit behavior is classified as either a physical, emotional or intellectual skill. This classification facilitates both client and treatment personnels' understanding of the diagnostic data and also provides a framework that encourages a comprehensive approach to assessment. A skill or behavior is classified as physical if the primary part of the skill performance involves some physical behavior. An intellectual skill is one in which the primary part of the behavior involves thinking or mental activity. A skill is characterized as emotional if the primary behavior involves relating or interacting with other people. For example, a psychiatric rehabilitation client can exhibit his or her physical skill of attendance by arriving at work daily, and demonstrate the physical skill of punctuality by arriving at work on time daily. Similarly, he or she can display his or her emotional skill in controlling his or her temper with coworkers or in accepting criticism from a supervisor. An example of an intellectual work skill or behavior might be remembering directions from day to day or the ability to make career plans and choices. Further examples of physical, emotional and intellectual skills related to work can be found in Table 1. This physical-intellectual-emotional categorization of work behaviors helps ensure that the diagnostician will examine a comprehensive range of client vocational behaviors.

One of the unique aspects of vocational assessment is its emphasis on an experiential component to determine present and needed level of skill performance (Nadolsky 1976a). Vocational diagnostic emphasis is on evaluation of the client through involvement in practical, realistic and concrete situations and tasks. The situations and tasks can be varied to allow the client to immediately and directly experience each different work situation and to react or adjust to its effects. Specific behaviors such as work skills, social interactions, self-evaluation, decision-making and planning related to work can be observed, measured and operationalized. Furthermore, with a strong emphasis on client involvement during the evaluation experience, the client has the opportunity for direct feedback, self-evaluation

Table 1 Sample Work Environment Behaviors

Physical	Emotional	Intellectual
Dress self for work	Telephone prospective employers	Identify three people to be used as references
Begin work on time daily	Request an appointment for a job interview	List career alternatives
Use public transportation	Maintain eye contact with interviewer	Fill out job application
Punch time clock at beginning and end of day	Introduce self to coworkers	Develop a resume
Maintain clean work area	Converse with coworkers	Compare similarities and differences of two jobs
Lift heavy objects	Listen to directions	Follow work schedule
Clean and store tools and equipment	Accept criticism from supervisors	Identify visual/auditory signals (fire alarm, work whistle)
Stand for long periods of time	Greet coworkers daily with "hello" or appropriate greeting	Read a diagram
Sort transistors by size and color	Ask for help when needed	Evaluate quality of work
		Follow safety rules

and exploration of new behaviors in a supportive, reinforcing environment.

Vocational assessment is a relatively new field among assessment approaches. Nevertheless, it has rapidly developed valuable measures to assess skills and abilities related to the client's vocational functioning. The skilled rehabilitation practitioner involved in assessment has many tools and techniques to assess client strengths, deficits and potentials (Task Force No. 2, 1975). These may be classified within the following categories:

1. Interviewing techniques
2. Work sample techniques
3. Situational assessment techniques
4. On-the-job evaluation techniques
5. Psychometric testing techniques

Interviewing Techniques

The interviewing skills of the vocational evaluator have received minimal and insufficient attention in comparison to the evaluator's other assessment techniques (Nadolsky 1976b). Very little attention has been directed toward using the diagnostician's interviewing or counseling skills to facilitate the goal of the assessment process. While much has been written about the evaluation experience resulting in self-exploration, self-understanding, decision-making, client involvement and so forth, a dearth of information exists as to how to achieve this type of client involvement in the evaluation process. Is it a natural or given result of the process? How can interviewing or diagnostic counseling facilitate the process and provide a framework within which the assessment experiences are explored?

Nadolsky (1976b) points out that in many ways the evaluator has a unique opportunity to utilize the interpersonal relationships between evaluator and client to assist the client in exploring and understanding his or her experience. By virtue of the evaluator's direct observations of the client's behavior, the evaluator can immediately explore with the client his or her skill performance and the client's reactions to the practical, realistic work tasks and demands. Rather than responding to client perceptions of what may have occurred within the past week or month, the vocational diagnostician is able to explore immediate performance, reactions and perceptions with minimal distortion of the experience.

The interviewing or interpersonal skills necessary to help the client explore, understand and assess his strengths and deficits have been researched and developed by Carkhuff (1969, 1971, 1972; Carkhuff and Berenson 1977). Although these interpersonal skills have been most often thought of as fundamental therapy skills, they are in essence the same skills needed by the diagnostician to help the psychiatrically disabled client explore, understand, and assess his skills and abilities (Anthony 1979). By using the interpersonal skills of attending, observing, listening and responding, the rehabilitation practitioner can initially begin to acquire an accurate assessment of "where the client is" in relation to his or her goal. Through using interpretive interpersonal skills, the practitioner can add to the client's level of understanding and identify the skills needed by the client to achieve rehabilitation objectives and goals (Carkhuff 1969).

The interpersonal skills of the evaluator can facilitate and promote client exploration, understanding and assessment through the phases of diagnostic assessment. Although a traditional objective of the assessment process is generally stated as the promoting and developing of client self-exploration and self-understanding, many psychiatrically disabled clients do not have the skills necessary to explore, clarify or give meaning to the evaluation experience. If they do, they are then often unable, to organize the information, assign values or priorities, or make decisions based on their exploration and understanding. The interpersonal relationship also serves a process evaluation function. The evaluator's interviewing skills assist him/her in deciding whether the client understands the goals, whether the evaluation process is assessing relevant abilities and adding to the client's level of knowledge, and/or whether the client understands how specific deficits hinder job performance.

In summary, by developing an interpersonal relationship which encourages client self-exploration, an assessment plan can be created to evaluate client interest, values and abilities. By assisting the client in attempting to understand the evaluation process, the client is encouraged to invest in the process and has increased motivation to perform the experiential activities. Through active client involvement and understanding of the assessment experience, the client is thus more readily able to accept the results as meaningful.

Work Sample Techniques

Although work sample batteries are relatively new evaluation tools, the development and use of work samples is increasing. Work sample techniques have become more complex, are highly sophisticated and include increasingly wider and wider ranges of occupational areas (Pruitt 1977). The usefulness of work samples for the psychiatric rehabilitation client relates to their close simulation of actual industrial job tasks. The client is involved in well-defined activities which include tasks, materials, equipment and tools similar to the work and work activity in many competitive work sites. Depending on the type and range of skill and ability being measured, work samples may be either simulations of a range of actual job operations or actual jobs replicated in the assessment unit. Another type of work sample, the trait sample, measures a specific ability or trait such as finger dexterity, upper extremity range of motion or discrimination ability. Other work samples, called cluster trait samples, measure a group of these specific traits to focus on a range of abilities required to perform a particular job. As a sample of work behavior, the work sample battery should approximate the range of work activities for the particular job as closely as possible.

Through flexible use of commercial work samples, the rehabilitation practitioner and client are able to make specific observations related to a wide range of different vocational behaviors. Obviously, most work samples are utilized to evaluate performance and skill in specific work tasks. However, work samples can also provide opportunity for vocational exploration. Commercial work sample batteries providing opportunity for vocational exploration activity are the MicroTOWER, Singer, and TOWER systems. Other work samples, such as the HESTER and VALPAR, may focus more specifically on the client's range of motion and physical ability to perform jobs. Behavioral observations during work performance are specified more clearly by the VALPAR and Singer systems. Exploration and understanding of work interest, values and needs are built into the group discussion procedures of the MicroTOWER system. The differential use of one work sample battery over another, then, may depend on the skills and behaviors the evaluator and the client want to measure.

By closely simulating work activities and behavior requirements, work samples yield particularly valuable diagnostic information about the psychiatrically disabled. As stated earlier, the diagnostic objective is a comprehensive, objective and measurable statement of the current and needed level of skill strengths and deficits. Involving the client in work sample assessment not only results in objective measures of work skill and ability, but can also provide information about work behaviors, work attitudes, needs, interests, and to a limited extent, psychosocial behaviors.

Although work sample evaluation takes place within a rehabilitation facility rather than an actual job site, a valid diagnostic picture of client's work skills and abilities can be acquired due to the strong reality orientation, simulation of work performance demands, and the exposure and experience with a range of jobs. It is the accurate and efficient measure of skills and abilities through direct and systematic observations of specific work behaviors that makes work samples a functional and valid tool in developing a diagnostic picture of the psychiatrically disabled client.

Situational Assessment Techniques

The situational approach to assessment originated around the middle of the 1950s (Neff 1966) and now is reportedly the most widely used approach in work evaluation (Dunn 1973). Of rehabilitation agencies surveyed, Sankovsky (1969) reported that 78% of the respondents utilized situational assessment and 24% ranked it as the primary evaluation technique. In reviewing the literature, however, it is evident that situational assessment lacks a unified theory as well as specific techniques and procedures (Dunn 1973). Several characteristics of the approach appear to be evident. Most situational assessment approaches place the clients in real (yet sheltered) work situations or job stations under the supervision of trained evaluators or work supervisors. The client typically works with other client-employees on contract jobs for real wages. The situational assessment site could be developed in workshop settings, institutional job sites or work evaluation units and is characteristically part of a rehabilitation facility.

It is generally agreed that while the emphasis in work sample evaluation is on concrete work skills or the ability to do a specific task, the focus of situational assessment is on the more comprehensive aspects of general work behavior, what Neff (1966, 1968) calls the "work personality." More consideration is given to the interpersonal and social behaviors than the technological skills necessary for the performance of a specific job.

It is the interpersonal, social and emotional behaviors, along with work adjustment skills, which are systematically evaluated in situational assessment. Evaluators observe how the client responds and relates to supervisors, relates on and off the job with coworkers, follows the "customs" or expected work patterns and rules for the specific work environments, and responds to the demands of an eight-hour day. The evaluator observes such characteristics as the client's response to distractions, noise, heat, humidity and other environmental factors. In addition, the evaluator has the opportunity to systematically alter elements of the work situation (tasks, location, amount of coworkers, supervisors, production demands) to provide behavioral observations of the client's strengths and deficits specific to various work settings.

On-the-Job Evaluation Techniques

The use of job sites in industries is one of the more recent approaches in work evaluation and holds much promise in assessment of the chronic psychiatric client. According to the Task Force of the Vocational Evaluation Project Final Report (1975), job site evaluation:

> usually means that evaluation takes place in an actual job setting outside of the rehabilitation facility. The evaluation is performed by the employer in industry or business. However, it can also mean the use of actual jobs, within the rehabilitation facility, which should conform to the Wage and Hour Regulations of the Department of Labor. The client is given the opportunity to fulfill the specific requirements of a particular job. He receives direction from a supervisor as if he were an employee of that industry. (pg. 53)

In essence, on-the-job evaluation techniques have the psychiatric rehabilitation client perform the job duties of a real job within competitive industry (Botterbusch 1978). The rehabilitation practitioner uses the job site evaluation approach to assess a wide range of skills and behaviors necessary for successful job acquisition and job performance. The evaluation process can include the client calling the employer for an interview, completing a job application and discussing qualifications with the "prospective employer." In this way, job seeking skills can be evaluated. Botterbusch (1978) identifies other significant behaviors to be assessed, including work performance skills, speed of learning, preferred learning mode and work adjustment skills. In a more realistic setting than provided by situational assessment, the rehabilitation practitioner can assess client behaviors in responding to environmental demands by, for instance, measuring work tolerance in response to the physical demands of the job and setting. As the job site is a competitive employment site in industry, the client is able to more realistically explore his or her interests and evaluate the job with respect to whether he or she can perform up to the standards required for successful employment.

The realistic nature of the job site is the main assessment advantage of on-the-job evaluation techniques. Although the behaviors and skills assessed are basically similar to those assessed by the situational approach, the situational approach usually takes place in a rehabilitation facility and can only approximate the competitive work employment environment. The level and consistency of work performance in a rehabilitation milieu does not necessarily generalize to the competitive employment site (Anthony 1979).

Job site evaluation holds much promise for being an effective and indispensable tool in the evaluation process. Industrial job sites promote valid concrete assessment in the most realistic setting available—the competitive work world.

Psychometric Testing Techniques

Objective paper and pencil tests and projective psychometric tests have been used extensively in traditional psychiatric diagnostic practices. Anthony (1979) has recently reviewed the literature relating the use of psychometric testing to subsequent outcome measures of recidivism and posthospital employment. His conclusions suggest that neither personality nor intelligence tests are very successful in predicting rehabilitation outcome. As the traditional personality tests and IQ measures have typically been developed and used for diagnostic labeling purposes, these findings are not unexpected. However, recent research in the area of measuring ego strength and self-concept has reported significant correlations with posthospital employment.

In developing a diagnostic picture of the psychiatrically disabled client which attempts to identify client strengths and deficits, useful psychometric tests are those that yield information about client skill behavior. As it appears that the measurement of skill and behavior is the critical indicator of future employability, psychometric tests that provide these measurements can be functional tools in skills-based diagnostic assessment.

IMPLEMENTING VOCATIONAL ASSESSMENT

To maximize client gains during rehabilitation, vocational evaluation and programming activities must be performed as integrated cooperative efforts. Diagnostic assessment should generate programming activity to increase or develop the skill levels objectively measured during assessment. For this to occur effectively and efficiently, evaluators must be aware of the resources, capabilities and skills of practitioners involved in programming, and conversely, training staff should be aware of the resources, capabilities and skills of the diagnostician.

Unfortunately, there are two factors that naturally function to restrict vocational evaluation services from being integrated with, and having impact on, the milieu of the rehabilitation facility, or more specifically, the training programs within the facility. First, the vocational evaluator is often seen as a professional specialist having a unique body of knowledge quite different from other rehabilitation practitioners (Sink and Porter 1978). Second, vocational assessment usually occurs in a separate and distinct unit within the agency, apart from the mainstream of the facility. Often the client is referred to another agency for evaluation services. The resulting professional and/or geographic distance breeds lack of communication. These practices often result in (1) a failure to receive feedback on the source of the vocational diagnosis, (2) inability to evaluate the impact of the diagnosis on the client's rehabilitation training program and (3) an inability to provide continuous client evaluation and update information.

While it is not the intention of evaluators to dissociate themselves from the rest of the rehabilitation process, strong measures must be taken to ensure close ties with all phases of the service delivery system. The integration of assessment into the overall rehabilitation process can be promoted in several ways: (1) all rehabilitation practitioners can develop minimal skills in vocational assessment; (2) rehabilitation evaluators can make sure that the assessment outcome relates directly to programming practices; (3) rehabilitation evaluators can actively pursue discussion and sharing of efforts with training staff; and finally, (4) they can build program evaluation methods into the assessment process itself.

Although program evaluation skills should be part of the skill repertoire of rehabilitation practitioners, it is unfortunate that vocational evaluation practices or models have not universally included program evaluation methods as a necessary, vital and integral part of the process. As with other techniques of vocational assessment, program evaluation methods should be considered as an ongoing, systematic function of the evaluation unit rather than a measure to be used occasionally. The effective and efficient delivery of assessment services is the primary goal and should be continuously evaluated by the assessment personnel. Both the process and outcome of assessment services are directly related to the benefits eventually received by the psychiatrically disabled client. For example, how well does the client understand his or her skills and abilities? Are the skills and abilities measured meaningful to the client? Will he or she, therefore, be more motivated to participate in training? Are the client's goals and the evaluation goals compatible? Were the goals understandable to training staff? Were they utilized? Program evaluation measures can yield information concerning the current level of program functioning as well as suggestions on how the assessment program might function in the future.

VOCATIONAL REHABILITATION PROGRAMMING STRATEGIES

An accurate vocational rehabilitation diagnosis is the key to the type of vocational training programs developed for the client. The product of the rehabilitation diagnosis is a description of the present and needed level of vocational skills and behavior. The goal of vocational programming is either to increase the skills necessary to succeed in the desired work environment, and/or to select a work environment that more closely accommodates the client's present skill level.

In examining the behaviors necessary to choose, seek, attain and maintain a job, it is evident that there is a wide and complex range of behaviors and supporting abilities in which the psychiatrically disabled client may be significantly deficient. Because of the range and complexity of training needs, it is imperative to begin vocational rehabilitation early in the overall treatment planning.

One way to better understand the complexities of the vocational programming process is to examine the various training intervention strategies or programs typically available. To establish a framework within which most vocational programs can be placed, the following program categories have been developed:

1. Work adjustment training programs
2. Career-counseling programs
3. Occupational skills training programs
4. Career placement training programs

Various vocational settings (e.g., sheltered workshops, transitional employment settings, sheltered employment sites, etc.) may have all or some of these programs.

Work Adjustment Training Programs

Work adjustment training programs are designed for those clients who lack basic work behaviors and social skills needed to maintain a job (Neff 1968). The goal of work adjustment training is to increase the physical, emotional and intellectual skills needed to function successfully on the job. Many psychiatrically disabled clients have never acquired or have lost such skills as, for example, arriving to work on time, attending to work tasks for a certain time, eliminating irrelevant verbalizations, wearing the appropriate clothing and so forth. They often lack the interpersonal and social skills to relate effectively with coworkers, take directions and criticism from supervisors, and give directions and assistance to those they work with or supervise. Work adjustment skill training is a critical programming area for the psychiatrically disabled, as it is often because of basic intellectual or interpersonal reasons that clients lose their jobs (Anthony 1979).

To be most effective work adjustment training should be initiated after the diagnostic process has developed a description of the client's assets and deficits and stated objectives. In this way the specifics of the work adjustment training program can be tailored to the client's actual needs.

Work adjustment training takes place in a work-training environment, usually, but not necessarily, in conjunction with occupational skills training. Work adjustment training can be performed in a variety of settings including a hospital ward, a sheltered workshop and a community setting. It is important to have a wide range of training sites available so that a variety of demands and responsibilities can be placed on the client. By having a range of work adjustment sites, the rehabilitation practitioner is able to deliver programs at the client's level of functioning. The client can receive skills training based on his or her unique pattern of skill and deficit behaviors in an environment most realistically suited to his or her ability to learn the new behavior. Additionally, when the individual has developed skills in one area, he or she can progress and receive training in more demanding and increasingly realistic work settings. This has the additional benefit of generalizing the previously learned behavior to an additional work environment, and using previously learned behavior as a foundation for new learning. Although work adjustment training sites have traditionally been primarily limited to hospital wards and sheltered workshops, new and innovative training and programming sites are being reported in the literature (Brown 1977; Lamb 1971).

Since work adjustment programs develop out of goal statements developed during the diagnostic process, the work adjustment process itself is goal directed and skill oriented. As the client increases his or her ability to perform specific skills, the rehabilitation practitioner must "move" the client into additional skill-oriented adjustment programs based on an ongoing diagnostic assessment. Unfortunately, too many times the work adjustment training ends up being an extended sheltered-employment placement. The goal orientation of work adjustment dictates that the client not stay in a training program without continual skill development.

Although Neff (1969) originally described work adjustment treatment settings as needing to be "realistic in terms of physical layout, kinds of work to be done, levels of compensation, quality of supervision, and hours of work," this does not appear to be true. Olshansky (1969, 1975) has observed that in many work settings the work being performed is tedious, often only "make work," with low-pay activities taking place in training environments that are drab, nonreinforcing and unappealing. It would not be surprising that behaviors learned in such an environment do not generalize to a competitive employment setting. To maximize functional skill acquisition and training effectiveness, work adjustment must take place in a realistic environment with relevant, meaningful tasks, and the client should receive pay comparable to the complexity of the work and the rate at which the work is performed.

In addition, work adjustment training must receive priority and emphasis as a treatment and training intervention strategy. Too often work adjustment training is one of the later treatment efforts utilized with insufficient time and attention given to the process.

Rehabilitation practitioners skilled in work adjustment programming must follow the client after vocational placement occurs. This is especially true when industrial or community training sites have not been utilized during training and clients are unfamiliar with the demands of a competitive environment. Some psychiatrically disabled clients only need support and reinforcement to generalize skills to a new work environment. Other clients may have to develop new skills and behaviors specific to the physical and interpersonal demands of the competitive work setting. The rehabilitation practitioner must continue to work with the client to learn any new skills and behaviors that are functional for that specific work setting.

Programmatic efforts should be skill oriented with clearly stated, observable and measurable goals. They should be explored, understood and developed between the practitioner and the client. For both practitioner and client to have a clear understanding of where he or she is in relation to the adjustment goal, the training program should be developmental in nature with clearly stated steps and stages. Work adjustment training is a relatively new field developed over the last 15 years with no generally accepted body of knowledge, theory or techniques (Ross and Brandon 1971). Thus, any new programming developments should be evaluated and reported within the field.

Career-Counseling Programs

The field of mental health has traditionally not emphasized the practice of teaching career choice and career development skills to psychiatrically disabled clients. This skill is particularly deficient in the chronic psychiatric client who has a history of job failure and inability to secure lasting employment, and who relies on hospital or mental health staff to find him or her a job. One of the greatest failures in traditional psychiatric treatment is the inadequate emphasis given to vocational intervention strategies in the overall treatment process, especially when compared to the value and significance placed on work as a therapeutic and normalizing activity. In particular is the failure to teach clients the skills necessary to choose occupations which relate to their interests, values and abilities, and to thereby give them some responsibility and control in making decisions concerning occupational choice.

Almost by definition chronic psychiatrically disabled clients have unstable work histories characterized by the inability to hold a job and unsuccessful attempts at a variety of different jobs. Conclusions they make about their work behavior may range from "work is not for me" to "I don't care where I'm placed next." Often this is a result of not exploring and understanding how their own values, interests and abilities, *no matter how limited*, interact with occupational areas. Consequently, vocational "placements" have little meaning or relevance and the client has no investment in the work activity. Work does not become a personally rewarding activity. What follows is a lack of involvement in the work activity and no responsibility in making decisions about future career plans. In fact, the concept of a career usually has little meaning.

A common cycle for the chronic psychiatric patient can be conceptualized as follows: Staff or others find a job for the client; he or she is then placed on the job, works for a period of time, meets with failure and returns to the hospital or simply remains unemployed. Self-statements about his or her inability to hold a job are reinforced, responsibility for failure can be placed on the staff, on others or on the job, but not on him or herself. At no time does the client really think he or she can effect change or have impact on the process. Decisions and choices are rarely based on a systematic decision-making process and do not consider the client's interests, values and abilities.

The purpose of career counseling is to promote exploration of the client's interest and value system; to develop an understanding about the relationship between the client's unique set of values and interests and those realistically expressed or demanded by employers in various occupations; and to develop an action plan to assist the client in the attainment of possible career choices. The overall goal, then, is for the client to develop the knowledge and skills which are needed to choose a career goal and develop a career plan (Pierce, Anthony, and Cohen 1980). As a result of the teaching and training process, clients are able to perform the career-counseling skills and activities either by themselves or with the practitioner's assistance. As a result, clients can gain more control and assume more responsibility for what happens in their vocational lives. Clients who have undergone a career-counseling process become less dependent on others for making significant decisions that affect major parts of his or her life.

Because of the importance and complexity of the problem, career counseling should begin early in the rehabilitation treatment phase, and optimally during the vocational diagnostic process. During the vocational assessment process the client has the opportunity to interact with a variety of occupational experiences and explore a variety of demands.

It is important to remember that even the chronically disabled can develop new interests and values as they are stimulated anew by various rehabilitation assessment and programming practices. As a result, clients can be helped to choose a career even though the choices may be between a number of different low level positions. Clients can even become involved in selecting a sheltered workshop setting or job site within the sheltered setting. Career counseling programs need not only be for the very skilled.

Occupational Skills Training Programs

The goal of an occupational skill training program is for the client to acquire the physical, emotional, and/or intellectual skills needed to perform a particular job or task. Conceptually, occupational skills training would take place after an individual has had adjustment skills training and has made a career and occupational choices. Practically, rehabilitation practitioners work on adjustment skills during occupational skills training, and many times the work environment is ideally suited for both purposes. The practitioner must continually monitor and evaluate adjustment skills as they relate to particular work performance and environment demands.

Occupational training takes place in environments which can be scaled according to the proximity with which the environment simulates *competitive work environments.* Table 2 demonstrates this range.

Traditional hospital and sheltered workshops (Level 2 and 3) are very familiar and widely used training concepts and practices, needing little further explanation. The interested reader is referred elsewhere for more specific coverage of sheltered workshops (Black, 1970; Nelson 1971). Level 4 is characterized by vocational training sites located directly in industry but under sheltered workshop status. Level 5 training is characterized by training sites where the client is employed by industry or business but is receiving additional programming support such as supervision and training by rehabilitation staff, individual counseling and/or peer support groups.

The mere provision of an occupational skills training site is not sufficient to effectively and efficiently train the psychiatrically disabled client to perform occupational tasks. Clients do not learn job tasks simply by association or modeling and are not usually motivated to acquire occupational tasks on their own. In addition to

Table 2 Occupation-Training Environments

Level 6	Competitive employment
Level 5	Fully integrated with supportive services
Level 4	Semiintegrated with some shelter
Level 3	Segregated work site—Prototype Workshop
Level 2	Hospital/ward work duties
Level 1	No institutional work demands

appropriate training sites, systematic occupational skills training programs must be developed. A rehabilitation occupational skills training program describes the specific steps which a psychiatrically disabled client must master in order to progress from his or her present level of occupational skill performance to a more advanced level of skill performance. A more detailed analysis and description of rehabilitation programming can be found in Anthony, Pierce and Cohen (1980b).

Career Placement Training Programs

Career placement skill training is the process in which the rehabilitation practitioner assists the client in developing the range of skills necessary to seek, acquire and maintain the best possible job available. Until recently career placement training has not been viewed as an important or valued activity for rehabilitation practitioners. Much more attention and interest has been given to the counseling or coordinating role. Placement activities have been left to a "job counselor," or the client has been referred to outside agencies for placement. However, rehabilitation practitioners are realizing that many chronic psychiatric patients fail to acquire appropriate work because they do not have the range of career placement skills required to seek the most suitable job available. For example, the chronic psychiatric client may be unable to identify possible job situations where he or she might want to work, and if the patient did find them he or she would lack the skills to identify his or her assets and/or relate them effectively to the job interviewer. Many chronic psychiatric clients simply do not have the physical and interpersonal skills to present themselves effectively to an employer.

The rehabilitation practitioner operationalizes the process of career placement by making each major step of the career placement process a clearly defined skill to be learned and performed. Clients must learn what job-related assets or strengths they have to offer the employer, how to find resources and develop a list of available jobs for their particular work skills, and how to present themselves in ways that best represent their qualifications for the job. Through actively involving the client in developing placement skills, the rehabilitation practitioner increases the client's motivation both to actively seek work and to learn to utilize the skills in the future. The client may also benefit therapeutically, as he or she does possess a list of strengths and skilled behaviors which others value. By listing strengths, skills and abilities, the client is establishing reasons why he or she is a desired person in the work world.

For all people, the task of job search or changing jobs is a highly stressful experience. Besides having to test the marketable worth of their abilities, people face possible changes in relationships, activities, status, and patterns of living. For the chronic psychiatrically disabled client the experience can be even more stressful. The client must challenge long term patterns of "patient" behavior, present him or herself face to face to an employer, account for and discuss hospitalization and poor employment histories, and perform other activities in which he or she may previously have failed. Often the job search is the culmination of many months of investment in skill development programs. It is a time to test the outcome value of these efforts and the acquired skills and abilities. Testing the value of this investment is an additional stress factor which chronic psychiatric clients often have a history of avoiding.

To not provide the client with skills necessary to successfully perform the activities of career placement is to leave a critical deficit in the client's rehabilitation program at a time when he or she needs intensive planning, training, support and reinforcement. The more skilled the client is in career placement activities, the better able he or she is to generate a number of suitable placement opportunities. To the extent that the client is able to find jobs that suit his or her needs and interests, the more motivated he or she will be to invest in the job and work hard to keep it. Placement skills are important, then, for both job acquisition and job retention purposes (Anthony, 1979).

As developed by Pierce, Cohen, Cohen, and Anthony (1980), a career placement skills program for psychiatrically disabled clients is comprised of three major steps. Initially the client must *explore* his or her past work and educational activity in order to identify and list assets related to work and educational experiences. The client can draw from his or her activities as explored during the assessment, training, and career counseling process. The assessment and training phases provide initial and current level of skill functioning ideally suited for listing the skills important at the time of career placement. The client must then work to *understand* specific job sites in industry, business or community which can utilize his or her own unique skills and assets. Many of the job sites explored during career development activities will serve as a place to begin this activity. After the client has determined the best available work site, he or she must *act* to present him or herself both orally and in writing. Completing resumes and application forms, dressing appropriately, learning transportation routes, developing answers to interview questions and being able to ask relevant questions are a few of the skills learned during this phase. In essence, clients must identify *what* they have to offer, *where* they have to offer it, and *how* to offer it, either in person or in writing.

Placement activities require time and skill to be performed effectively. Rehabilitation practitioners use group support, problem solving techniques, decision-making skills, and programming skills to successfully train the client. The practitioner may also spend time visiting employment sites, practicing job interviewing skills, "walking" the client through transportation routes and introduction to the work site, co-workers, and supervisors. The rehabilitation practitioner must also creatively explore new placement avenues such as group or homebound employment (Fairweather et al., 1969; Lamb, 1967) or develop extended employment programs within industry (Burger, 1978). Effective placement activities require specialized and particular skills and should not be relegated to unskilled professionals. Research into the training of career placement skills has shown that psychiatrically disabled clients can learn various career placement skills (Anderson, 1968; Kerl & Barbee, 1973; Prazok, 1969; Pusso, et al., 1966; Safieri, 1970), and that these skills do impact on job outcome (Keith et al., 1977; McClure, 1973).

SAMPLE ASSESSMENT AND TRAINING PROGRAMS

Assessment and training strategies have been presented as separate entities for ease of understanding; yet in practice assessment techniques are often integrated with various programming strategies within the same comprehensive rehabilitation setting. For example, work adjustment training can take place concurrent with situational assessment or other assessment techniques (Hoffman, 1971). The exploration phase of career counseling can likewise be facilitated by the use of work samples or situational assessment techniques. Typically, various rehabilitation settings such as sheltered workshops and sheltered employment sites utilize both programming strategies and assessment techniques. Several innovative programs which are described in this section have combined systematic assessment strategies with training programs in community and industrial settings.

Workshops Without Walls

Vash (1977) has observed that irrelevant training performed in inadequate sheltered workshops or similar training sites is undoubtedly one of the most tragic practices occurring in rehabilitation. Unrealistic work environments do not develop the skills necessary to function in competitive employment. Clients who do learn skills may subsequently find that jobs for which they have been trained do not exist. In addition, because workshops rely primarily on assembly, inspection, coding, packing, and other bench work training activities, clients interested in service jobs, working with people, or business jobs relating to data, are hard pressed to find adequate training sites. Clearly an expanded model of sheltered training is needed.

The "Workshop Without Walls" concept has been explored as a means to expand sheltered training into the private sector and provide realistic vocational evaluation, work adjustment, and occupational training in an industrial yet sheltered setting. Brickey (1974) describes a workshop without walls concept as a workshop with job stations in community businesses and industries. He notes that with this improvement and expansion of the workshop model, assessment and training situations then resemble the employment goal (competitive employment situation) as closely as possible.

During diagnostic assessment, the level of skill performance and the description of vocational objectives relate directly and immediately to easily observable criteria—performance in an industrial setting. Clients easily understand how vocational objectives relate to job success. As a result, clients view the training activity as valid and have increased motivation to work toward the objective. Furthermore, the work tasks involved in occupational training are not "make work," but saleable services or products. Consequently, the client values him or herself as a worker and is able to make positive self-statements about skills, productivity level, and the product or service resulting from his or her efforts. This is in direct contrast to many of the stigma-related responses clients might have made had their evaluation and training been with typical hospital or institutional sheltered workshop training tasks.

Reports of the Industrial Therapies Organization in England (Early 1975) demonstrated further support to the claim that "groups working under supervision in open industry are superior to sheltered workshops" in training psychiatrically disabled clients. As the training program closely resembles competitive employment settings, transition to competitive employment has less of a "culture shock."

One additional but important development resulting from community- and industry-based training sites is that the community becomes more aware of rehabilitation programming, goals and efforts. The reputation of successful sheltered work training sites can open doors for additional community sites. Rather than being limited to subcontract work of traditional workshops, relevant training opportunities in service and business fields can continue to be developed.

Transitional Employment Programs

Fountain House in New York City has developed a program which provides transitional employment experiences for chronic psychiatrically disabled clients who have difficulty making the transition from hospital to competitive employment (Bean and Beard 1975; Beard, Schmidt, and Smith 1963; DeSimone 1974). Through the program, members work either individually or in groups in commercial or industrial job slots allocated to Fountain House by the employer. Members usually work for four hours a day, from a period of three to six months. For the rest of the day members take part in a prevocational day program which provides varied opportunities for involvement in work-oriented activities.

The purpose of the training and transitional employment is not to learn specific occupational skills, but to assess and strengthen work habits, attitudes and additional work adjustment skills necessary for working competitively. A primary emphasis of the employment program is that jobs are entry-level positions, often below the skills or potential of the worker, and are therefore likely to ensure successful job performance and increased self-confidence. As the emphasis is on work adjustment training, employers are hiring workers who are less than work ready. Attention is given to the benefits gained by employees. Supervision and training is provided by Fountain House staff; the employer saves benefit payments by hiring part-time staff; Fountain House provides reliable coverage for high turnover, entry-level jobs; production standards are maintained. The benefits to the client, as noted by Bean and Beard (1975), are that "money is earned, a job reference is secured, self-confidence and esteem are strengthened, and independent employment on a job of one's own becomes a realistic objective."

A number of transitional employment programs containing many of the same ingredients of the Fountain House program are being developed around the country. In Massachusetts, the Transitional Employment Program (TEP), a component of the Placement Project, Inc., is one such program. The program developed from a Governor's Special Project, but has since become a nonprofit organization. Modeled after the Fountain House program, TEP serves clients needing a gradual supportive employment experience to develop skills necessary for full-time permanent competitive employment. TEP provides adjustment and occupational skills training through placement in competitive job sites. Like Fountain House, the job tasks are routine and low pressure to ensure success. TEP placement specialists work alongside clients to ensure that job skills are learned and performed correctly, and that production standards are maintained.

The client has the opportunity both to learn and to try out skills and abilities in an industrial setting. Through experience and accomplishment in meeting production demands, the client increases self-confidence and is able to feel more valuable as a worker.

The client also participates in peer support meetings and has almost daily contact with TEP personnel. The client is provided with feedback and support and an opportunity to develop additional behaviors to adapt to the work environment and interpersonal situations. The TEP placement specialist provides progress information to the referring agency on client skill level and discusses possible training or reinforcement approaches. The close communication functions to aid the referring rehabilitation practitioner, TEP personnel, employers and the client.

Projects with Industry

Projects With Industry (PWI) programs constitute a major effort to involve government, industry and rehabilitation to meet the employment needs of the disabled. They are large-scale contracts funded by the federal Rehabilitation Service Administration to state vocational rehabilitation agencies to promote job training and placement of disabled clients directly in industry (Brubeck 1974). The emphasis, then, is on direct placement in community industry or business rather than on utilizing a sheltered workshop model. Three model PWI programs have emerged (Burger 1978) including (1) a work adjustment model, where the client is provided a specific period of time in the industrial setting to develop the behaviors and skills necessary for competitive employment, (2) a job skills training model, which trains clients in the technical occupational skills necessary for job performance, and (3) a job placement model, which seeks permanent competitive employment for clients who are job ready. There are over 50 PWI projects across the country in what appears to be a strong commitment at the federal level to actively integrate industry, unions and community with rehabilitation efforts (Burger 1978).

From a skills-training framework, PWI's increase training and employment opportunities, ranging from unskilled to highly skilled and technical jobs. From the employer's point of view, there is an opportunity to hire experienced and skilled employees, who have been trained in an industrial or business setting often not unlike their own. Psychiatrically disabled clients have been included in client population groups served by PWI programs, but most PWI programs have been developed to provide training for many disability groups. The Fountain House program is an exception to this, as it was originally started as a PWI program, demonstrating success in involving the psychiatrically disabled in industrial training programs. As an example of a Projects With Industry program, the Menninger Foundation's Center for Applied Behavioral Sciences (1977) has developed a comprehensive PWI emphasizing the needs of the psychiatrically disabled, while also serving other disability groups. The project provides many program components to train and place individuals in competitive jobs and ensure that they maintain the jobs. Programming strategies include vocational assessment, training in occupational and job-seeking skills, job placement programs, including job modification to adapt the task to the particular skills of the individual, and a support system after the individual has been placed. Support services vary but are aimed at assisting the employer or worker in making any adjustments that are necessary. Traditionally, they have included work adjustment training, further academic education and/or counseling to assist the individual in maintaining the training or employment site. In addition, the project recognizes the need of the employees and coworkers to better understand the worker. Consequently, a major program thrust is to change employer and coworker attitudes about the disabled through seminars, workshops and consultations.

FUTURE DIRECTIONS

1. All too often assessment efforts are characterized by random administration of psychometric tests and/or unsystematic placement and observation of the client in a hospital ward or sheltered workshop setting. Vocational evaluation efforts must derive from a model which integrates the various tools of assessment into a systematic, purposeful process that yields functional information about the level of skills and behaviors of the individual. Furthermore, rather than functioning as separate and distinct processes within psychiatric rehabilitation, vocational assessment and vocational programming efforts should be functionally related. The observable and measurable description of present and needed levels of behavior obtained during assessment clearly relate to program direction. Vocational assessment should have an impact on the training programs subsequently developed, and they in turn should provide feedback to assessment professionals about the utility and validity of assessment results.

To promote this relationship, program evaluation methodologies should be developed as ongoing and necessary functions within the rehabilitation process. In this way program evaluation efforts can provide functional information to improve both the process and outcome of assessment and training services. As the process and results of assessment focus on observable measures of behavior, program evaluation methodologies can be easily developed within the process.

2. Vocational evaluators must make better use of their interviewing skills in the vocational assessment process. By using his or her interpersonal skills, the evaluator can encourage client self-exploration and involvement in the evaluation process. In this way the vocational diagnostician can select the evaluation techniques and settings based on the client's unique vocational situation. For example, evaluator-facilitated client exploration may result in the assessment that the client has limited understanding of his or her range of occupational skills and limited understanding of the range of occupations that may be of interest. It is through specific interviewing skills that the client is able to understand how these deficits hinder vocational choice. Specific work samples can then be chosen to explore these deficits and provide information about a wide range of potential job skills within a relatively short period of time. The client is invested in the work samples as he or she is able to see how they relate to his or her occupational objective and overall rehabilitation goal. The

evaluator would then assist in clarifying the client's performance and organizing the occupational information into meaningful data for the client. In this way the client is able to establish direction for additional exploratory activity. At the same time, the evaluator is indirectly teaching the client how to evaluate experiences, organize information and make decisions.

Similarly, situational assessment approaches may be used to assess the frequency, duration or intensity of specific work adjustment behaviors. By means of interviewing skills the evaluator can facilitate client understanding of how these behaviors hinder or assist successful job performance. In essence, evaluator's interviewing skills can be used to provide direction in planning the assessment, to assist the client to explore and personalize the experience so that the experiential activity and results are meaningful, and to communicate in an understandable manner a skills-based description of the client's present and needed level of skills. To the extent that the client is helped to personalize or "own" his or her involvement in experiential assessment activities, he or she will view the diagnostic process as meaningful and will be able to "own" the results. To the extent that the client is able to "own" the results and view them as accurate descriptions of his or her present and needed level of skill, the client will be able to participate in the prescribed vocational training programs and accept them as meaningful programs relating to rehabilitation goals.

3. The foundation for collaborative vocational training programs between rehabilitation and community or industrial settings has been well established, but now requires further expansion. Innovative ideas must continue to be developed. Such considerations as wage incentives and payments to industry for providing training and job sites (Nelson 1971), and the development of sheltered employment in industry must be examined and explored. The regulations governing Section 504 of the Rehabilitation Act of 1973 may have influence on this last suggestion. In addition, rehabilitation practitioners must develop the knowledge and skills to work with community and industrial sites to creatively develop additional innovative training opportunities.

Training placements in industry have fostered a closer relationship between government and industry and rehabilitation. These training placements can no longer be considered as a "straw in the wind" approach (Black 1970), or as experimental or pilot projects. They are viable efforts that have demonstrated positive results.

What is indicated for hospitalized psychiatrically disabled clients is a continuum of vocational training opportunities from hospital to community and industrial sites. Equally as important is the availability of realistic training models for the chronic psychiatric client already in the community. The availability of community training could reduce the need to be hospitalized for many.

Riscalla (1974), noting the increase and benefits in community-based training opportunities, asks, "Can workshops become obsolete?" Although traditional workshop sites provide valuable training opportunities for some individuals, innovations in programming techniques and training environments demonstrate that at the very least, there is no longer a need for the client to be returned to the institution for vocational training.

4. The psychiatric rehabilitation model and its supporting research has as much implication for the rehabilitation practitioner as for the chronic psychiatrically disabled client. It appears that the initial level or degree of client skill deficiency does not appear to correlate that highly with the ability to learn or develop skills (Anthony 1979). However, the level of client skill deficiency does place demands on the technology of program development. That is, the level of client skill deficiency relates to the complexity of the training techniques and technical skills necessary for skill development—but not necessarily the outcome. It appears that it is not the degree or level of disability that correlates with successful functioning, but the skill level, or technology, of the rehabilitation practitioners. As a result, the focus of improving the efficacy of psychiatric rehabilitation should be on the expertise of rehabilitation practitioners rather than on the "symptomatology" of the client.

5. To the extent that the success of psychiatric rehabilitation depends on the skill level of rehabilitation practitioners, rehabilitation educators must design curricula to increase the practitioners' expertise in skill areas that seem capable of affecting client outcome. Just as the skills needed by the chronic psychiatrically disabled client to function in the community must be defined as objectively as possible, so too must the skills required for the practitioner to *practice* in the field of psychiatric rehabilitation be equally so defined. The rehabilitation educator must develop performance or competency-based training programs whereby the student will have an objective measurement of his or her skills relative to the fundamental skills needed to practice rehabilitation (Anthony and Carkhuff 1977; Anthony, Cohen and Vitalo 1978).

6. Finally, as reflected by the high recidivism rates of psychiatrically disabled clients (Anthony et al., 1972), many chronic psychiatrically disabled clients are not able to function adequately in the community. Although work, as both a training activity and an outcome measure, has a significant impact on the success of the client, he or she must also develop the skills necessary to perform a range of behaviors required to function in other community environments. Community programs must be on a broad scale to attend to the wide range of concerns associated with chronicity. Although much emphasis has been placed on developing community residential facilities (Mannino, Ott, and Shore 1977), these residential settings must also develop effective diagnostic and programming efforts. Skills-based diagnostic and training programs can be effective in improving not only the client's vocational functioning, but also the client's ability to live more independently in the community (Anthony 1979).

REFERENCES

Anderson, J. A. The disadvantaged seeks work—through their efforts or ours? *Rehabilitation Record* 9: 5-10 (1968).

Anthony, W. A. Psychological rehabilitation: A concept in need of a method. *American Psychologist* 32: 658-662, 1977.

Anthony, W. A. *The principles of psychiatric rehabilitation.* Baltimore, MD: University Park Press, 1979.

Anthony, W. A. and Carkhuff, R. R. The functional professional therapeutic agent, in *Effective Psychotherapy: A Handbook of Research*, Gurman and Razin, eds. Oxford: Pergamon Press, 1977.

Anthony, W. A., Buell, G. J. Sharratt, S., and Altoff, M. E. The efficacy of psychiatric rehabilitation. *Psychological Bulletin* 78: 447-456, 1972.

Anthony, W. A., Cohen, M. R. and Vitalo, R. The measurement of rehabilitation outcome. *Schizophrenia Bulletin* 4: 365-383 (1978).

Anthony, W. A. and Margules, A. Toward improving the efficacy of psychiatric rehabilitation: A skills training approach. *Rehabilitation Psychology* 21: 101-105 (1974).

Anthony, W. A., Pierce, R. M., and Cohen, M. R. The skills of diagnostic planning. *Psychiatric Rehabilitation Practice Series: Book 1.* Baltimore, MD: University Park Press, 1980(a).

Anthony, W. A., Pierce, R. M., and Cohen, M. R. The skills of rehabilitation programming. *Psychiatric Rehabilitation Practice Series: Book 2.* Baltimore, MD: University Park Press, 1980(b).

Bachrach, L. Deinstitutionalization: An analytical review and sociological perspective, DHEW Publication No. (ADM) 76-351, Supt. of Documents, U.S. Government Printing Office, Washington, D.C., 1976.

Bean, B. R., and Beard, J. H. Placement for persons with psychiatric disability. *Rehabilitation Counseling Bulletin:* 253-258 (June 1975).

Beard, J. H., Schmidt, J. R., and Smith, M. M. The use of transitional employment with rehabilitation of the psychiatric patient. *Journal of Nervous and Mental Disease* 136: 507-514 (1963).

Becker, P., and Bayer, C. Preparing chronic patients for community placement: A four-stage treatment program. *Hospital and Community Psychiatry* 26: 448-450 (1975).

Berk, R., and Rossi, P. Doing good or worse: Evaluation research politically reexamined. *Social Problems* 23: 337-349 (1976).

Black, B. J. Principles of industrial therapy for the mentally ill. New York: Grune and Stratton, 1970.

Bockoven, J. S. *Moral Treatment in American Psychiatry.* Springer Publishing Co., 1963.

Botterbusch, K. F. *A Guide to Job Site Evaluation.* Menomonie, Wisconsin: Materials Development Center, 1978.

Brickey, M. Normalization and behavior modification in the sheltered workshop. *Journal of Rehabilitation* 40: 44-46 (1974).

Brown, B. S. Responsible community care of former mental hospital patients. *New Dimensions in Mental Health. NIMH,* Rockville, MD. (1977).

Bubeck, T. They come to work. *Social and Rehabilitation Record* 8: 18-22 (1978).

Burger, G. *Program Model for Projects with Industry.* Chicago, Illinois: Chicago Jewish Vocational Service, 1978.

Carkhuff, R. R. *Helping and Human Relations.* Vol. 1 and 2. New York: Holt, Rinehart and Winston, 1969.

Carkhuff, R. R. *The Development of Human Resources.* New York: Holt, Rinehart, and Winston, 1971.

Carkhuff, R. R. *The Art of Helping.* Amherst, MA: Human Resource Development Press, 1972 (Third Edition, 1977).

Carkhuff, R. R., and Berenson, B. G. *Beyond Counseling and Therapy.* New York: Holt, Rinehart and Winston, 1977.

DeSimone, A. Industries commitment to VR. *Social and Rehabilitation Record,* 1: 23-27 (1974).

Dunn, D. J. *Situational Assessment: Models for the Future.* Menomonie, Wisconsin: Research and Training Center, No. 22, 1973.

Early, D. F. Sheltered groups in open industry: A new approach to training and to employment. *Lancet:* 1370-1373 (June 21, 1975).

Fairweather, G., Sanders, D., Maynard, H., Cressler, D., and Bleck, D. *Community Life for the Mentally Ill.* Chicago: Aldine Publishing Co., 1969.

Hoffman, P. R. Work evaluation and adjustment: The relationship. *Journal of Rehabilitation* 37: 19-22 (1971).

Jacobs, M. K., and Trick, O. L. Successful psychiatric rehabilitation using an in-patient teaching laboratory. *American Journal of Psychiatry* 131: 145-148 (1974).

Keil, E. C., and Barbee, J. R. Behavior modification and training the disadvantaged job interviewee. *Vocational Guidance Quarterly:* 50-56 (September 1973).

Keith, R. D., Engelkes, J. R., and Winborn, B. B. Employment — seeking preparation and activity: An experimental job-placement training model for rehabilitation clients. *Rehabilitation Counseling Bulletin:* 159-165 (December 1977).

Kirk, S. A. Effectiveness of community services for discharged mental hospital patients. *American Journal of Orthopsychiatry* 46: 646-659 (1976).

Lamb, H. R. *Rehabilitation in Community Mental Health.* San Francisco: Jossey-Bass, 1971.

Levine, M., and Levine, A. *A Social History of Helping Services: Clinic, Court, School and Community.* New York: Appleton-Century-Crofts, 1970.

Mannino, F. V., Ott, S., and Shore, M. F. Community residential facilities for former mental patients: An annotated bibliography. *Psychosocial Rehabilitation Journal* 1: 1-43 (1977).

McClure, D. P. Placement through improvement of client's job seeking skills. *Journal of Applied Rehabilitation Counseling* 3: 188-196 (1973).

Menninger Foundation. Jobs for the handicapped. *Menninger Perspective:* 22-23 (Fall 1977).

Nadolsky, J. M. The experiential component of vocational evaluation. *Vocational Evaluation and Work Adjustment Bulletin* 9: 3-7 (1976a).

Nadolsky, J. M. The counseling function in vocational evaluation. *Vocational Evaluation and Work Adjustment Bulletin,* 9: 39-45 (1976b).

Neff, W. Problems of work evaluation. *Personnel and Guidance Journal* 44: 682-688 (1966).

Neff, W. *Work and Human Behavior.* New York: Atherton Press, 1968.

Nelson, N. *Workshops for the Handicapped in the U.S.: An Historical and Developmental Perspective.* New York: C. C. Thomas, 1971.

Olshansky, S. Changing vocational behavior through normalization, in *Normalization: The Principles of Normalization in Human Services,* W. Wolfensburger, ed. Toronto, Canada: National Institute on Mental Retardation, 1975.

Pierce, R. M., Anthony, W. A., and Cohen, M. *The Skills of Career Counseling. Psychiatric Rehabilitation Practices: Book 4.* Baltimore, MD: University Park Press, 1980.

Pierce, R. M., Cohen, M. R., Cohen, B., and Anthony, W. A. *The Skills of Career Placement. Psychiatric Rehabilitation Practices: Book 5.* Baltimore, MD: University Park Press, 1980.

Prazak, J. A. Learning job seeking interview skills, in *Behavioral Counseling,* Krumboltz and Thoreson, eds. New York: Holt, Rinehart and Winston, 1969, pp. 414-424.

Pruitt, W. A. *Vocational (Work) Evaluation.* Menomonie, Wisconsin: Walt Pruitt Associates, 1977.

Pumo, B., Sehl, R., and Cogan, F. Job readiness: Key to placement. *Journal of Rehabilitation* 32: 18-19 (1966).

Retchless, M. H. Rehabilitation programs for chronic patients: Stepping stones to the community. *Hospital and Community Psychiatry* 18: 377-378, (1967).

Riscalla, L. Could workshops become obsolete? *Journal of Rehabilitation,* 40: 17-18 (1974).

Ross, D., and Brandon, T. In pursuit of work adjustment. *Journal of Rehabilitation* 34: 6-8 (1971).

Safieri, D. Using an educational model in a sheltered workshop program. *Mental Hygiene* 54: 140-143 (1970).

Sankovsky, R. *State of the Art in Vocational Evaluation: Report of a National Survey*. Pittsburgh, PA: Research and Training Center in Vocational Rehabilitation (Rt-14), 1969.

Scoles, P., and Fine, E. Aftercare and rehabilitation in a community mental health center. *Social Work* 16: 75-82 (1971).

Sink, J. M., and Porter, T. L. Convergence and divergence in rehabilitation counseling and vocational evaluation. *Vocational Evaluation and Work Adjustment Bulletin* 11: 5-20 (1978).

Task Force No. 2, The tools of vocational evaluation. *Vocational Evaluation and Work Adjustment Bulletin* 8: Part I, Special Edition, 49-64 (1975).

Turner, J., and Ten Hoor, W. The NIMH Community Support Program: Pilot approach to a needed social reform. *Schizophrenia Bulletin* 4: 319-344 (1978).

Vash, C. L. *Sheltered Industrial Employment.* Washington, D.C.: Institute for Research Utilization, 1977.

Walker, R. Social restoration of hospitalized psychiatric patients through a program of special employment in industry. *Rehabilitation Literature* 30: 297-303 (1969).

Weinman, B., Sander, R., Kleiner, R., and Wilson, S. Community based treatment of the chronic psychotic. *Community Mental Health Journal* 6: 12-21 (1970).

CHAPTER 9

THE PLACE OF THE PARTIAL HOSPITAL IN THE TREATMENT OF CHRONIC PSYCHIATRIC PATIENTS

STEPHEN L. WASHBURN

In the past several years the political ferment focused on the increasing presence of long-term mental hospital patients in the community has stirred thoughtful reactions by many professional as well as political groups. The report in 1977 of the President's Commission on Mental Health, as well as the official position statement of the American Psychiatric Association in 1978, focused on the systems defects in the country's attempts to make effective care available to chronic patients throughout the country. Ironically, these very issues had been previously addressed in the Community Mental Health Centers Act of 1963. This act mandated the structures needed for the care of chronic and acute psychiatric patients. Since that time, clusters of inpatient and outpatient units, as well as day, evening and night care programs, have been established in increasing numbers. Some, such as the Day-Night unit at the Allen Memorial Institute in Montreal or the Day Hospital at the Massachusetts Mental Health Center, had been functioning effectively years before the landmark federal legislation had been passed. Grouped under the name of partial hospitalization, these units developed a capacity for treating both acute and chronic patients. By 1968 there was one partial hospital patient for every 40 psychiatric inpatients in the U.S. This trend has continued. By 1976 the ratio had increased to one in 10 and day treatment units had increased to 1,458 in 3,495 mental health facilities of all types.

These part-time units were able to avoid the hazards of the social breakdown syndrome commonly associated with patient life in the large mental hospital. On the other hand, some investigators, who have followed the course of mental patients in the community for long periods of time, have empirically documented patterns of social and treatment factors expected as a result of the progression of a chronic illness. Segal and Aviram (1978) observed a large cohort of former mental patients in community care who have never been integrated into society, either before or after their illness began. Hogarty and Goldberg (1974) have noted the failure of psychotropic drugs and/or psychotropic social outpatient treatment to definitively prevent relapse. Morgan (1979) has reported failure of an extensive rehabilitation program, as intensive as the patients could tolerate, to alter the social and cognitive disabilities of chronic schizophrenic patients in community settings. None of these studies however, give a balanced picture of the way hospital-related or free-standing day treatment centers have been able to offer a stable base of operations for increasing numbers of chronic or deinstitutionalized mental patients. These vulnerable people need the sophisticated multidisciplinary treatments available in large hospital centers, but do *not* need the isolation and infantilizing overprotection and unimaginative, repetitive patterns of interaction to which large institutions unwittingly become accustomed. The partial hospital does not offer a cure-all for major chronic, psychiatric illness. It is uniquely situated to view and use treatment patterns from the best of two worlds—the intensive, elaborate 24-hour care of inpatients, and the 1-hour-per-week care which most outpatient clinics offer to their clientele. This paper will discuss how this synthesis is becoming increasingly available for patients in the U.S. today. It will also indicate how the effects of the day hospital have been validated and how these effects can be maximized in the future.

WHY USE PARTIAL HOSPITALS?

This question can be answered from several viewpoints: Philosophically and politically, there is greater appeal to living in one's community where life is not constricted by the regulations and barriers found necessary for the organization of large numbers of people in institutional life. The potentially degrading experience of being unduly controlled by others, the interference in family and intimate life intrinsic in hospital routines, the potential loss of affective stimuli—all lead to a barrenness of human interaction which constitutes the *social* reason for using the "partial" alternative to full hospitalization.

Other practical justifications—the *feasibility*, clinical *efficacy* and *cost*—will be spelled out below.

The landmark study of Zwerling and Wilder (1964) at Bronx Municipal Hospital convincingly demonstrated the feasibility of a day hospital program, as an alternative for approximately two thirds of all emergency room patients, both chronic and acute, who required intensive, psychiatric treatment in the form of inpatient hospitalization. Some of these required one or two nights of "boarding" at the inpatient service before being able to sustain the program of up to 8 weeks at the day hospital, which was located in a municipal health building one or two miles away. For the most part, patients suffered from schizophrenia, affective psychosis, and personality and neurotic disorders. Patients with organic brain disease or serious physical disability were not successfully randomized because of the difficulties in navigating the daily transportation from their homes to the day hospital. Although the day hospital concept had been in use since first established by the Russians outside of Leningrad in the 1930s, this was the first demonstration of the extent to which mental hospital patients could be assigned to an alternative community program. The results strikingly demonstrated that not only could the large spectrum of patients be managed, but that by and large they fared as well as the inpatients at a two-year followup.

In a prior study involving only chronic schizophrenic patients, Kris (1961) had demonstrated the feasibility of the day hospital as an alternative treatment location for relapsing former state hospital patients. A few years later, the diagnostic characteristics of a day hospital sample were described in great detail by Hogarty et al. (1968) in the study of an urban day hospital in Baltimore. The full range of personality and psychotic disorder managed in the day hospital tended to have more affective psychopathology than the range of those who were treated in the alternative inpatient service.

WHO IS IT FOR?

From the above studies and from clinical experience in many settings, a rationale with specific criteria has evolved to determine appropriate patients for participation in a partial hospital treatment system. First, patients with most types of psychopathology, with the exception of the minimally and extremely ill patients, are eligible. In addition, the abnormalities to be addressed should be of such severity that they cannot readily be treated in an outpatient office setting.

They usually require a combination of psychological, social and biochemical therapy sustained over a number of weeks or months. Second, whatever range of cognitive impairment, conceptual aberration, mood disturbance or behavioral abnormality the patient demonstrates, he or she must have sufficient intact ego functions to ally at least minimally with the day or evening hospital staff. A patient is engaged and supported and induced to participate by interpersonal means alone, as restraint or other limit setting by physical structures is not possible in a partial hospital program. Third, a corollary of this is a capacity to attend the center with some regularity, to use the transportation available and to return to some domicile—home, halfway house, dorm, sheltered apartment—where reasonable needs for shelter and social contacts can be met during the majority of the hours when the patient is not attending the treatment setting. Fourth, threats to human existence such as suicide, externally directed aggression and uncontrolled abuse of drugs cannot be effectively managed in the partial hospital setting. Some suicidal tendency or symptoms of drug abuse can be tolerated, provided the patient can communicate sufficiently with staff so that measures to prevent major bodily harm can be implemented. This is especially important since the partial hospital milieu has limitations on the stresses which its staff and patient participants can absorb. Fifth, although not an absolute requirement, the presence of a significant other, such as a spouse, a halfway house manager or a close friend provides welcome support in helping the patient to attend regularly or to work with the staff in time of crisis. This added assistance can greatly expand the range of psychopathology and social aberration which the day hospital can tolerate.

Given these criteria, conditions usually treatable in these settings include: chronic or acute schizophrenia, childhood schizophrenia as seen in adult life, borderline, hysterical, compulsive, schizoid and passive-aggressive personality disorders, as well as chronic depression and bipolar affective disease [excluding mania, suicidal depression, and alcoholism (except for acute intoxication)].

DIVISIONS AND STAFFING OF PARTIAL HOSPITAL PROGRAMS

Day programs typically run on a 9:00 A.M. to 5:00 P.M. schedule. Staffs often meet before patient hours to hold review conferences or organize for the day's activities. Some programs close to patients earlier than 5:00 P.M. so staff may regroup and plan for the next day or the forthcoming evening program.

For the patient who is not able to manage effectively at home or in some work setting due to acute exacerbation of illness or chronic symptomatic impairment, attendance at a day program five days a week is a logical alternative to a shift into 24-hour care. Ideally, the patient could be referred to such a program early in the emergency or recurrence of symptoms, so that a modest increase in psychosocial support might curtail the extent of the disability.

For the inpatient who is in partial remission, the day setting serves as a natural bridge to the fuller pressures of community life. Such patients can visit the day hospital from the inpatient unit and, as appropriate contacts are made, move to their community domicile and continue the intensive transitional day program for as many weeks or months as is necessary.

For persons from the community whose strengths allow them to continue at work or school, or for former inpatients who are able to return to their usual vocation, the evening program from 6:00 P.M. to 10:00 P.M. is uniquely available for treatment. In addition to core psychological and biological treatment, a comprehensive program includes a range of social and recreational therapies, as well as a spectrum of prevocational and vocational discussion groups. Naturally, the evening program is more likely to have a greater need for the latter, as its members are often struggling with the return to and continuation at their usual job.

Staffing of the typical day program includes the professional spectrum of psychiatrist, social worker, psychologist, psychiatric nurse, mental health worker, vocational counselor and occupational therapist. Day program staff/patient ratios of 1 to 4 are usually found in programs which offer intensive treatment to a wide range of diagnostic categories. This ratio is analogous to what is seen during the daytime hours on any active inpatient treatment unit. Because the ego function of evening program patients is usually somewhat higher than day patients, staff/patient ratios in that program may be somewhat less, at 1 to 5 or 6. This latter ratio is also typical of programs which serve less acutely symptomatic or chronic patients.

In addition to the core day or evening programs, most networks have access to an ad hoc overnight boarding or night care system by which the partial hospital treatment team may briefly employ 24-hour care. These overnight units tend to be primarily supportive and do not provide specialized treatment experiences per se, as the patient continues to receive these in the day or evening programs.

Although partial hospital programs may emphasize one of two main models, most are, in fact, an intermixture of an individualized, medically oriented treatment program with a milieu-based, social, educational, behavioral model. This usually includes a problem-solving ego growth component, a role-modeling ego identification component and some degree of straight-forward behavior modification with components of positive reinforcement and aversive deconditioning in them. As with inpatient settings, there seems to be little justification for the unit settling exclusively for one of these theoretical models. Any one might be optimum for some aspects of the huge range of aberrant symptoms or behavior with which an active partial hospital unit can be faced.

PARTIAL VERSUS INHOSPITAL PLACEMENT

In his study of the Baltimore Psychiatric Day Center, Hogarty (1968) observed that the intensity of psychopathology of day patients fell between those in inpatient and outpatient settings. The schizophrenic patients, a large portion of the day center population, demonstrated a greater tendency to mood disturbance and less of the cognitive disorganization characteristically seen in the state hospital inpatient population. The Bronx Municipal Hospital study (Zwerling and Wilder 1964) demonstrated that patients with organic brain syndromes characterized by severe confusion and physical impairment were found unfeasible for the day hospital setting. Other studies (Washburn et al. 1976; Herz et al. 1975; Krowinski and Fitt 1980) have indicated that intense suicidality, impulsivity, extreme disorganization and unremitting addiction were the psychopathological dimensions which ruled people out from the day hospital alternative. Not more than 31% of patients referred for inpatient hospitalization at Washington Heights Community Mental Health Center in Manhattan and only 25% in the McLean (a private nonprofit hospital) study (Washburn et al. 1976) were found to be clinically ineligible for the day hospital. (In the latter study, this percentage was arrived at after 2 to 6 weeks of inpatient evaluation.) The major nonclinical factors which interfered with the partial hospital referral were inexperience or lack of familiarity with partial hospitalization by the evaluating psychiatrist, inability to finance the day hospital alternative or unavailability of a suitable supporting domicile. These factors were particularly applicable to the middle range of all patients who were considered to need more inpatient stay. At the same time, psychopathologically speaking, they were considered eligible for treatment in either the day or inpatient setting. On the other hand, it was a highly selected, very sick population that required intensive, sustained hospitalization as the only viable alternative.

From the above studies one is able to conclude that about 70% of a seriously ill population referred for inpatient care can, within 1 day to 6 weeks, be effectively managed in a non-inpatient program. However, one half of these will require the intensity of a day hospital. This is not to say that other community alternatives such as home visiting, as described by Pasamanic (1967), treatment apartments, as described by Pollock and Kirby (1976), or training in community living, as described by Stein and Test (1976), could not be employed in lieu of the day hospital. Each of these alternatives could serve as the core or base for the treatment, depending on the balance of chronic patients and the treatment units available in a catchment area. The common denominator in all, however, is the organized treatment team in a nonhospital setting, in which each patient has an identified clinical administrator—a psychiatrist or other qualified mental health professional—who orchestrates a program for which the goals and process are actively negotiated with the patient. None of these alternatives can achieve the management of 95% of all mental hospital referrals, which was eloquently prophesized by Winston and Crowley in a paper at the American Psychiatric Association Meeting of 1970. In fact, considerable creativity and activism is necessary to achieve the 70% estimation mentioned above.

Consider the following case: I have observed the long-term management of an adult, impaired with schizophrenia since childhood, in a day program with many community adjuncts. This patient lived at home with companions employed by the family to be with him around the clock. Periodic excitements have been controlled by use of no more than 4 or 5 hours of inpatient structure, and more recently through the effects of a very clear-cut behavior modification program. Periods of individualized therapy, special education activities, prevocational training, speech therapy, medications, etc., have all been used in a coordinated program for limited periods. I have been asked many times by colleagues who viewed this patient on the hospital grounds, "Why is he not in the disturbed male unit?" Given his slow but perceptible progress, the fact that his life has been lived at home within the neighboring community and the fact that he knows his family and his family values his presence, there is no demonstrated program, inpatient or otherwise, which could offer more.

Thus, if the support system is adequate and the family and the community are willing to tolerate the inconvenience and disruptions and stress of seeing psychopathology in their midst, some extremely impaired chronic patients can be advantageously managed in a community-based day hospital.

Before viewing partial hospital treatment and outcome in more detail, let us note the expectations and attitudes of the referring professionals. A study by Grob and Washburn (1976) noted that the referring persons referred to the inpatient service when they were looking for relief for the disruptive stress of acute disorganization or antisocial behavior on the part of the patient. In contrast, they tended to refer to the day hospital to help a regressed person reorganize and rehabilitate in a clearly defined and structured program over a sustained period of time. Persons referred to the inpatient service in fact showed a greater frequency of acute symptomatology and recent changes in their immediate environments. Those initially referred to day hospital from the community tended to have experienced less hospitalizations, and fewer had evidence of cognitive dysfunction. On the other hand, day hospital patients referred from the inpatient service for aftercare were characterized by more serious pathology as well as chronicity. The majority of the patients in the inpatient and day hospital samples studied were schizophrenic. In contrast with samples described in prior reports, the day sample was not predominantly female, but rather, was equally divided between the sexes.

The range of specific and milieu treatments, as well as the variety of professional staff, are analogous to those seen in inpatient settings. The outstanding difference, of course, is that day hospitals' treatment periods are usually for only 4- to 8-hour intervals. The openness of the physical setting requires the partial hospital staff to constantly attend to the state of interpersonal relationships with any patient. A formal "visiting period" may serve as patient introduction to this system, to give an estimate as to whether the patient can cope and to assess whether sufficient relationships with the treatment team can develop. Similarly, at times of stress, when impulsivity and gross aberrant symptomatology begin to reappear, the supportive aspect of the interpersonal relationship based on positive ties is the primary tool which can be brought to bear to guide the person through a tumultuous period. Previous creative negotiations called forth both by patients and staff offer a form of constructive alliances which, in the subsequent periods of stress, make it possible for the patient to accept the discomfort of sustained attendance or structuring in the program as an alternative to 24-hour hospitalization.

DOES THE PARTIAL HOSPITAL HAVE A UNIQUE CLIENTELE?

There is not a clear answer to this question, especially when the clientele of the partial hospital is compared to some other settings. If a person has a diagnosis of appendicitis and requires abdominal surgery, it is clear that only an inpatient hospital with operating room facilities would be sufficient. Similarly, for the treatment of moderate anxiety neurosis or reactive depression, the simplest setting, such as the private office of an outpatient clinic, is clearly appropriate. Placement in the day hospital appears more complex. The history of mental hospitals in the last one hundred years documents the overcontrol and the undertreatment of the major chronic illnesses, especially chronic schizophrenia. The day hospital is uniquely structured to deliver sufficient psychopharmacological and psychosocial treatment in concert with sheltered community living, so that the patient is not overstimulated into relapse, or understimulated and allowed to drift into a social breakdown syndrome period.

The placement of patients in a day hospital is done with confidence, or not at all, depending on the referers past experience with such a setting. It has been well documented by Mendel and Rapport (1963), Washburn (1976) and others that psychiatric trainees tend to overrefer to an inpatient setting for the management of a psychiatric emergency. Familiarity and experience with less intensive levels of care are necessary factors in fostering their actual use. Once given a real option, it is a rare patient or family member who regrets having opted for partial care. There is a strong appeal for the opportunity to receive intensive psychiatric care without having to live in a 24-hour hospital and especially without having to live behind locked doors. Not only does the patient maintain a major element of responsibility for his own life management, but he continues to be a factor in the family life. Thus, any capacity to serve as a companion, sexual partner, or a functional role as cook or household maintenance person is continued. "The waters never completely close over his spot," and emotionally he cannot be forgotten. Naturally, these matters which pertain to the quality of life are less powerful as influences in patient referral patterns if solid partial hospital or other inpatient alternatives are not available. In situations where such facilities exist, the life quality issues are further supported by the therapeutic advantage, which has been repeatedly demonstrated. This will be further documented in detail in the section on patient outcome.

To deal with the question of proper fit of patient to partial hospital setting, most units have made provision for a "visiting" process. This occurs after initial screening by a pre-admissions social worker in which it is determined that the patient has a need for more than office treatment but is not so impulsive or self-destructive that community tenure is clearly impossible. Usually the patient spends some time familiarizing himself for several days with the program. Simultaneously, the partial hospital staff begins some initial engagement and fitting of the patient to the spectrum of social and educational groups available. Experienced staffs comfortable with this modality can make the judgment rapidly. It should be emphasized that the patient's capacity to develop a meaningful relationship to the staff is the primary vehicle for therapeutic engagement and social stability. The development of this requires time to evolve. An empirical assessment as to the rate and capacity for this relationship is of great value to all concerned. If the patient cannot so engage the day or evening program in a reasonable length of time, it is logical to refer to a higher-intensity 24-hour care. At the initiation of the Fort Logan program in the early 1960s (Glascote et al. 1969), all patients were referred to the day hospital. It soon became clear that for a day hospital load of some 50 to 70 patients, an inpatient unit of 5 or 6 beds was initially needed for those who could not be sustained clinically in the day hospital. Ultimately more beds were required.

CLINICAL OUTCOME

In the past two decades the psychiatric partial hospitalization movement has been strengthened by validation through outcome studies. These have often taken the form of naturalistic longitudinal followups of a cohort of day hospital patients during or after treatment exposure. Sometimes they have involved the assessment of two or more comparison groups observed over similar periods. The former method is basically an extension of the clinical case method in which the individual's mental state is diagnosed, treatment is carried out and the patient's condition is observed months or years after treatment. In the case method, it is assumed but not proven that alterations in the patient's condition following exposure to specific treatment or treatment settings are related to the imposed treatment factors. The observation of a cohort of cases, rather than a single case, gives the opportunity to observe trends in larger numbers. This yields more credence to the proposition that clinical change following exposure to an identified treatment variable is related to that variable. This, of course, becomes even more believable if relapse occurs when the treatment is removed, and if improvement occurs in individual or multiple cases when treatment exposure is renewed. On the other hand, the introduction of a true comparison group gives the possibility of a much more convincing case that the independent treatment variable, or treatment setting, is the factor responsible for the differential longitudinal outcome observed. A crucial dimension, of course, is to make explicit the degree of similarity of the groups being compared.

The clinician informally draws on various combinations of patients in various groups that he has treated through his career and makes conclusions regarding these rough groups without any scientific estimate of their similarity. Although a rough comparison of the outcome of cohorts of patients from different studies has traditionally been carried out in the past, the results of this process are becoming more quantifiable with the beginning of the use of standardized scales of symptom intensity and social and vocational role functioning. More specifically, the Global Assessment Scale of Spitzer et al. (1976) and the Functional Baseline Scale of Krowinski and Fitt as applied by Davenport (1979) are now making intercohort comparisons between different settings possible. These scales give a quantitative rating which can be used as a "generalizable marker" of the type of clinical pathology being addressed. Nevertheless, the more convincing type of comparison methodology continues to be that in which cases are matched by important demographic and clinical variables. The cases are even more convincing when they fall into the comparable groups achieved by random assignment. The groups are then seen by statistical comparison to be similar except, of course, for the effects of independent treatment variables to which they are exposed.

The past two decades have witnessed the completion of large numbers of controlled studies in which the day hospital has been compared not only with inpatient treatment but with other outpatient settings as well. I will now proceed to briefly review the most important of these studies.

The 4- to 7-year followup study of the first hundred patients in the day hospital of a nonprofit private psychiatric hospital (Washburn and Grob 1973) indicated that 79% of all patients showed improved "current adjustment," 8% were unchanged, and 12% were worse. Current adjustment was a global rating which included mental status, interpersonal functioning and social role effectiveness. The fact that data for this rating was obtained by independent interviewers added to their credibility. The population consisted of chronic and residual schizophrenics, as well as patients with affective disorders and personality-disordered patients. They were compared with long-term inpatient followups from the Chestnut Lodge (Schulz 1963) and/or Hillside Hospital (Levenstein et al. 1966) studies. These comparisons suggested that the superior day hospital outcome might be due to differences in setting. On the other hand, the likelihood that the inpatient samples were a sicker group to begin with could not be refuted.

When clinicians argue the pros and cons of the one setting over another, a good deal of heat may be engendered. One of the reasons for this is that clinicians in either setting may be observing an overall improvement of their patient population from one time period to another. In the study by Washburn et al. (1976) of a day and inpatient population, this was clearly the case. Either across both samples, or within each sample, there was significant improvement from one time period to the next at 6, 12 and 18 months. Thus, enthusiasts of any setting are not just expressing their bias when they say patients definitely improved when exposed to their program.

Now let us look at some of the more convincing comparisons, "harder data" which has accumulated regarding partial hospital effectiveness. The patient mix at most day hospitals and, thus, in the studies discussed, are predominantly schizophrenic, and within the schizophrenic category the majority of patients are chronic schizophrenic. Thus, they either have had symptoms for long periods of time or repeated hospitalizations which attest to the severity, if not the absolute chronicity, of the problem. Wilder et al. (1966), in his 2-year followup of patients randomly assigned at point of entry to a municipal hospital emergency unit, found overall that there was no difference in the outcome of those whose treatment consisted on the average of 2 months of inpatient stay versus those with 6 weeks in the day hospital. In terms of personal satisfaction, patients and families generally preferred the latter. Based on a global 10-point outcome measure, schizophrenic women generally fared best in the day hospital; paranoid schizophrenic men showed little advantage in that setting. However, it is important to note that over the 2-year followup period, relapse rates reflected in rehospitalization were high, approximately 40% in both settings. Consequently, the authors concluded that extensive aftercare, after the initial intense treatment, was essential to maintain the improvements and to prevent such frequent rehospitalizations.

The extensive studies of Herz and colleagues (1971, 1975) at an urban community mental health center used two different study methodologies. In his initial study, patients on the same ward were randomly assigned to the day or inpatient mode after evaluation for 1 or 2 overnights in the emergency unit. Those randomly assigned to day treatment returned home at night. In the early months of comparison, the day treatment sample had a clearly superior outcome in terms of symptom control and role functioning. These differences tended to wash out at the 2-year mark, but some social role advantages were still maintained. In the second design, he randomly assigned all patients referred for treatment as inpatients in the mental health center to three groups: one received the usual inpatient treatment; one received a brief inpatient stay of 10 to 20 days plus outpatient followup; a third received a brief inpatient stay with the option of day hospital followup, an opportunity which was used by about half of that group. In each time period up to one year, the results tended to favor the brief inpatient–day hospital sample. However, at 18 and 24 months, the differences again tended to "wash out." Although schizophrenic patients in the study tended to be readmitted more frequently than other diagnostic groups, there was no difference in this across the three samples studied.

In her study of matched cases treated in a State Hospital inpatient unit versus those of like pathology assigned to the day hospital, Michaux et al. (1973) reported an initial advantage in the treatment of schizophrenic patients in the inpatient setting, particularly in the dimension of "intropunitiveness." In the followup phases of 12 and 24 months, this difference diminished. On the other hand, the greater improvement in social role functioning in the day patients continued throughout.

In a most recent study the day hospital was used as an initial alternative to inpatient care. At the General Hospital of Reading, Pa., Krowinski and Fitt (1980) found that the initial outcome advantage at discharge in terms of role functioning was sustained at 2 years, and there was no symptom disadvantage for the day hospitalization group.

Although it seemed to have little impact at the time, the first convincing study of the use of the day hospital as an alternative to rehospitalization at time of relapse was carried out by Kris (1960) at the Manhattan State Hospital. The relapsing chronic patients were randomly assigned to the day hospital or state hospital receiving unit. The average stay of the former was 7 weeks, whereas those who became inpatients experienced the then-average stay of 9 months. About twice as many day hospital patients as inpatients were able to return to work in the one-year followup, although social adjustments were the same.

These studies, by and large, show essentially equal outcome in terms of symptom remission, but a definite advantage in social role capacity for the day patient samples.

Now let us look at the studies where the day hospital has been used primarily to serve as an aftercare function following a brief period of inpatient care. In a study involving middle and upper socioeconomic class patients, Washburn et al. (1976) randomly assigned patients requiring further inpatient hospitalization after a 2 to 6 week period to the day or inpatient units. This study had the advantage in that all major areas of patient behavior were assessed. Thus, the outcome differences were not subject to the often heard criticism, "different results would have been noted if only the omitted alternate behavior had also been studied." Clinical change was evaluated through the use of the Psychiatric Status Schedule and Psychiatric Evaluation Forms of Spitzer and his colleagues (1977) and on rating scales for family and community adjustment adapted from Meltzoff and Blumenthal (1966); scales of burden on family, social roles and days of attachment to the hospital, etc., were assessed. Although there was no difference between settings by major diagnosis, day patients fared equally as well as the inpatients at 18- to 24-month followup on most measures, and they fared specifically better in the areas of subjective distress, community functioning, burden on the family, cost and days of attachment. In another study done at another private nonprofit setting, when the day hospital was used as an initial alternative to inpatient care or as a means of earlier discharge from inpatient care, the outcome (Fink et al. 1978) from matched cases in both symptoms and role functioning variables was similar.

Looking at all these aftercare studies, one naturally asks the question, is there any difference in the use of day hospital as aftercare compared with the employment of psychotropic drug treatment in an outpatient clinic? Fortunately, an extensive study of chronic schizophrenic patients in 10 VA hospitals carried out in the late

1970s by Linn and coworkers (1979) addressed that question. Patients in 10 hospitals were randomly assigned after discharge to receive day treatment plus psychotropic drugs or psychotropic drugs alone. There is no main effect difference in terms of community tenure for the two treatment conditions. However, the day treatment group produced significant social improvement compared with the outpatient drug maintenance group. Six of the day centers significantly delayed relapse, reduced symptoms and changed attitudes. These results seemed compatible with the study by Meltzoff and Blumenthal (1966) of chronic schizophrenic patients randomly assigned to day hospital or outpatient clinic. They found that the lower-adjusted patients improved significantly more in day hospital as compared to outpatient in terms of interpersonal adjustment, family adjustment and self-concept. Similarly, Guy et al. (1969) at the Baltimore Psychiatric Day Care Center found that schizophrenic patients improved, whereas a neurotic group did better in the outpatient clinic.

At this point, it would be timely to comment on the question as to why patients do as well or better in the day hospital than in other standard settings. Washburn et al. (1976) postulated that the superior outcome in the day hospital as compared with the inpatient setting was due to a *systems effect*. The patients' expression of psychopathology tends to keep the day hospital staff as well as the family in a state of unbalance, which calls for creative support, resolution of tension, the opportunity for more venture into community life with subsequent stress, some degree of decompensation, and then further creative support and resolution. The usual inpatient setting on the other hand, especially if it is locked, has a patient–staff interaction which is much more focused on the setting of controls, privileges and goals, with tensions set around these issues rather than around those related to the realities of everyday living. Furthermore, families continue to experience the day patient as an important part of the family circle.

Some quantitative validation of the systems theory was seen in the data collected as to the use of social work contacts by family members (Vannicelli et al. 1976). In general, families of day hospital patients were seen as needing more assistance, as being less capable of coping with the situation at certain time periods. All of this was congruent with the notion that the professional workers were kept on edge by the realities of the families whose patient was in their midst. They were stimulated to be more alert, more on guard and creatively more on edge than those professionals working with the families of inpatients.

In addition to these social role and systems effects, other etiological factors may include: less personal stigma associated with partial hospital attendance, less exposure to the "regressive pull" of inpatient care and avoidance of initial conditioning to its use.

COSTS

The basic cost advantage of any partial hospital service is contained in the fact that round-the-clock coverage is not needed. One shift is required for a day program, a half a shift for an evening program, etc. Moderate-intensity backup can be offered by the use of a night program, which, as with the other services, is open for one shift—i.e., 10:00 P.M. to 7:00 A.M.—but with only a third of the usual staff of a full inpatient unit. For more intensive backup, the brief treatment unit of a psychiatric specialty hospital or a general hospital is appropriate. Anything more intensive would require the use of a 24-hour mental hospital unit already in place.

Another source of cost advantage is the simple structure needed to house a partial hospital program. Any medium-sized home, on a hospital grounds, nearby, or even free-standing in, the community can be converted to service an overall census of 25 to 30 patients with a daily attendance of about half that number. For a day program which aims to serve as an intensive treatment alternative for inpatient hospitalization, the staff/patient ratio would be analogous to that of a well-staffed inpatient unit, i.e., 1 to 4. For a slower-moving chronic population, this can be lessened to a ratio of 1 to 6 or 7 based on the actual daily attendance.

Validation of this theoretical cost advantage has been demonstrated by well-controlled studies carried out in a variety of settings. At the Washington Heights Community Mental Health Center, this was true for the brief inpatient–day patient sample compared with the usual inpatient sample. The advantage in cost for the former for hospital services for 2 years after admission was less than one half that for the inpatients. Endicott et al. (1978). Fink et al. (1978) demonstrated at Butler Hospital in a collaborative study with Blue Cross/Blue Shield that when day hospital was used as an alternative to inpatient for a wide spectrum of psychiatric patients, the initial cost advantage of the less-expensive day hospital alternative was maintained in the 1-year followup at a level of slightly more than one half the inpatient cost. Another collaborative study with Blue Cross/Blue Shield done at the Reading Hospital by Krowinski and Fitt (1980) demonstrated a cost advantage for the day hospital randomized patients of 20/27ths of that for a similar inpatient sample at 6-month followup. In our 24-month followup of the randomized comparison groups in the McLean Hospital Study (Washburn et al.), day patient costs were 8/11ths of that for inpatients for the first 6 months, and one half for the study as a whole. Comparison by Guillette et al. (1978) of day hospital costs to the Aetna Insurance Company with projected costs of the usual inpatient alternatives gave a cost ratio of 16 to 41. It can be argued that the lesser cost reported for day hospital treatment does not always include the costs of room and board or living in a halfway house, etc. Conversely, it does not reflect the income achieved by day or evening patients who are able to work on a part-time basis while continuing their treatment, or the nonpecuniary benefit of community living. All in all, this adds up to a generalization that day-hospital-based treatment is approximately half as expensive as that at the 24-hour hospital. This has lead to the practice in some settings of allowing the clinician and patient the option of converting inpatient hospitalization days in their insurance coverage to day hospital care on a basis of 2 days of day hospital for 1 of inpatient. Insurers unfamiliar with this mode of care delivery always object to this concept, especially when they are unfamiliar with its actual advantages to the patient. However, the concept has worked well in a number of settings such as Blue Cross/Blue Shield in California, United Auto Workers nationwide and the MIT Health Plan. Currently, a bill in the Massachusetts legislature would mandate this type of conversion in all health policies in Massachusetts. This bill has been achieving backing from groups such as the Massachusetts Psychiatric Society, the Massachusetts Medical Society, the Massachusetts Hospital Association and the Massachusetts Association for Mental Health.

Although there has been no controlled study of cost comparisons for a purely chronic population, generally, the lower staff/patient ratios required for the single-staff day program as compared with the round-the-clock 24-hour program assure at least the same comparative cost advantages as those seen in services provided for more acute or subacute patients.

CONSIDERATIONS IN STARTING A PARTIAL HOSPITAL PROGRAM

There should be a perceived and documented need for intensive care for persons on the sick end of the psychopathology spectrum. Data from an outpatient or private practice setting might indicate that a large number of inpatient referrals was customary. Day hospital "places" could be developed in lieu of additional inpatient beds to meet this need. A medium or large inpatient service without an aftercare network could appropriately use partial hospital places for 20% to 30% of its patients after a brief (2 weeks) or moderate-length (6 weeks) hospitalization. An even larger proportion of the long-stay inpatients could be expected to appropriately use the day hospital to make the community transition without relapse and for further rehabilitation. The least expensive way to house a partial hospital service is to begin it on an inpatient ward. Thus, the same living room, office and group meeting areas, backup activity therapies facilities can be used at scheduled times dovetailing or overlapping with inpatient groups. An inpatient unit with a census of 20 could accommodate a day patient census of 10 to 15 patients, especially if they do not attend every day. The crucial element in such an arrangement is to be sure that staff are designated specifically to administrate, support and plan programs with the day patients. Inpatient personnel are naturally most concerned with the lives and treatment of those acutely disturbed persons assigned for 24-hour care, and unless the day patients are realistically assigned staffing hours for their program, it will be of poor quality.

A second, relatively inexpensive arrangement is to develop the day and/or evening program in an existing residence or home on the hospital grounds. An average-sized dwelling can house a day program with a census of up to 25 patients of which presumably about 15 would be present each day. This has great appeal for people who are frightened by the concept of attending a mental hospital and is a definite rehabilitative plus for persons using the day hospital as aftercare. Housekeeping and food-processing chores can readily be used as important patient/staff activities, both for support and in the development of skills of everyday living.

Another model is that of conversion of a portion of an inpatient unit to make places for day patients. This has been done in many state hospitals. The painting and refurbishing to some degree can be carried out by patients and staff as an initial collaborative project which can inexpensively get the unit under way. This service should of course be located near public transportation and should have easy access to other rehabilitative and medical resources on the grounds.

When the need is clear and likely to continue for the next decade, a new facility should be built which includes the best location and space for triage, long-term care and rehabilitation as required by other ingredients of the mental health network. Such a partial hospital unit should relate readily to activity therapies and prevocational and sheltered vocational programs, and should have easy access for and to the community. Day, evening, weekend and special aftercare programs can, in rotation, use the facility for appropriate time spans.

The last model is the free-standing day hospital, located by itself in the community. The successful facilities of this type have had to put a strong emphasis on referral lines with inpatient services and on easy access to a general hospital for brief stays or boarding. Because they are usually not clearly part of a medical setting, free-standing day hospitals have even more trouble than hospital-related units in obtaining insurance coverage by third-party carriers. Of course, this would not necessarily be true for those eligible for funding by a department of mental health or Medicaid.

Nearness to public transportation is essential to facilitate the continuing rehabilitation and autonomy of the individuals using the program. A free-standing partial hospital unit should be especially accessible to patient population areas it serves, as it does not have the built-in referral source which a unit located on an inpatient hospital grounds enjoys.

The sources of funding for patient services must be carefully considered. Most Blue Cross/Blue Shield policies do not include coverage of day or evening hospital care. Nevertheless, there are many types of insurance vehicles that cover these services to some degree, and some cover it very well. For example, Medicare refunds 80% of day program for the seriously disabled who qualify. CHAMPUS formerly covered 75% for relatives of government employees for partial programs in hospital settings. In Massachusetts, Medicaid will refund patient care in settings which have met the Medicare standards and accept the reimbursements of the State Rate Setting Commission. Federal Blue Cross/Blue Shield has covered 70% for a limited period. Of course, many community mental health centers have the capacity to offer day programs through government funding grants. As mentioned previously, the United Auto Workers offers a 2 to 1 conversion of inpatient coverage. General Electric's plan covers 80%. Only the federally funded community mental health centers offer day or evening hospital on a parity with inpatient or outpatient clinic services. Thus, it is extremely important to assess the types of insurance coverage offered to large groups of public or private employees in the area where one is considering the beginning of a new partial hospital program.

One should consider the state of familiarity of mental health professionals in the community with the partial hospital modality. Although patients and families have little problem in grasping the value of the partial hospital concept, many inexperienced professionals react with alarm and anxiety at the presence of a disorganized individual in a day hospital setting. It is crucial to have the explicit backing of the training program director to give trainees in psychiatry, psychology, social work and nursing an exposure to treating a large range of psychiatric patients in these community-based settings. Conceptually, it is initially simpler to assign patients to outpatient or inpatient settings alone. By definition, the partial hospital addresses the range of patients between these two extremes, and thus there is always a matter of experience and judgment in deciding just where the cutoff of this middle third of patients should be.

If adequate transportation is available, a rural setting should be no contraindication to the use of partial hospitalization. A variety of creative models have been successfully used. In one setting, the day hospital is on the first floor of a residence on Main Street, and the night care unit is on the second floor. In another, the treatment team comes to town two days a week, and the patients gather by bus from surrounding communities. In urban settings the time of transportation for practical purposes should be no more than an hour and a half one way. On the other hand, patients may come from a greater distance, experience an afternoon of day care, spend the night on night care, the next day on day care, and then return home. Another option is for the patient to stay in a motel or with a friend for the night. For example, in Newfoundland, at one time, patients came from all parts of the island and stayed in boarding houses while they attended a central day hospital in the main city.

There are a number of sets of standards which have been developed for partial hospital systems and which address particularly the qualifications of staff, the staff/patient ratios for intensive and less intensive levels of care, the importance of easy, reliable access to hospitalization, night care and physical assessment, and criteria for adequate medical record keeping. All require medical management of the treatment programs, but there is variation as to who the chief administrator of the unit may be. The more prominent sets of standards are those established by the American Association for Partial Hospitalization, the Aetna Insurance Company, Medicaid as promulgated in Massachusetts and, of course, the Joint Commission on Accreditation of Hospitals. Currently, JCAH outpatient medical record keeping criteria seem quite appropriate for use in a partial hospital service. The JCAH does not stress specifics of professional utilization of staff/patient ratios as do the other sets of standards. Any new program should address the criteria of the standards which relate to them in their local region, especially those of the third party payors.

Lastly, and perhaps most importantly, are the personality requirements for staff working in a partial hospital setting. Within the standards of good psychiatric practice, a capacity to flexibly meet the disturbed or the stably chronic but limited patient "where he is" is an essential for the initiation and maintenance of a lively and viable partial hospital program. By its very nature, the precise boundaries inherent in office or inpatient practice are not available in partial hospital. It has no locked doors; people can come and go at their own will. In the early phases of program explorations, many patients cannot accept full participation. The staff has to tolerate initially their tentativeness and their reluctance to engage. On the other hand, as patients experience the stimulation of meaningful relationships, it is the social structure of the program which gives both support and strength to the patient to cope with the concomitant internal and external stresses. If staff reacts too rapidly or promptly to move a patient to an inpatient service, the opportunity for mastering life's stresses in an empathetic interpersonal environment may be lost. On the other hand, when aggression, either externally or internally directed, is about to be unleashed, or if it is already out of control, the staff must act promptly and vigorously to limit impulsive expression. Because of the range of psychopathology which is optimally treated in a partial hospital program, it is very helpful if the majority of the staff have had experience on inpatient disturbed units, where the extremes of symptomatology and behavior have been experienced and managed. Without this experience, it is hard for a staff person to realize just how tumultuous things can be without necessarily requiring immediate closure or removal of the disturbing individuals. It is the creative dealing with these trying stresses that indeed may be the factor which gives the partial hospital setting its therapeutic advantage.

CONTINUING SUCCESS OF A PARTIAL HOSPITAL PROGRAM

Once a program has been established and the advantages of newness and innovativeness, the release of creative energies, and unusual teamwork and esprit have passed, what are the principles which ensure a continuing effective service? A way must be found to reenergize the vigor and creativity of the staff on all levels. This can be done by continuing education, by periodically revising in a major way the format of the program and by bringing in outside resource people. The most important factor to prevent burnout is to sustain a sense of importance and integrity for every member of the staff and to develop some method of rewarding staff for creative alignments with difficult patients and for moves towards innovative programming for these patients. Secondly, if there is a parent institution, it is essential that there by administrative support for the appropriate flow of aftercare from an inpatient service. This is, of course, a two-way street, and the referring inpatient service should be used when day patients require a more intensive, round-the-clock level of care. If trainees are involved, the leaders of those programs must be kept up to date in supporting the students to become familiar with the special anxieties and uncertainties that treatment of sick people in a community program entail. Similarly, efforts must be made to involve attending psychiatrists and other persons in the referral network, either as consultants or as participants in an updating educational program regarding the partial hospital. Lastly, the financial difficulties of patients in paying for such services out of pocket and their insurance opportunities must be actively matched. At the same time, the cost effectiveness of these services justify the degree of sacrifice that the out of pocket investment may require, and these advantages have to be communicated to prospective patients and families.

REFERENCES

American Psychiatric Association. Position Statement adopted by the Assembly of District Branches, October 13-15, 1978, and Board of Trustees, December 9-10, (1978).

Davenport, B. A cost-effective model for psychiatric day treatment, in *Proceedings of the Annual Conference on Partial Hospitalization: 1978*, R. Luber, J. Maxey, and P. Lefkovitz, eds. Boston: Federation of Partial Hospitalization Study Groups, Inc., 1979, pp. 149-158.

Davenport, B. Personal Communication, 1980.

Endicott, J., Herz, M. I., and Gibbon, M. Brief versus standard hospitalization: The differential costs. *Amer. J. Psychiat.* 135(6): 707-712, 1978.

Fink, E. B., Longabaugh, R., and Strout, R. L. The paradoxical underutilization of partial hospitalization. *Amer. J. Psychiat.* 135(6): 713-716, 1978.

Glascote, R., Kraft, A. M., Glassman, S., and Jepson, W. Partial hospitalization for the mentally ill. *American Psychiatric Association* (1969).

Grob, M., and Washburn, S. L. Factors effecting referral to inpatient and day hospital services. *Proceedings of the Annual Conference on Partial Hospitalization.*, R. F. Luber, J. T. Maxey, and P. M. Lefkovitz, eds. Federation of Partial Hospitalization Study Groups, Inc., Atlanta, Georgia: 1976.

Guy, W., Gross, M., Hogarty, G. E., and Dennis, H. A controlled evaluation of day hospital effectiveness. *Archives of General Psychiatry* 201: 329 (1969).

Herz, M. I., Endicott, J., and Spitzer, R. L. Day versus inpatient hospitalization: a controlled study. *Amer. J. Psychiat.* 127: 1371-1382 (1971).

Herz, M. I., Endicott, J., and Spitzer, R. L. Brief hospitalization of patients with families: initial results. *Amer. J. Psychiat.* 132: 413-418 (1975).

Hogarty, G. E., Dennis, H., Guy, W., and Gross, G. M. Who goes there?—a critical evaluation of admissions to a psychiatric day hospital. *Amer. J. Psychiat.* 124: 94-104, (Jan. 1968).

Hogarty, G. E., Goldberg, S. C., and Schooler, W. R. Drug and sociotherapy in aftercare of schizophrenic patients II: Two-year relapse rates. *Archives of General Psychiatry* 31: 603-608 (1974).

Kris, E. Prevention of rehospitalization through relapse control in a day hospital, in *Mental Patients in Transition,* Milton Greenblatt, ed. Springfield, Ill: Charles C. Thomas, 1961.

Krowinski, W. J., and Fitt, D. X. On the clinical efficacy and cost effectiveness of the psychiatric partial hospital versus traditional inpatient care with six-month followup data. *Community Mental Health Journal* (1980).

Levenstein, S., Klein, D. F., and Pollack, M. Follow-up study of formerly hospitalized voluntary psychiatric patients: the first two years. *Amer. J. Psychiat.* 122: 1102-1109 (April 1966).

Linn, M., Caffey, E., Klett, J., Hogarty, G., and Lamb, H. R. Day treatment and psychotropic drugs in the aftercare of schizophrenic patients. *Archives of General Psychiatry* 36: 1055-1066 (1979).

Meltzoff, J., and Blumenthal, R. L. *The Day Treatment Center: Principles, Applications and Evaluation.* Springfield, Ill.: C. C. Thomas, 1966.

Mendel, W. M. and Rapport, S. Outpatient treatment for chronic schizophrenic patients. *Archives of General Psychiatry* 8: 190-196 (1963).

Michaux, M. H., Chelst, M. R., Foster, S. A., Pruim, R. J., and Dasinger, E. M. Postrelease adjustment of day and full-time psychiatric patients. *Archives on General Psychiatry* 29: 647-651 (1973).

Morgan, R. Conversations with chronic schizophrenic patients. *British Journal of Psychiatry* 134: 187 (1979).

Pasamanic, B., Scarpette, F., and Dinitz, S. Schizophrenics in the community, an experimental study in the prevention of hospitalization. *Sociology Series.* Appleton-Century-Crofts, 1967.

Pollack, P. R., and Kirby, M. W. Followup evaluation of an inpatient alternative program in a Symposium in *Followup Studies of Community Care*, M. Greenblatt and R. Budson, eds. *Amer. J. Psychiat.* 133(8): 916-921 (1976).

President's Commission on Mental Health, Volume 1, Stock No. 040-000-00390-8, U.S. Government Printing Office, Washington, D.C. (1978).

Schulz, C. G. A follow-up report on admissions to Chestnut Lodge 1948-1958. *Psychiat. Quart.* 37: 220-233 (1963).

Segal, S. P. and Aviram, U. *The Mentally Ill in Community-Based Sheltered Care.* New York: Wiley Interscience, 1978.

Spitzer, R. L., Gibbon, M., and Endicott, J. Global Assessment Scale (GAS), in *Resource Materials for Community Mental Health Program Evaluation,* H. A. Hargreaves, C. C. Attkisson, and J. E. Sorenson, eds. DHEW Publication No. ADM 77-328, U.S. Government Printing Office, Washington, D.C. (1977).

Stein, L. I., and Test, M. A. Training in community living: one year evaluation, in *Followup Studies of Community Care,* M. Greenblatt and R. Budson, eds. *Amer. J. Psychiat.* 133(8): 916-921 (1976).

Taube, C. A., and Redick, R. W. Provisional data on patient care episodes in mental health facilities, 1975. *Mental Health Statistical Note No. 139,* DHEW Publication No. (ADM) 77-158, Washington, D.C., (Aug. 1977).

Vannicelli, M., Washburn, S. L., and Scheff, B-J. Partial hospitalization—better but why and for whom? *Journal of Community Psychology* 6: 357-365 (1978).

Washburn, S. L., and Grob, M. Psychiatric day care patients—four to seven year outcome. *Mass. J. Mental Health IV:* 16-36 (1973).

Washburn, S. L., Vannicelli, M., Longabaugh, R., and Scheff, B-J. A controlled comparison of psychiatric day treatment and inpatient hospitalization. *J. of Consulting and Clinical Psychol.* 44(4): 665-675 (August 1976).

Washburn, S. L., Vannicelli, M., and Scheff, B-J. Irrational determinants of the place of psychiatric treatment. *Journal of Hospital and Community Psychiatry* 27(3): 179-182 (March 1976).

Wilder, J. F., Levin, G., and Zwerling, I. A two-year follow-up evaluation of acute psychotic patients treated in a day hospital. *Amer. J. Psychiat.* 122: 1095-1101 (April 1966).

Winston, H., Crowley, R., McCormack, J., Goldberg, D., Meng, R., Nardini, J., and Levensohn, Z. Ariadne's spool: the independent day hospital. *Scientific Proceedings of the 123rd Annual Meeting of the American Psychiatric Association,* p. 246, California, (May 1970).

Zwerling, I., and Wilder, J. F. An evaluation of the applicability of the day hospital in treatment of acutely disturbed patients. *Israel Annals of Psychiatry and Related Disciplines* 2: 162-185 (1964).

CHAPTER 10

PSYCHOSOCIAL REHABILITATION CENTERS: OLD WINE IN A NEW BOTTLE

SAMUEL GROB, Ph.D.

I. INTRODUCTION

The President's Commission on Mental Health in the Report to the President in 1978, 17 years after the landmark report of the Joint Commission on Mental Illness and Health in 1961 to President Kennedy, reaffirmed with the hindsight of experience the need for correction of the deficiencies in deinstitutionalization and in community-based services for the chronically mentally ill population as *a national priority* (1). Though much progress is noted as having taken place since the first report, continued neglect of this population in the establishment of services is acknowledged as a recalcitrant problem bedeviling the country. The fact that this problem was a primary motivating factor for the first study only underscored the need, problem and failure. Detailed specifications of these deficiencies were amply documented in the 1976 report of the Senate Subcommittee on Long-Term Care (2) and the 1977 GAO Report to Congress (3). At the same time, the National Institute of Mental Health began to respond to this widespread criticism by a somewhat belated, agonized reappraisal of the role of community mental health centers. These considerations and resulting recommendations constituted much of the material which finally entered into the report of the Commission's special, if less well-known, Task Panels on Community Support Systems and Deinstitutionalization, Rehabilitation, and Long-Term Care. Though these reports now provide a comprehensive and far-reaching reevaluation of this problem, high priority was given to redefining concepts and methodology for new social approaches for effective implementation. A review of the background may provide insight into some original oversights and, concurrently, a better perspective for a redirection of effort.

Buried among the voluminous reports of the Joint Commission on Mental Illness and Health in 1961 is reference to a 1958 study of ex-mental patient organizations (4). Only 70 such organizations were found; California was the state with the greatest number—14. Of these 70, the largest number could be classified as *social clubs* whose activities were essentially social and recreational in nature. A smaller number could be classified as *therapy groups*, which were generally smaller in size than the social clubs and oriented to verbal interaction of a more therapeutic nature under professional leadership. A variant of this development was Recovery, Inc., which claimed 250 groups alone (5). However, this movement, like Alcoholics Anonymous, offers a somewhat ritualized and limited form of group therapy under lay leadership, compared with the more informal, broadly based socialization activities of the social club or the more professionally led therapy groups. Some note is made of the existence of eight *social rehabilitation centers* in North America, of which Fountain House, Inc., in New York City was the best known, and whose schedule of activities was divided between a day vocational program for those not yet able to work and an evening program for expatients who worked full-time. This latter program was the first sign in this country of the need for programs in the community based explicitly on the concept of the schizophrenic patient as suffering from inadequate socialization, or as it came to be called "the social breakdown syndrome" (6) Almost as an afterthought, an imaginative suggestion of the Task Force on Social Approaches to Mental Patient Care to the Joint Commission (7) was that a departure from the mental health center medical model could be a socialization center model for dealing with problems conceived as psychosocial disabilities rather than as "mental illness." The program would be designed to reeducate and resocialize persons by way of interpersonal and group interactions in specified milieus. Further, this model was conceived as a combination of home, school, and community center, oriented toward the resocialization of its trainees through relationships in peer groups, such as workshops, classes, activity groups, and social-recreational and cultural programs. In this social training model, trainees could experiment with new roles, learn new values and norms, and participate in meaningful and satisfying relations conducive to mental health. Unfortunately, although support and research was recommended for this model in the final report, this note had little impact on subsequent developments.

II. HISTORICAL ANTECEDENTS TO SOCIAL APPROACH

Early in the 1930s, Sullivan, the neoFreudian famous for his work with young schizophrenic patients, concluded that his positive results came from his use of a sociocultural approach. He saw his patients improve in *social* insight rather than in personal insight into the roots of behavior as Freud had believed. He came to strive for the path to *social* recovery through the medium of a sympathetic environment. Intimations of both Adler and Skinner may be seen in his formulation: "Given the correct situation, the 'social' recovery goes far towards a 'real' recovery and certainly includes much of a true reorganization of the disordered personality. . . . The sympathetic environment to which I refer is a group of persons, some 'psychotic' (patients), some relatively 'sane' (personnel); in the latter of whom there is conscious formulation of *community* with the more disordered ones, and a deliberate, rather than a good-naturedly, unconscious purpose to enter into the life of the patient to a beneficial goal. . . . the situation is one of education, broadly conceived, not by verbal teaching but by communal experience . . . good tutoring." Of parenthetical interest is his foresight in predicting an increase in the relapse rate without the intervention of "convalescent camps and communities for those on their way to mental health" (8).

A development parallel to the psychoanalytic tradition and destined to play a significant role in psychosocial rehabilitation of chronic schizophrenic patients is the group psychotherapy movement (10). Although claims to its paternity conflict, the first conscious and deliberate application of the principles of group psychotherapy was not made in the treatment of psychoneurotic or psychotic patients, but in tubercular patients. Pratt, an internist at the Boston Dispensary, discovered as early as 1905 that when his tubercular patients met in a class for instructions from him, they seemed to derive mental stimulation, encouragement and satisfaction from the company of their fellow patients. As a result of this experience, he extended the application of this method to include patients suffering from other chronic illnesses (9). It was not long before classes were organized for diabetics, cardiacs, postpartum patients, hypertensives, ulcer patients, etc.

The first conscious application of group psychotherapy to mental disorders may be attributed to Moreno. In 1921 he opened a spontaneity theater in Vienna which also came to be used in the treatment of mental patients. Later he brought psychodrama to the States. The first theater for this purpose was built at Beacon, New

York, in 1936 exclusively for the treatment of psychiatric disorders and for research (11). St. Elizabeth's Hospital, Washington, D.C., became the first public mental hospital in the United States to introduce Moreno's psychodrama in 1940.

An early, though less known, American psychiatrist, Trigant Burrow, having studied with Freud and Jung, gradually became dissatisfied with the emphasis psychoanalysis placed upon an individualistic assessment of human behavior. As early as 1923, he saw behavior disorders as essentially social or interrelational, requiring observation and study in a more natural dynamic group setting. Actually, he learned this from a patient in the process of analyzing him (12). He spent the next thirty years of his life, at the cost of a successful analytic career, developing the theory and practice of group analysis with this patient—now an associate—and a small group of coworkers, professional and lay. The history of this group, outside the mainstream of official psychoanalytic thought and practice, is the history of the Lifewynn Foundation. Burrow's work does fit into the early history of group psychotherapy though with some notable idiosyncratic features (13). He described his approach as phylobiology, the application of the scientific method to the field of human relations, and phyloanalysis, the method of his particular form of group analysis and research. The basic goal of this research was an understanding of man as a species and the development of unbiased functioning in relation to the real world around him. It should be clear that Burrow conceived and applied this method as a tool of research into generic man's basic nature, his feelings and motivation as part of a group, rather than as a therapy specific to any individual. Through this method he aimed at no less than a science of social behavior, transcending psychoanalysis and embracing biological and social psychological concepts.

Marsh approached group therapy by applying it to patients in mental hospitals by means of group expressive and inspirational techniques almost revival-like in nature. He stated, "I use the crowd psychology to bring their emotional interests into squad formations to discipline and direct them toward life. The aim is to extrovert all energies at the social level" (14). It is interesting to note that he already envisioned at that time institutions for mental patients as schools rather than as hospitals, reeducating rather than treating. Even more striking is his advocacy of an organization of expatients on a national basis in order to help remove the stigma of mental illness. Many of the elements found in psychosocial rehabilitation centers today and considered innovative may be found in Marsh's pioneering work at Worcester State Hospital in the 30s.

Slavson, another pioneer in group psychotherapy during the 30s, began his work with problem children in the care of the Jewish Board of Guardians, New York City. Utilizing psychoanalytic theory, and coming from a background of progressive education popular in the 20s, he believed in the passivity of the therapist and the permissive atmosphere of the group. He summed up his aim as "the modification or elimination of egocentricity and psychological insularity" (15). He subsequently founded the American Group Psychotherapy Association, which has exerted a profound educative influence on developments in psychiatry, community mental health and psychosocial rehabilitation.

The years during World War II and after saw an expansion of group therapy programs in hospitals and clinics of the armed forces and Veteran Administration to meet the needs of large numbers of casualties with limited available personnel. Though often employed as an expedient, this method more often than not surprised sponsors by its unique contribution to the therapeutic enterprise. Although Klapman favored didactic forms of group therapy such as exemplified by Marsh, Lazell, Low, Harris, Hadden, Hamilton and others, more analytically oriented forms of group psychotherapy began to prevail during the war and postwar years, initiated by Wender, Schilder, Slavson, Wolf and Foulkes.

In England Joshua Bierer introduced independently a form of group psychotherapy in a mental hospital. His orientation was Adlerian and had no affinity with group analysis such as practiced by Burrow or Foulkes. He preferred a more leader-centered and more active method. He pioneered a therapeutic approach to the community of the hospital, including day hospital and therapeutic clubs, and great flexibility in the use of situational treatment.

Maxwell Jones began with didactic class and discussion methods, but became more analytic in his orientation after the war. He was particularly known for his institutional work with the "therapeutic community," which consists largely of work with groups in a deliberately therapeutic way. It is a grim irony of history that much of Jones's pioneering work in the 40s and after was presaged by the beginning of milieu therapy in Germany during the late 20s prior to the Hitler period. It was the early work in Germany which influenced people like Marsh and Myerson in Massachusetts in their "total push" treatment and the Menninger brothers in Topeka, Kansas.

Social interaction thus began to be used consciously and planfully as a useful therapeutic experience sui generis. This approach differed from therapeutic community in adhering more strictly to a medical prescriptive model in its use of social interactive process, whereas the therapeutic community model emphasized group treatment and decision making in which patients were participants in the process (16). Bierer suggests that the fortuitous circumstance of his inability to speak English in the mental hospital to which he was attached in 1938 led to his conception of a therapeutic club with participation in leadership and decision making by patients. Subsequently, the shortage of manpower in institutions during World War II had the effect of encouraging the group trend more by default than by design and aided by the work of neoFreudian practitioners and social scientists such as Sullivan and his associates in America.

The gradual incorporation of rehabilitative thinking and practice in the care and treatment of the chronic mental patient adds the final ingredient to our current recipe. Due largely to the influence of psychoanalytic theory and practice since World War II, too much emphasis was placed upon intrapsychic problems alone, to the relative exclusion of social problems of adaptation to prevailing norms of behavior in American life. We had forgotten the lessons of history, and experience from as far back as the late Middle Ages in Gheel, Belgium, and the moral treatment era following the Enlightenment of the late eighteenth century, when social training humanely applied demonstrated positive results while psychiatry as such was only in its infancy.

Rehabilitation gained conceptual clarity twenty-five years ago when Williams defined it as "that form of therapy which is primarily concerned with assisting the patient to achieve an optimal social role [in the family, on the job, in the general community] within his capacity and potentialities" (17). Whatever one's persuasion concerning the cause and cure of mental illness, neither of which is actually established as yet, there is agreement that such illness is usually accompanied by a serious disturbance in the patient's interpersonal behavior. Since we do not know yet how to prevent this form of illness, rehabilitation addresses itself to what is considered in public health terms as tertiary prevention, which aims at control and reduction of disabilities resulting from the illness. One peculiar effect of mental illness, more characteristic of the past, was the widespread use of hospitalization that induced iatrogenic effects of dependency disabilities, secondary to institutionalization. It is not easy to separate these disabilities from those consequent upon the illness alone.

Until World War II, vocational rehabilitation was a small agency in the federal government whose function it was to stimulate appropriate services to the physically disabled. Created initially in 1917 to aid the wounded veterans of World War I, enabling legislation was passed by Congress in 1943 to widen the scope of the agency's efforts to include service to the mentally retarded and the mentally disordered. During the following decade, the funds made available to the agency were greatly expanded and diversified. It was authorized in 1955 to launch an extensive program of grants-in-aid for research and demonstration projects.

This was the period during which this writer and his associates conducted the studies which led to the development of the Psycho-Social Rehabilitation Center in Boston, now known as The Center House. These studies exemplify the introduction of rehabilitation theory and practice into the care and treatment of the mentally ill, both in the institution and in the community. In our first study, we stated (18), "It is generally recognized in the rehabilitation field that the proper employment or placement of the employable ex-patient constitutes an essential part of this recovery process, especially in our work-oriented culture. It is perhaps the first major link in reintegrating the expatient into normal community life. It is basic to both his self-acceptance and social acceptance. It symbolizes his acceptance in a productive role, that is, of contributing value to society as well as receiving some in return." Our conclusion (19) supported by subsequent studies was that only about 10% of the total released population would require vocational rehabilitation services, and for these, "counseling and guidance, *most broadly conceived*, and not traditional vocational rehabilitation services, would be the major service required by expatients, and for long periods of time." The lack of self-esteem and social acceptance appeared to be at the root of the disability presented by this population (20).

The term "rehabilitation" has come to imply a many-sided and multidisciplinary process for the chronic psychiatric patient. The goal is an optimal life adjustment within the limits of continued mental or emotional impairment. Sociocultural norms and attitudes imposed from without, and the subjective perception of the degree of handicap induced by mental illness define the scope of the problem and outcome prospects. Finally, work is conceptualized as part of the socialization process, assuming different forms according to the subculture in which it is embedded (21).

The state vocational rehabilitation agency is showing increasing recognition of social variables. The reorganization of the Department of Health, Education, and Welfare in 1967, establishing the social and rehabilitation services, served to stimulate the incorporation of broad rehabilitation philosophy, goals and practice in mental health programs within hospitals and communities. New rehabilitation professionals are emerging who are trained to bridge the gap between traditional clinical and vocational personnel (22).

III. EARLY BEGINNINGS OF SOCIAL REHABILITATION CENTERS

The Russian Revolution and spread of Marxist thought during the bohemian 20s and depression 30s lent a special enchantment to the importance of social, economic and cultural determinants of individual and social behavior. Alfred Adler was a psychoanalytic offshoot of this influence, an early disciple of Freud who broke away because of his belief in the overriding importance of the social factor. Joshua Bierer, an Adlerian, and a refugee from Nazi Germany, started the first therapeutic social club in Great Britain shortly after he arrived there from Vienna in 1938. Because of the circumstances of his time, he adopted a simple social-psychological model for his therapeutic practice.

The key concept of this model was socialization, by which Bierer meant that process in which the individual acquires behavior appropriate to constructive participation in his society. By contrast, psychoses involved deficiencies in the individual's basic socialization skills within one or more of the following areas: (1) family (2) occupational environment (3) some aspect of general interpersonal relationship. Bierer increasingly centered his efforts on the idea that treatment of the mentally ill should remain within the natural community as much as possible. He was the first to suggest the use of social club therapy as a deliberate treatment modality for mental illness. He defined the aim of the club as the preparation of the patient to adapt himself to everyday social life and participate in normal social functions (23). He predicted that the next steps in psychiatry would be on sociological levels of application and saw such forms as the therapeutic group, the therapeutic club and the community clinic as the milieu therapies of the future that would replace mental hospitals.

We have described the beginnings of new social methods of treatment in our discussion of historical antecedents. A cumulative change in attitudes toward mental hospitals has developed since the

30s in America from growing reaction to traditional forms of seclusion and physical restraint and with the advocacy of open-door policies and the therapeutic community. The term "therapeutic community" was actually coined by Main in describing the pioneering work done at Northfield Hospital, Birmingham, during the latter part of the Second World War (24). The main developer, however, was Maxwell Jones, who in 1946 took over a wing of Belmont Hospital as a treatment unit for semiderelict men. At first it was called the Industrial Neurosis Unit, then the Social Rehabilitation Unit. The program consisted largely of meetings and discussions throughout the day in the form of workshop groups, domestic groups, small psychotherapy groups, staff sensitivity groups and assessment sessions—all designed to increase the individual's awareness and understanding of what he was doing to himself and to other people (25). Many of these ideas and practices have been widely implemented in this country as good social therapy for a wide range of clinical psychopathologies. World War II, by its large-scale utilization of group structure and function, facilitated the use of social therapeutic modalities in psychiatric care systems, which were set up within the armed forces and the Veterans Administration following the war years. The more flexible employment of varied professional disciplines and skills in these systems further encouraged greater experimentation with these new psychosocial approaches.

IV. CURRENT STATUS OF SOCIALIZATION IN THEORY AND PRACTICE

Angyal once defined psychiatry as the application of a science which does not exist (26). A pluralistic universe of models exists today with reference to the etiology and treatment of schizophrenia, including: (1) genetic (sociobiology), (2) biochemical (drugs), (3) psychological (psychoanalysis), (4) learning theory (behavior modification), (5) family dynamics (family therapy), and (6) sociocultural (sociotherapy). Like the elephant and the blind men, each advocate of a special school sees the phenomena from his/her point of view. While this approach may have heuristic value for science, it does not do justice to the complexity and totality of the problem. Throughout history, we have seen emphases fluctuate from one end of the continuum to the other. Having been exposed to all these models at one time or another, and having tested them in the crucible of experience, my associates and I gradually arrived at an eclectic attitude and pragmatic approach as most appropriate to the state of the art. We settled on the common denominator of all theoretical possibilities: namely, socialization, whether curative or meliorative, as a basic therapeutic value sui generis, and as a necessary, if not sufficient, condition of therapy for the chronic psychiatric population. Coleman has given the best nonschematic description of this group: (27)

"If they can be characterized in any way, one may think of them as people who are more vulnerable than others, more easily hurt, less resilient in the face of stress and rejection . . . with a long history of severe characterological problems . . . suffering from a chronic ingrained disturbance. There are many such people in communities and they do not all become patients in mental hospitals. Their relation to others is often tenuous, lacking in closeness, and peripheral. Often, too, they are socially isolated, particularly in terms of their own feelings and need of acceptance which does not impose pressure or demands for emotional response. By and large, these are the most neglected patients in our society, not only because it is so difficult for them to make known their distress but also because, made known, it is often likely to arouse little response of sympathy or concern."

It is estimated that 10-15% of patients become chronic after an acute episode. Klerman has warned that "one of the unintended consequences of decarceration and deinstitutionalization may be new forms of anomie and isolation for the schizophrenic in the community" (28). Research studies by Pasamanick, Zwerling, Gruenberg, Fairweather, Stein and others since the 50s have provided considerable evidence in support of socialization as a crucial factor in the success of deinstitutionalization. While socialization may be broadly conceived as inclusive of areas of work and living arrangements in community life, I will address myself to the basic aspect of socialization encompassed by the relatively new development of what are known as psychosocial rehabilitation centers.

Socialization or resocialization comprise those aims and practices by which former mental patients are enabled to reenter the community and function in socially adaptive ways. The aspect to which I am refering is the socialization process in its purest form, apart from the treatment, residential, vocational and educational components with which it may be associated, but from which it is analytically separate. For the most part this development grew in a spontaneous way out of the needs of mental patients as they were expressed either in self-government attempted while in the hospital or in voluntary associations started after discharge. The first expression of this process had its origin in the early 40s when patients in Rockland State Hospital, N.Y., began meeting on the steps of the New York Public Library. They went under the name of WANA, "We Are Not Alone," without any professional or financial backing other than the help of some volunteers. These informal meetings gradually assumed the form of a social club for mutual aid and emotional support. This is the true founding spirit and basis of the large, multifaceted *Fountain House* as it exists today in its spacious home on 47th Street.

Horizon House, in Philadelphia, was begun in 1953 by a former mental patient and a group of interested citizens mostly from the Society of Friends, also with little psychiatric sponsorship and financial support, but responding to group self-help impulses of expatients in an alien society. This elaborate, diversified program as it exists today is a far cry from these humble beginnings.

Council House, in Pittsburgh, Pennsylvania, began in 1957 as an expatient club sponsored by the local chapter of the National Council of Jewish Women and inspired by the example of Fountain House. Their ground plan was to establish a resocialization program that would serve as a bridge to the community, utilizing existing community resources as sites for program activities.

Thresholds, in Chicago, was founded by the local chapter of the National Council of Jewish Women in 1958 to provide socialization experience to discharged mental patients.

In Massachusetts, the first social club was known as the *103 Club* because of its address near the Boston Psychopathic Hospital, now the Massachusetts Mental Health Center. This club grew out of a patient-government program in 1948. Discharged patients met weekly at club quarters under indigenous leadership with the help of volunteers and hospital staff from across the street. Though not entirely self-governing because of its proximity to the hospital, it enjoyed a surprisingly long life, so long as it maintained charismatic leadership. When the *Center Club* was formed in 1959 by a group of expatients meeting with this author and some volunteers under the sponsorship of the Massachusetts Association for Mental Health, the old 103 Club merged with us at the suggestion of Jack Ewalt, then superintendent of the Massachusetts Mental Health Center.

Comparable programs have proliferated throughout the country, such as Friendship House, Prospect House, The Club in New Jersey, Hill House in Cleveland, Portals House in L.A., Fellowship House in Miami, and many others. Though no two programs are exactly alike, and show variations according to local circumstances, they are in essential respects alike in origin, purpose and program development. Furthermore, over the years they have shown a vigorous growth rate in size and diversity of program, staff and budget, testifying to social need, program effectiveness and staff creativity. New support from NIMH for the development of community support systems for chronic psychiatric patients, reinforced by the report of the President's Commission on Mental Health during the Carter Administration, promises to provide further stimulus to the socialization process as a vital therapeutic component in the network of community mental health modalities.

In 1975 leaders in this development decided to formalize their affinity by organizing the International Association of Psychosocial Rehabilitation Services, the fourth annual conference of which was held in Miami, November 1978. The comprehensive, multi-service rehabilitation agencies into which the early social approaches have grown, now usually allied to community mental health centers, continue to thrive to the extent that they maintain their original social base of consumer input, cooperation and planning within a deeply resistive society.

V. PROGRAM STRUCTURE: MODAL ELEMENTS

The underlying premise of this paper is that socialization as a therapeutic approach for chronic psychiatric patients is not to be considered as a lesser element in the logically compartmentalized package of a rehabilitation-oriented skills-training kit (29). While this is the trend in the process of rationalizing a system of aftercare, the danger is one of sacrificing substance for form, a substitution dear to the heart of the technician, bureaucrat and fiscally minded expert. The inevitable consequence of this trend is to exclude the very patients for whom the system is presumed to care. As psychosocial rehabilitation centers continue to grow into large, multiservicecenters across the country, it is not unlikely that the social impulse which inspired their inception will be subordinated to the economic and bureaucratic pressures traditionally associated with the process of institutionalization.

The elements of socialization outlined below, if adhered to, will serve to immunize us against such contingencies (30). The invisibility and informality of the socialization process makes it difficult to identify and quantify as a general factor underlying and conditioning the long-term success of psychosocial rehabilitation in its various forms. However, these elements are found in most successful centers of this type and reflect qualities rather than quantities of expression implicit, if not explicit, in the structure and function of every program, whatever the nature and degree of skills involved. They have appeared recurrently throughout history and have survived the most rigorous tests of survival. These elements transcend any particular school of thought or discipline:

1. *Culture* Base: Rooted in Judeo-Christian and democratic tradition
2. *Community* Base: Freeing mental patients from a segregated and isolated role in society
3. *Normalization* of Function: Maximizing involvement and participation in natural community activities
4. *Ego Enhancement:* Affirmation of individualism, voluntarism and freedom of choice
5. *Group Therapy:* Exploiting the potentialities of group experience in any modality as the principal vehicle of change
6. *Staff Roles:* Emphasis upon competency, flexibility and diversity, rather than upon status and credentialism, in staff, volunteer and client roles
7. *Planning:* Orientation to process rather than product in program planning
8. *Temporal-Existential:* Primary attention to here and now rather than past or future
9. *Praxis:* Providing varied opportunities for social and self-governance
10. *Rehabilitation Philosophy:* Adapting rehabilitation ideology as a conceptual and instrumental tool.

It is suggested that only to the extent that we legitimate and incorporate these elements in the structures of any community mental health programs will we be enabled to provide effective community support to chronic mental patients. Final validation of results will rest upon the availability of research funds and the capability for mounting definitive, controlled studies (31).

SUMMARY

Throughout history, the mentally ill have been the pariahs of society—rejected, punished, segregated and excluded. A few bright spots have illuminated this otherwise bleak landscape, such as the story of Gheel, Belgium in the late Middle Ages, moral treatment in early nineteenth century America and possibly the current era of community mental health. However, we are slow to learn the lessons of the past.

Since the bold new approach to mental health was inaugurated in 1961, a vast movement of deinstitutionalization has begun, with the result that in ten years the hospital census has been reduced by 60% or better across the country. Yet, as various government reports have pointed out, the care of chronic mental patients, including those remaining in the institution as well as those released to the community, continues to be less than adequate in both quality and quantity relative to the volume of resources now being poured into new systems of care and treatment. True to our historic record, the chronic mental patient provides the main justification for reform in our mental health practices, but gains few of the promised benefits.

A respectable body of theory and practice concerning the care and treatment of the chronic mental patient, dating from the beginning of the twentieth century, forms the knowledge base now available to correct this bias in history and humanity. The core of this knowledge is embodied in the recent development of a psychosocial rehabilitation model for application to this population. Eclectic in theory and pragmatic in adaptation, this model and approach revolve around the fundamental concept of socialization and the utilization of practical techniques for enabling the client to adjust to the requirements of modern life in a socially productive and satisfying manner, despite the residuals of mental illness. This approach has been tried and tested in bits and pieces throughout time, and everywhere found effective. These bits and pieces have also been combined and integrated during the last thirty years to constitute what are now known as psychosocial rehabilitation centers. Examples of this development can be found in all the major cities of America—for instance, Fountain House, N.Y.; Horizon House, Philadelphia; Center House, Boston; Threshold, Chicago; Hill House, Cleveland; Fellowship House, Miami; Portals House, L.A.; and many others.

The heart of these centers is seen to lie in the essential socialization process underlying and connecting, but analytically separable from, the structured services provided, which are specifically social, vocational, residential, educational, cultural, recreational or whatever. This unique process arose spontaneously out of the expressed needs of patients in patient government and has continued to emerge in the community in the form of voluntary associations of expatients, usually called social clubs.

The comprehensive, multiservice, community-based psychosocial rehabilitation center of today requires this social base if it is to fulfill its mission to this population. It is suggested that history will be repeated if a rationalization of this development imposes a new form of institutionalization and bureaucracy, with concomitant fiscal imperatives, to erode the natural social base and deny the basic social needs of this particular patient. As immunity against such an unhappy contingency, ten principal elements are conceptualized for incorporation in any program structure designed specifically for this patient population.

REFERENCES

1. *The President's Commission On Mental Health,* Vol. I and II. U.S. Govt. Printing Office, Wash., D.C. (1978).
2. *Nursing Home Care in the U.S.: Failure in Public Policy.* U.S. Senate Special Committee on Ageing: Subcommittee on Long-Term Care. U.S. Govt. Printing Office, Wash., D.C. (1976).
3. *Returning the Mentally Disabled to the Community: Government Needs to Do More.* U.S. GAO, Wash., D.C. (1977).
4. *Action for Mental Health.* Final Report of the Joint Commission on Mental Illness and Health. New York: Basic Books, 1961.
5. Wechsler, H. The self-help organization in the mental health field: Recovery, Inc., a case study. *J. Neur & Mental Disorders* 130: 297 (1960).
6. Gruenberg, E. M. The social breakdown syndrome. *Am. J. Psychiatry* 123: 1481-1489 (1967).
7. Schwartz, M. S., and Schwart, C. G. *Social Approaches to Mental Patient Care.* New York: Columbia Univ. Press, 1964, pp. 2-9. *Ibid.* pp. 307-8.
8. Sullivan, H. S. Socio-psychiatric research: Its implications for the schizophrenic problem and for mental hygiene. *Am. J. Psychiatry* 87: 977-991 (1930-1).
9. Pratt, J. H. The principles of class treatment and their application to various chronic diseases. *Hosp. Soc. Service* 6: 401 (1922).
10. Klapman, J. W. *Group Psychotherapy.* New York: Grune & Stratton, 1946.
11. Moreno, J. C. Who shall survive? *Nerv. & Ment. Dis.* (1934).
12. Syz, H. *A Summary Note on the Work of Trigant Burrow in Group Psychotherapy and Group Function,* M. Rosenbaum and M. Berger, eds. New York: Basic Books, 1963, p. 159.
13. Burrow, T. The social basis of consciousness. A study in organic psychology, in *The International Library of Psychology, Philosophy, and Scientific Method.* New York: Harcourt Brace, 1927, pp. XV-XVII.
14. Marsh, L. S. Group treatment of the psychoses by the psychological equivalent of revival. *Ment. Hyg.* 15: 328-49 (1931).
15. Slavson, S. R. *An Introduction to Group Therapy.* New York: Commonwealth Fund, 1943.

16. Almond, R. *The Healing Community.* New York: Jason Aronson, 1974, pp. XXI–XIVI.
17. Williams, R. H. Psychiatric rehabilitation in the hospital. *Pub. Health Reports* 11: LXVIII (1953).
18. Olshansky, S., Grob, S., and Malamud, I. T. Employers' attitudes and practices in the hiring of ex-mental patients. *Ment. Hyg.* 42: 391–401 (1958).
19. Olshansky, S., Grob, S., and Ekdahl, M. Survey of employment experiences of patients discharged from three state mental hospitals during period 1951–1953. *Ment. Hyg.* 44: 510–521 (1960).
20. Grob, S. Making the vocational rehabilitation of the mentally ill more effective, in *Report of OVR Region V Conference,* Madison, Wisconsin, pp. 63–4 (March 1960).
21. Neff, W. S. *Work and Human Behavior.* New York: Atherton, 1968, pp. 252–257.
22. Cubelli, G. E., and Havens, L. L. The expanding role of psychiatric rehabilitation, in *Progress in Community Mental Health,* Vol. I, L. Bellak and H. H. Barten, eds. New York: Grune & Stratton, 1969, pp. 167–178.
23. Bierer, J. A self-governed patients' social club in a public mental hospital. *J. Ment. Sci.* 87: 419–26 (July 1941).
24. Main, T. F. The hospital as a therapeutic institution (Bull. Menn. Clinic 1946, 10 p. 66) in *Psychosocial Nursing,* E. Barnes, ed., Tavistock, 1968, pp. 5–11.
25. Jones, M. *Social Psychiatry: A Study of Therapeutic Communities.* Tavistock, 1952.
26. Angyal, A. *Foundations for a Science of Personality.* New York: Commonwealth Fund, 1941.
27. Coleman, J. Adaptational problems characteristic of returning mental hospital patients, in *The Community Social Club and the Returning Mental Patients,* S. Grob, ed. NIMH Conf., Boston (1963).
28. Klerman, G. L. *Community Treatment of Schizophrenics.* New Eng. Conf. on the Chronic Psychiatric Patient in the Community, Boston (1976).
29. Glasscote, R. M. *Rehabilitating the Mentally Ill in the Community.* Study of Psychosocial Rehabilitation Centers, Joint Information Service, APA and NAMH, Wash., D.C. (1971).
30. Grob, S. Psychiatric social clubs come of age. *Ment. Hyg.* 54: 129–136 (1970).
31. Klerman, G. L. *Ibid.* pp. 1–29.

CHAPTER 11

RESIDENTIAL CARE FOR THE CHRONICALLY MENTALLY ILL

RICHARD D. BUDSON

At its best community residential care for the chronically mentally ill provides both sheltered housing and a sustained rehabilitative orientation. This requires careful individual program planning to help the resident grow both within and outside the residence. The entire program is organized with the recognition that it plays a central role in facilitating the resident's development at different psychological, psychosocial and behavioral levels. It encourages individual psychological growth; it fosters socialization by creating an internal social system within the residential milieu; and it enables the resident to play meaningful roles in a variety of external systems—vocational, family, avocational and others. Thus, the community residence not only provides a potentially rich inner life, but it also interacts with an entire spectrum of services outside of its immediate confines which are vital to the successful rehabilitation of the resident. Although this network of community treatment is generally conceived of solely in medical terms, the entire program can in fact be considered to be the fulfillment of normal family function. Thus, as in the normal family, the program insures maturation, socialization, education and vocational preparation for its member (Budson 1978a).

The accompanying figure represents a schematic depiction of the various components of the community residence program. The reader can readily grasp the multifarious system into which the resident enters. Many of the modalities which a resident will encounter

---

A portion of this chapter is reprinted with permission from *The McLean Hospital Journal* 4: 140-157 (1979).

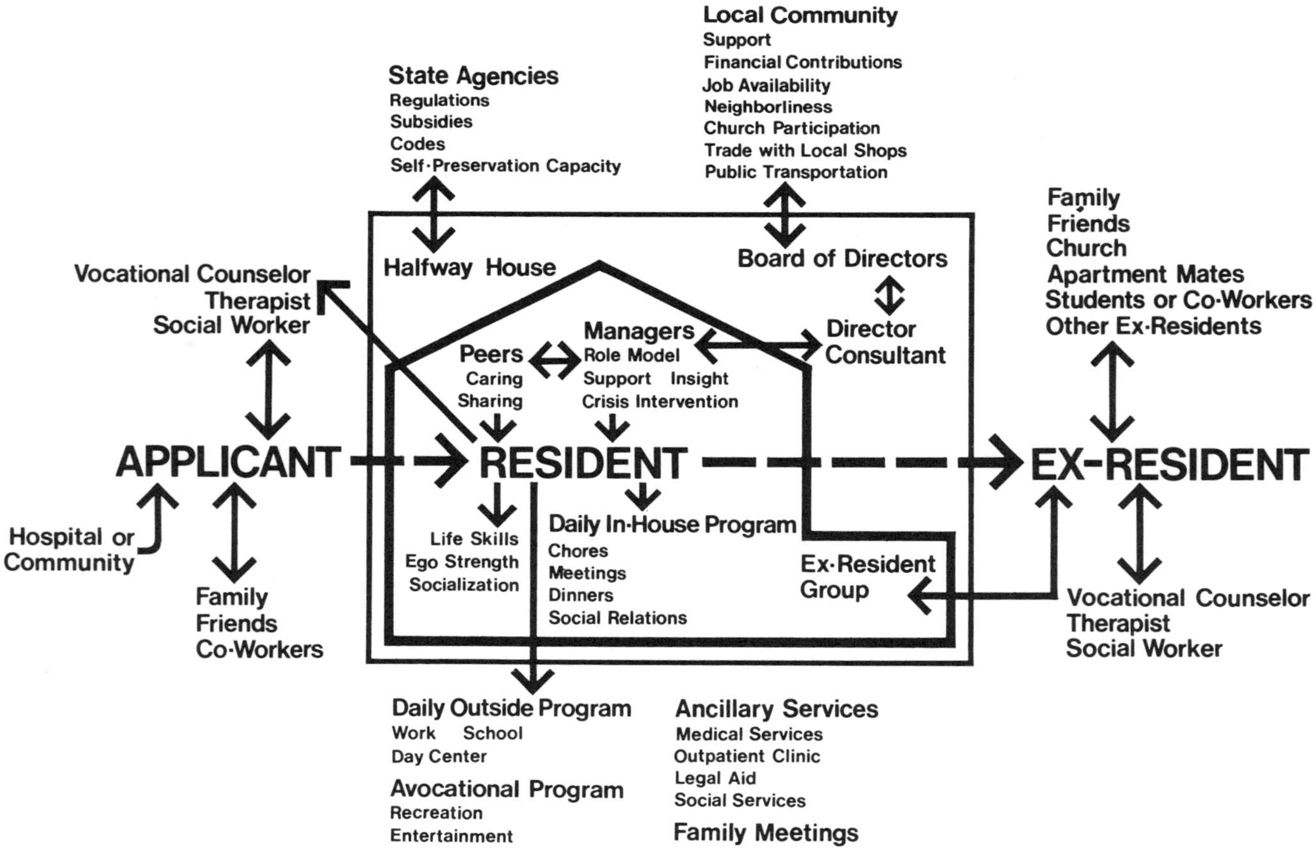

Figure 1. The Community Residence Program. Reprinted from R. D. Budson, *The Psychiatric Halfway House: A Handbook of Theory and Practice*, by permission of the University of Pittsburgh Press. Copyright © 1978 by University of Pittsburgh Press.

during his stay in the community residence are described in accompanying chapters within this book. Thus, through the emerging social network of peers sharing meals, chores and meetings, a caring milieu evolves which enhances the development of life skills and ego strengths. The staff of the program, well versed in the essentials of good psychotherapeutic management, provides role models, support and insight. Crisis intervention is a frequent practice designed to prevent rehospitalization. The social club, day center or vocational setting of the resident makes up his daily program. Medical and outpatient clinic services are part of the normal schedule for monitoring pharmacotherapy. Legal aid and advocacy of social services are available. Family meetings are a frequent part of the program as well. This coordinated program interacts with the local community, purchasing services and goods and receiving various municipal benefits. The quality of the program is assured and community credibility enhanced through the acquisition of the state's regulatory credentials.

Unfortunately, this ideal of a rich and comprehensive program is not representative of all programs. Although many of the community residential facilities currently available nationwide are carefully planned, staffed and operated under professional supervision, an increasing concern of responsible mental health planners is the inadequacy of other housing to which many thousands of patients have been discharged in the name of progress. Often in declining urban areas, these facilities are neither purposefully planned nor adequately supervised, and they represent little improvement over a custodial hospital. This erratic quality of care is partly a reflection of the spontaneous and sometimes chaotic origins of the community care movement.

THE SETTING—THREE DECADES OF CHANGE

Dramatic pharmacological, social and legal changes have shaped community living programs for the chronically ill patient. In the 1950s a revolution in the care of these patients was made possible by the discovery of antipsychotic medications. Under the influence of the phenothiazines and other drugs, previously disoriented patients demonstrated a renewed capacity to care for themselves. This, then, set the stage for the possibility of community care for patients who had been receiving only minimal care in large public hospitals.

Simultaneously, there were several attempts to improve the hospital care itself. Maxwell Jones (1953), Stanton and Schwartz (1954) and Cumming and Cumming (1963) all attempted to approach the hospital as a uniquely responsive psychosocial milieu in an effort to make it more therapeutic. However, the total success of these models was hampered by the isolated nature of the "communities" on the hospital wards and by irreconcilable differences between the classic medical model of hospital psychiatry and a newly emerging antipathy to large institutions in general.

Within the broader social context of America in the 1960s, there developed a general feeling that primary social institutions had outgrown their human constituencies. Bigness became synonymous with unresponsiveness. Upheaval and protest against the federal government and its Vietnam policy, the university and its arbitrary curriculum and the big city and its unresponsiveness were the rule. The large state hospital was certainly not immune to scrutiny of a similar social consciousness. It was becoming clear to many mental health workers that there were better housing alternatives to those "human warehouses."

Coupled with this reaction against bigness and remoteness in the 1960s was a reaction to a unique development in American family life—the isolated nuclear family. Corporate mobility policies, which shuttled employees and their families hither and yon, contributed to this phenomenon, as did the migration to the suburbs and a "culture of narcissism" that discouraged family and community association and obligation. The geographically intact extended family, living in a stable neighborhood, became a rarity. The move to establish cooperative and communal living arrangements that developed in the late '60s was clearly an attempt to recreate the ethos of the extended family and concerned community of the past.

The community resident movement was clearly influenced by these attempts of social reformation. Experiencing the impersonal bigness and isolated smallness as a sign of society's decay, and a detriment to the rehabilitation of the mentally ill, small groups of workers began, largely on their own, to develop the first psychiatric halfway houses in different locations across America. Very often these community residential facilities began as experiments, defined as much by an antiestablishment tone as by common programmatic factors. Certainly there was no directed, unified policy coming from a high-level bureaucracy. About the deficits of the traditional large public psychiatric hospitals, there was considerable agreement: they were too large, were limited by a universal medical model and functioned as a closed society—they were isolated, like a penitentiary, from society at large. Community residences, by contrast, were to be small, family-modeled living arrangements, functioning as open social systems that existed within, rather than isolated from, the community (Budson 1978a; Budson 1973). These new facilities survived and began to proliferate. In 1960 there were only 7 professionally conceived programs in the entire country (Wechsler 1960); by 1973 there were 209 (U.S. NIMH 1973); and there are surely many more by now. Ultimately these highly motivated, carefully planned, transitional halfway houses were well described in the literature by Landy and Greenblatt (1965), Rothwell and Doniger (1966), Raush and Raush (1968), Glasscote et al. (1971) and Budson (1978a).

If the psychotropic drug revolution of the 1950s and the tendency in the 1960s to experiment with human-scaled institutions contributed to the development of the community care models, the proliferation of these models was given enormous impetus by the courts of the 1970s. In addition, the large institutions, the local communities and the state governments were all affected by these judicial decisions. A tragic irony, however, is that these judgments in the name of patients' rights too often had the effect of forcing many patients into the community before adequate rehabilitative facilities were there to receive them.

The first class-action suit "brought against a state's entire mental health system" was *Wyatt* v. *Stickney* (325F, Supp. 781 M.D. Ala. 1971), now known as *Wyatt* v. *Anderholt.* Here the court "affirmed the constitutional right to treatment for those mentally disordered persons who were involuntarily civilly committed" (Kopolow et al. 1975). In this decision, specific, legally binding and often very expensive standards of care were set forth, such as substantially increased staff/patient ratios. As fewer patients in the hospitals required fewer staff and less state appropriations, what followed were large-scale, economically motivated discharges. In place of the old custodial-care arrangements, which had previously been funded by the states, discharged patients were now offered federal supplemental security income. Unfortunately, there were simply too few formally organized community residential facilities to receive these incoming patients. Uncounted numbers drifted into proprietary boarding homes and single occupancy hotels into a kind of isolation that was little better than that of the hospital wards. Lack of daily programs also contributed to patient deterioration.

In 1975 the United States Supreme Court issued a landmark ruling that further contributed to the rising pressure to discharge patients. In *O'Connor* v. *Donaldson* (43 *U.S. Law Week*, 4930, June 24, 1975), the Court ruled for the first time that a mentally ill person could not be held against his will in a state hospital if he was not dangerous to himself or others, if he was not being offered treatment and if he was able to survive on his own in the community. The option of release to a halfway house if the patient was not able to survive independently in the community was not addressed. This was an irony, as denying the plaintiff the right to move to a halfway house was a precipitating issue in the case.

Another class-action suit, this one against the federally operated St. Elizabeth's Hospital in Washington, D.C., helped define the treatment issue in terms favorable to community residences and other forms of sheltered housing. In its decision, the Federal District Court ruled that mental patients were guaranteed "suitable care and treatment *under the least restrictive conditions*, including placement of patients in community-based facilities" (italics mine) (*Dixon* v. *Weinberger*, #74285 D.D.C., February 11, 1974). Although this decision helped move public mental health policy toward a legislative requirement for the least restrictive alternative, it neither identified these facilities specifically, nor did it define criteria for appropriate patient placement. The implementation of this decision is still in some turmoil because of these omissions.

More recently, one state, Massachusetts, has agreed to establish explicit community residential alternatives (*Brewster* v. *Dukakis*, U.S. District, Dist. of Mass., Civil No. 76-4423-F, final consent decree signed 12/06/78). As these carefully designed community residential facilities are developed and hospital patients placed in them, the hospital population will decline until, over time, the state hospital theoretically is able to close. Whether *all* patients ultimately can be managed outside of a closed hospital setting is doubtful, however.

On the legislative side, it should be noted that the United States Congress, when enacting the Community Mental Health Center Law in 1963, ignored the community residence entirely. It wasn't until 1975, when the act had to be renewed, that Public Law 94-63 included the community residence as an essential service of the community mental health center for the first time.

Thus, in the space of three decades, powerful medical, social and legal forces moved the locus of treatment for the severely mentally ill from the state hospital to the community. Attempts to reform the old custodial system produced in their turn a complex and often contradictory set of demands—that patients not be incarcerated without treatment; that patients not be released into the community before adequate community care programs exist; that large, expensive institutions not continue to drain dwindling state coffers; that unscrupulous private entrepreneurs not victimize again the vulnerable population of discharged patients. In many instances, the pace of reform and demolition of the old have outstripped creation of the new; and while the past decade of intensive development has, indeed, produced a broader spectrum of community care facilities, these facilities vary not only in function and philosophy, but often, unfortunately, in quality of care as well.

DIFFERENT TYPES OF HOUSING

At least ten different types of housing are currently in use in the United States: 1) transitional halfway houses; 2) long-term group residences; 3) cooperative apartments (satellite housing, landlord-supervised apartments, post-halfway-house accommodations); 4) lodge programs; 5) total rural environments (work camps); 6) foster care (family care); 7) crisis centers; 8) nursing homes; 9) board and care homes; 10) hotels.

While most of these entities (depending, of course, on individual variations in quality of service) are bona fide components of comprehensive mental health programs (nos. 1–7), others are often not (nos. 8–10). Irrespective of either the locale or the level of care for which the program was conceived, one of the minimal requirements for program adequacy is the maintenance of a sustained rehabilitative orientation. Involvement with a mental health agency, either directly as part of a mental health center's spectrum of services, or indirectly through regular consultation, is an important way of attaining this rehabilitative goal.

The National Institute of Mental Health has defined the transitional halfway house as a "residential facility in operation seven days a week with round-the-clock supervision (often a staff member living on the premises) and providing room, board, and assistance in the activities of daily living." Nonprofit, private corporations usually operate these facilities, in large old houses, with 15–20 residents, who generally participate daily in a planned program outside the dwelling. Whereas some facilities are increasingly acting as an alternative to hospitalization, the "halfway house" has conventionally been used as just that—a transitional facility from hospital to the community. Quality programs usually provide individual counseling, house meetings and recreational activities with emphasis on mutual support and understanding among house residents. The transitional halfway house is likely to have a relatively younger population, whose problems are of more recent onset, and whose potential for reentry into the community and total independent living is quite high (Budson 1978a; Landy and Greenblatt 1965; Rothwell and Doniger 1966; Raush and Raush 1968; Glasscote et al. 1971; Budson 1978b; Cannon 1975; Cannon 1973; Beigel et al. 1977).

Although the long-term group resident resembles the transitional halfway house in many particulars, its residents are usually sufficiently lacking in living skills, or sufficiently symptomatic, to require a higher on-site staff/resident ratio. In addition, the duration of residence in these facilities may exceed one year, in contrast to the transitional facility where the average stay may only be six to eight months. This facility, however, is designed to care for those most difficult patients who otherwise would be detained in a psychiatric ward.

Cooperative apartments are distinctive in that they have no on-site staff and are usually comprised of groups of two to four per unit. There is a regular staff visit from the sponsoring mental health agency to oversee the living arrangements as well as the required outside daily program. Landlord-supervised apartments are similar to other cooperative apartments, except for the fact that the landlord is in a contiguous dwelling and oversees, as a quasi-staff member, implementation of some programmatic goals—such as insuring that residents leave for their daily program in the morning, that they are properly dressed when they do so, that they are eating well and in good health and that their premises are adequately maintained. In this program, the landlord as well as the resident are helped by consulting visiting staff from the sponsoring agency. Cooperative apartments are often developed as outward community extensions—or satellites—of staffed residential programs. These programs may be designed not only to broaden the scope of these core community care programs, but also to avoid various constraints—to minimize start-up costs, lower operating costs, avoid community opposition and circumvent special restrictive building codes (Budson 1978b; Goldmeier et al. 1978; Sandall et al. 1975; Chien and Cole 1973).

It has been found that patients known to each other in the hospital can more easily move into the community as a group. George Fairweather (1969) developed such a model, the group establishing economic independence by organizing itself to operate a self-sustaining business. The hospital staff prepares the group for both the living and business aspects of the community program prior to leaving the wards. "Patients function together as a cooperative, communal society, running the household and working together to earn money" (Mannino et al. 1977; Anthony 1972; McDonald and Gregory 1971).

Total rural environments are nonhospital residential facilities which offer total supervised living including daily on-premises farming chores. In general, total enveloping milieus should be avoided to prevent repeating the isolative, closed society of the custodial institution. The focus here, however, is that of an operational farm which provides on-going reality-based responsibilities with high attention to the fulfillment of rehabilitative goals. Such facilities are particularly suitable for those clients who, although not needing a hospital, cannot reliably or safely manage in a more independent urban community setting. Gould Farm in western Massachusetts and Spring Lake Ranch in Vermont were pioneers in this area (Huessy 1966; Wechsler 1961).

Foster or family care, one of the oldest community placements, entails the location of expatients in private homes. The Veterans Administration has relied more heavily upon foster care than the state systems. Up to four residents may be placed in one foster home. The patient is supervised by the family caretaker, who is in turn supervised by a visiting social worker from the referring institution. Whereas the state systems formerly funded such homes, they now tend "to carry former patients on foster care rolls only long enough to transfer financing arrangements to other sources of funding such as Supplemental Security Income. Long-term arrangements are seen as more and more falling within the welfare or housing sectors" (Goldmeier 1977). One continuing problem about foster home care is the concern that it provides primarily a custodial function. A significant study on foster homes in Canada by Murphy et al. (1976) showed that there was no, or only minimal, improvement in social functioning or community participation (Morrissey 1967; Chouinard 1975; Fields 1974). A more recent study by Linn et al. (1980) showed that foster care serving Veterans Administration Hospitals in Alabama, Arkansas, California, Kentucky, and Massachusetts provided better social adjustment.

Nursing homes are a major community residential site to which thousands of chronically mentally ill who are elderly or physically handicapped are sent. The nursing home was one type of supervised residential facility which was readily available when the pressure to discharge patients mounted. Indeed, nursing homes doubled from 10,000 in 1964 to almost 20,000 in 1969. The Medicare/Medicaid Programs becoming available in these years accounted for much of this growth. However, these facilities continue to play a controversial role in the rehabilitation of the chronically ill in the community. In addressing this problem, Goldmeier (1977), for one, had the opinion that "nursing homes appropriate for the patient's level of functioning have a definite role to play in a continuum of community mental health services." He felt that ideally these facilities "should serve those requiring a relatively high degree of personal, medically oriented attention. . . ." As part of the whole continuum of service, he felt they provided the "most closely supervised of residential facilities." At the same time, it must be noted that various other investigators have suggested that more developed activity programs were needed in nursing homes in order to prevent physical and self-care decline (Dobson and Patterson 1961; Epstein and Simon 1968; Gaitz and Baer 1971; Goldstein and Rogers 1973).

A recent concept is the prevention of a full-blown psychosis in a rapidly deteriorating clinical situation by the use of a "crisis center." This alternative residential facility would allow the patient to leave a noxious home situation without having to go to a psychiatric hospital. Such a facility would have a higher staff/patient ratio, would be small and would have a capacity for around-the-clock care. There would usually be a time limit on the stay of a week or two, following which the patient could go to longer-term residence, home or, if necessary, a hospital (Smith 1974).

Board and care homes have been the recipients of uncounted numbers of discharged chronic patients. Their use has stimulated much controversy, which will be reviewed more fully in the next section. These are generally proprietary rooming houses which provide a wide range of care, depending upon the interest and motivation of the proprietor. Some of the facilities provide little more than room and board in dingy surroundings, with no semblance of a rehabilitative program whatsoever. Other programs, although deficient in many services, have well-kept, pleasant surroundings, and close alliance and consultation with referring mental health agencies. In the larger metropolitan areas the size of such facilities can be so large—up to several hundred beds—as to make much more difficult any meaningful program. Serious efforts are being made to try to improve this important area of community care because it involves such a large number of patients (Reich and Siegel 1973; Shadoan 1976; Lamb and Goertzel 1971; Tunakan and Schaefer 1965; Fields 1975; Murphy et al. 1972; Roberts 1974).

PROBLEMS OF APPRAISAL AND CURRENT DEBATE

Given the antiestablishment, civil libertarian origins of the community residence movement, and the host of different models which have evolved in different settings, it is not surprising that one encounters disarray and controversy when evaluating the state of the art. Indeed, Leona Bachrach (1978), one of the most astute observers of the deinstitutionalization scene, has noted that to appraise at this time is "difficult because we lack historical perspective." After recently reviewing fully 60 evaluative studies of community residential care, Mary Carpenter (1978) concluded that "little is known . . . about factors which contribute to the success or failure of these community residences." In support of this conclusion she cited the difficulties in evaluation due to the great unevenness and variability of the programs studied and the differences in the populations served, as well as the problems of different dependent variables being used and the paucity of controlled studies (Gumrukcu 1968; Gibson et al. 1972; Weinman et al. 1970; Lamb and Goertzel 1972). To further complicate the picture, the discrepancy in the goals set by the different programs studied determined a variety of different outcomes to be measured. What may be considered a success in one program may be seen as a failure in another. It is apparent that there are enormous disparities from program to program in the socioeconomic class of the residents, their age, their sex, and the onset, nature and severity of their illness, as well as the size of the facility, its location, the services offered and the training and size of the staff.

Generalizations are difficult to make in such a sea of variables. However, it is clear that there has been a mounting number of concerns about the community residence movement. One concern was that there was too much emphasis on location and not enough on appropriate programs geared to the needs of a specific population. For example, Chu and Trotter (1974) suggested that the community treatment movement had simply resulted in "more of the same" being given in different locations. Koltuv and Neff (1968) similarly warned that without a new technology, the only accomplishment of community treatment will be to move the "locus in which the emotionally disturbed (individual) vegetates and experiences personal misery."

At issue, in particular, was the concern in the early 70s that the board and care homes were becoming the new dumping grounds for the undesirable, indigent, chronic schizophrenic patient. Initial studies of this problem clearly concluded that halfway houses were more therapeutic than boarding homes for this population—a point of view which would not survive the decade. Lamb and Goertzel (1971), comparing boarding homes to high-expectation halfway houses, described boarding homes as characterized by an assumption that "guests" will "remain regressed and dependent indefinitely," whereas high-expectation halfway houses facilitate a "process of delabeling—the residents (being) less segregated, less likely to be labeled as deviate, and experiencing less stigmatization—with the individuals seeing themselves as functioning members of the community." Reporting on the problems in New York, Reich and Siegel (1973) described proprietary homes with as many as 285 beds that failed to provide any day programs, rehabilitative services or systematic psychiatric care.

Clearly, the initial implication was that the board and care homes were to be shunned. However, it became increasingly apparent that there had to be an accommodation to the reality that extremely large numbers of patients were nevertheless living in those very facilities. In response to this fact, Shadoan (1976) suggested ways to make the board and care homes more therapeutic. Most important was his attention to the proprietors, for whom he set up consultation and training programs. He also suggested the direct involvement of professionals on a regular basis to work with problems of the individual residents and to help the homes incorporate therapeutic community principles into their everyday operation. These tenets included a "high expectation atmosphere," weekly house meetings, having residents assume important positions in the management of the home and teaching residents how to care for themselves.

A number of recently published studies indicate that Shadoan's (1976) suggestions have been implemented with some apparent success. Dubin and Ciavarelli (1978) believe "boarding homes are a viable place to house former patients. . . ." They organized in Philadelphia a "Cooperative Boarding Program" with 80 boarding home proprietors who took from 1 to 6 residents into their homes. These operated essentially as landlord-supervised apartments as previously described by Chien and Cole (1973). Crucial to their point of view is their recognition that the proprietors of the homes can "successfully be incorporated into a team treatment approach." They drew the proprietors into the treatment program through close contact with professional staff and through a formal inservice training program as well as monthly meetings to take up practical issues. The group also felt that certain myths about boarding home proprietors were dispelled, including the notion that they stood to gain much monetarily. It was noted that the proprietors themselves were often lonely, had no family and generally seemed to be fulfilling their own desire for family. There was some regressive aspect of this with the proprietors often noted as being like "good mothers" to their "children." Though there were no formal followup studies, there was a general impression that there were fewer missed clinical appointments, that medication was able to be decreased and that the need for rehospitalization was lessened.

A group from the Hillside Division of the Long Island Jewish Hillside Medical Center led by Abbie S. Burger developed a program of apartment living for discharged patients with no more than 2 apartments per highrise building in order to prevent "a psychiatric ghetto." An aftercare team visited the patients in their apartments monthly. It also functioned as a crisis intervention team arranging "emergency meetings with patients, landlords, or both as necessary." Parents, families, patients and staff were also involved in a monthly meeting. Only 30 of the 92 patients involved were able to be retrieved for followup. However, there was a general impression that the program was a useful one in that "for many patients the period of apartment living coincided with the period of highest functioning in their lives" (Burger et al. 1978).

It would appear that two crucial factors highlight these studies: first, the landlords are incorporated into the treatment team; second, the programs are small.

In contrast to these reports, facilities that are just too large continue to be described. Melick et al. (1978) studied 1,999 residents in 26 "private proprietary homes" for adults in New York City. It is telling that fully 45% of the residents lived in "homes" each of which housed more than 150 residents. This group made no comment about the basic premise of whether such large facilities were appropriate to provide adequate services. Rather they assumed that they were capable of caring effectively for a certain kind of patient. When they tested that hypothesis against the population sample studied, they concluded that as many as 45 out of 100 referrals would be inappropriate—with 21 needing a lower level of care, and 24 requiring a higher level of care such as a nursing home or a halfway house.

Van Putten and Spar (1979) have taken a somewhat unique position on the matter of board and care homes. These authors concluded that the "schizoid-compliant pattern of outcome . . . characterized by blunted affect, passivity, and lack of initiative, interest and spontaneity . . . are the negative symptoms of schizophrenia, mistakenly attributed to the presumed inadequacies of the board-and-care environment." It is this fact, the authors contend, that has given the board and care home a bad press both in the newspapers and in the psychiatric literature. They feel that the schizoid-compliant schizophrenics are naturally selected to live in the board and care homes.

In variance to the literature of the early 70s, we see that there is now increasing support for the notion that board and care homes, in contrast to halfway houses, may be a preferred site for the severely chronically ill. Changing his original position, Lamb (1976) didn't "really see halfway houses as being much of an answer to the problem of the long-term, severely ill mental patient." He complained that halfway houses "require around-the-clock staffing, are difficult to set up and maintain, and when they are professionally run, they wind up frequently excluding the long-term severely ill, either by high expectations which are not realistic for these patients, or by the preferences of the staff who'd rather serve other kinds of people." Shadoan (1976) had already coined these preferences as the YAWIS syndrome, "an acronym referring to a preference for young, adult, white, verbal, intelligent, sophisticated patients."

Clearly, we are observing a process of delineation of different kinds of programs for different types of patients. In addressing this issue, Segal (1979) draws upon two sets of psychological assessments—"*psychological disturbance*," which is considered "gross symptoms or deviant behaviors such as motor retardation, hallucinating behavior, grandiosity, mannerisms, and posturing," and "*psychological distress*," meaning the ability to verbalize one's internal discomforts. He found that these two types of problems differed importantly in terms of the characteristics of the population in need of sheltered care. He concluded that "the environments in which we find the psychologically distressed are more likely to be halfway houses. The psychologically disturbed are more likely to be found in board-and-care homes. The severely psychologically disturbed population constitutes approximately 19% of those living in community-based sheltered-care facilities in California. However, half of the total sheltered-care population in California is showing serious psychological distress." From these conclusions there is clearly a need for adequate facilities and programs for both types of populations. Budson (1978b), comparing cooperative apartments to halfway houses, has recently documented such a division of facilities in Massachusetts as they appeared in 1976. "The cooperative apartment served a more chronic, older population with fewer vocational skills, and community ties. The [halfway house] population, on the other hand, is more likely to be a younger, more vocationally able population, with retention of their ties to the community to which they return, usually within a year." In addition, Lamb (1980) has recently reported a study of 101 board and care home patients which also showed that the younger, more goal-directed patients with more recent illness did *not* remain, but rather moved on.

The author's clinical experience has led to the conclusion that it is shortsighted to consider community residential care only for the chronic schizophrenic patient. The halfway house is particularly useful as well for the management of severe affective disorders (especially the recurrent relapsing manic-depressive) and the difficult borderline patient. In particular, it is clear that repeated hospitalizations can be avoided for the regressed, panicky, suicidal or destructive borderline patient by providing a safe "holding environment" in the halfway house.

We are clearly in the infancy of a new era in mental health care. It appears that a carefully designed range of residential rehabilitative alternatives is required to serve the spectrum of disability with which we are presented. We have already noted some attempts to match patients to specific program models. However, the science of client/milieu matching is not yet fully developed. We do not yet have the ability to authoritatively predict which patient should go where, even assuming the resources were available. More study and experience are needed, and premature closure on this issue would be a serious mistake. To be considered are such client factors as life skill attainment, inappropriate or bizarre behavior, social skills and available social network, daily program, suicidal potential and motivation to function. It would appear that the more difficulty a given patient has in any of these areas, the more intense the overall program that is required. Programmatic/milieu issues include staffing patterns, staff sophistication and training, degree of supervision available, staff stability and commitment, number of clients per program, the location, the intensity of planning and structure, and the interrelationship of the program with other rehabilitative services. Clearly, the more thorough a clinician's knowledge of both client and program, the greater the likelihood of a beneficial referral.

Some basic principles are emerging which are receiving some general acceptance. Test and Stein (1977), in addressing their concern over inadequate residential placements, specify that first, the "special support system should be adequate to assure that the person's unmet needs are met." Secondly, they urge that at the same time the special support system "not meet needs the person is able to meet himself." In addition to this vital concept to avoid either over- or underprovision of services, Budson and Jolley (1978) have suggested that all community programs are enhanced if they are able to enrich the extended psychosocial kinship system of their clients. In particular, they have shown how a community residence can be instrumental in providing such a social network, which, they suggest, enhances health and sustains successful community tenure.

ISSUES IN DEVELOPING A NEW PROGRAM

Irrespective of the type of community residence program to be developed, it is important that the organizing group setting up the new program review carefully a series of steps most often required to establish a new program. These include: forming a sponsoring organization; evaluating the types of clients in need of community residential services who are to be served by the new halfway house; determining the scope and size of the facility that will meet the specific needs of the clientele; planning the program components; establishing a network of ancillary services off the premises that is available to the clients; defining staff requirements, job descriptions, staffing patterns and policies, and hiring procedures; finding a suitable location and building; planning and implementing a "community entry" strategy; developing budget (seed money and capital) for the building, initial staffing and operating expenses; securing sources of funds; drafting a comprehensive statement suitable for public information that describes the results of the completed preparations and the projected operations of the facility.

In establishing the sponsoring organization, it should be recognized that a wide variety of special skills will enhance successful completion of the task. Thus, it is helpful to have a legal expert to facilitate compliance with zoning and other regulations; a fiscal expert, such as an accountant, to assist in preparation of a sound budget; a banking specialist to help in obtaining a loan for start-up costs; an architect or contractor to assist with building-code compliance and structural renovations; and a real estate expert to inform the group of new listings of appropriate houses or apartments. A mental health professional's presence on the corporate board will facilitate the coordination of program planning and the maintenance of clinical integrity in the face of a multitude of administrative decisions. In addition, significant community leaders, such as a respected business man, a local politician or a local minister, can help in the process of community entry by representing the program to other community members as an asset to the community.

For planning purposes, there should be a clear understanding of client characteristics for which special program components may be needed. For example, residents suffering from schizophrenia will usually need a supportive environment which enhances socialization. Manic-depressive patients who are prone to hypomania will require a highly structured program to prevent deterioration into a serious mania. The facility's primary responsibility to the depressed resident is the maintenance of alertness to situations that are likely to precipitate suicidal feelings and acts. Depressed residents must feel safe at the halfway house so that they will be willing to inform the house parents, other staff or fellow residents when they experience self-destructive impulses. Patients with personality disorders require a strong peer group able and willing to exert a rehabilitating influence on them. The use of illicit drugs is forbidden in community residences. In addition, unscheduled urine checks must be arranged with an outside clinic to impress the former drug addict that staff is neither gullible nor naive and well understands how difficult it is for the exaddict to abstain in times of stress.

All residents with major superego defects, such as antisocial personalities, present special problems for a community residence. Such behavior can be destructive to the entire program, both within the facility and in relation to the external community. The rules and expectations of the program must be made very explicit to such persons, and the consequences resulting from violations must be clearly delineated.

To care for young adolescents, the community residence must be small—not exceeding twelve youngsters. Adolescents are often action oriented, with a propensity for rapid, intense mood swings. Running away is a common form of acting out. An appropriate program must be carefully structured and enriched, with a firm, cooperative high school environment, where appropriate. Skilled house parents for this group should foster positive cohesion to prevent outbreaks of rebellion. A capacity for family intervention and liaison is also desirable for adolescent programs.

Serving the elderly requires a program with increased staff, special safety precautions and appropriate social and activity programs.

Chronic patients, in particular, frequently suffer a loss of social and other life skills, develop considerable dependence on the program and show slow progress. They may require a long-term group residence with staff who can maintain a therapeutic stance over the long haul. The program must stress gradualness—but it must nevertheless be rehabilitative rather than custodial. Interactions with the "real world" through shopping, entertainment and work (even if "sheltered") should be maximized. Whenever life skill development is a major need, the use of community volunteers should be considered. They can be very helpful in providing one-to-one community training in basic skills, including use of public transportation, use of money, shopping, use of community recreation and entertainment resources, working with community social service agencies, and learning how to obtain emergency medical attention.

When planning a new group residence, one must not forget the importance of the character of the building and its location. Ideally, it should have a homelike quality. There should be adequate space, including public rooms for dining, socializing and recreation as well as adequate bedrooms. Adequate lighting and windows, soft textures and warm colors, the generous use of fabrics and rugs—all may contribute to give the residents the feeling of a comfortable family setting. Victorian homes found in both urban and rural areas are often very suitable.

Community entry strategy is a vital part of starting a new program. It can be considered to be operational in two distinct arenas: one is political, the other is legal. There are similarities between the two sectors, but it is important that the differences be understood. There are arguments for both publicly announced as well as covert entry. To some extent, zoning laws will determine which alternative should be pursued. The key questions are: Is a public hearing required? Does a special permit have to be granted by an official body? Low-profile entry is only feasible when no hearing or permit is required. The political task is to convince the governing body to grant a required permit. If this fails then legal approaches have to be explored and pursued.

Factors that influence the local governing body must be assessed. If the agency is composed of elected officials, then it will be responsive to the electorate. Gaining the electorate's support then becomes the primary political goal. Several general principles should be considered. First, the program should be presented as offering a service to the community, not imposing a burden. The impression of a foreign intruder can thus be avoided. Second, explicit standards must be established for both the behavior of residents and the maintenance of the property. This helps to reassure the community that its norms will not be violated. Third, influential community leaders should be involved. Fourth, the immediate neighbors must be considered as a very special group. They will feel most threatened about property values and personal safety and are likely to become the best-organized opponents of the community residence. Recruiting respected immediate neighbors as allies can therefore do a great deal to ensure successful entry.

SOME SELECTED CLINICAL CONSIDERATIONS

The entire clinical operation of a community residence is a very complex matter. However, only several critical points will be discussed here. Careful and thorough work during the evaluation and admission phase will enhance the ensuing quality of care for any given resident and facilitate a smooth-running clinical operation for the staff. A clearly defined admissions meeting should be organized. It is advisable that the clinical team that referred the applicant be present along with some representatives of the ancillary services. Thus, in addition to the community residence staff, the applicant's therapist, representatives of the inpatient back-up facility, the applicant's social worker, the vocational counselor and representatives of day care or sheltered workshop facilities should meet together. Discussion should air any disagreements among the staff involved in prior treatment, as well as differences that may crop up during the meeting between these prior care givers and the community residence staff. A list of critical issues to be reviewed include: history of the prospective resident; the dynamics that contributed to the acute illness; the family's relationship to the applicant; the house's approach to the applicant's family; the role of continuing therapy; the status of medication; services required to ensure that medication is maintained and monitored; the applicant's physical health; his proposed outside daily program and transportation to the program; his history of peer relationships and interpersonal difficulties; arrangement for potential inpatient back-up if necessary; the applicant's special talents, interests and strengths; and planning the applicant's transition into the community residence. It is important in relation to the issue of relapse prevention that the community residence staff try to find out two key pieces of information: 1) Does the prospective resident have a particular stress which frequently and commonly tends to precipitate an exacerbation of symptomatology. 2) Is there a prodromal phase before a frank psychotic relapse which is characterized by certain changed behavior patterns and portends the forthcoming difficulties. The acquisition of such knowledge can be crucial in facilitating early staff intervention to avert unnecessary relapse.

The admission meeting establishes personal contact among all clinical participants in the applicant's rehabilitation program. This face-to-face discussion familiarizes the participants with one another's roles and points of view, and opens communication lines among them. Phone numbers should be exchanged to ensure mutual availability in the event that anyone believes the resident is doing poorly and beginning to slip. Again, this expedites rapid intervention in the face of impending relapse.

Experience has shown that it is wise that there be no more than one significant change in the applicant's life at any time in three key areas. These areas are: the residential circumstances, the job situation and therapy. Changes in these areas subject the vulnerable applicant to significant stress and require careful preparation and support. Change in more than one area at a time is likely to be intolerable. Turmoil and risk of relapse may be the consequences of the violation of this important principle. Experience has shown that a two-week interval between changes in the various life sectors is the minimal period to secure adequate adaptation.

Finally, long-range future disposition should be addressed. Post-residence social housing, where appropriate, should be planned far in advance. Some residents may move out with fellow residents into independent apartments. Other residents may need a more sheltered living arrangement for an indefinite period.

In general, the community residence clinical staff decides collaboratively with the applicant's clinical team whether the applicant is suitable for the program. The residence may have specific admission criteria. Conditions that usually disqualify an applicant for admission include: poorly controlled destructive impulses toward the self, others or property; ongoing narcotic addiction; unremitting abuse of alcohol; and sexual promiscuity. Other characterological problems may or may not disqualify an applicant. Negativistic, stubborn applicants who refuse to get up and go to any meaningful activity may be taken on by some halfway houses as a therapeutic challenge. Such persons pose special problems which ought to be clearly understood from the outset. If accepted, they might undermine the group expectation that all residents must engage in meaningful daily activity off the premises; they might demand unreasonable attention and staff time; and they might breed resentment toward themselves that would further promote their negativism.

Once the resident has moved in, the value system of the program should be apparent in all aspects of the milieu. The fundamental principle is that each resident has both healthy and troubled parts of his personality, and that the healthy parts can increasingly understand and master the areas of difficulty. The acquisition of new skills and insights strengthens healthy functioning and contributes to an inner sense of mastery. Ideally, the resident increasingly feels himself to be competent and capable—a person of value. The old concept of the self as defective and valueless slowly withers in response to this growth force. No less than the residents, the staff support this growth ethic through their own commitment to it. All members of the milieu are expected to look honestly at themselves to recognize their weaknesses and to address themselves to improvement and growth. Although the staff are presumably at a more advanced level of growth, they participate in and benefit from this process. Smug, self-satisfied, patronizing staff have no place in a community residence.

These goals and values saturate the whole residence, and they are obvious to the resident from his first contacts with the program. From the program's brochure, to the first admission meeting, and throughout the moving-in process, the resident is valued as a whole human being, not just a specimen of psychopathology. The managers' careful nurturing of a trusting relationship prepares the resident for the future task of developing self-awareness, mastery and new executive and social skills.

Each setting in the community residence program can provide opportunities for learning and growth. Both house routines and informal socialization can foster the growth ethic. Dinners, shopping, working, chores, avocational activity—all of these are settings where growth can occur. The resident learns that growth is sustained and that reality is tested in relation to communication with significant others. The house managers set the tone by establishing a relationship based on trust and self-disclosure. Improved peer relationships in the house should follow. Newly established friends in the house share leisure activities, support each other in times of stress and confront distortions when they arise. An authentic reality sense is thus sustained through continual interplay with peers.

Occasionally, a resident experiences a crisis. To approach the problem rationally, the precipitating event must be explored and the reasons for the resident's particular vulnerability to this event investigated. Then the best method of dealing with the resident's strong reaction must be discussed. Sometimes, the very recognition that the precipitant reactivated an old rage or grief, understandable in relation to the past but unreasonably strong in relation to the present, will alleviate the upset. In other circumstances, the situation might call for some action on the resident's part, for example, confronting one of the persons allegedly causing the disturbance or dealing with noxious situations in some other constructive manner.

Minor crises can often be dealt with by staff and the peer group alone. If they fail, the residence consultant can be asked whether administration of antianxiety or antipsychotic medications is indicated, or whether an adjustment in the dosage of ongoing medication may help the resident weather the crisis. Sometimes a crisis can be alleviated by enlisting the support of a resident's family and significant others in a joint meeting to identify the nature of and solutions to the crisis.

If the resident, in spite of these efforts, remains agitated, psychotic or seriously depressed, requiring continuous attention by staff, and especially if sleep is disturbed, inpatient back-up for short-term night care may often shorten the duration of the disturbance. Whenever possible, such action should be taken with the cooperation of the resident, with the explicit understanding that the bed at the residence will remain available for immediate return.

After a successful rehabilitative tenure in the facility, a resident's leaving the program represents another critical instance requiring careful planning. Ideally, the resident who leaves should still retain an established program, with a functioning psychosocial network. The postresidence program should have several important features. Exresidents should optionally move into a living arrangement with known others, not live alone. They should have a daily program of familiar activities. They should maintain a therapeutic relationship with someone—a psychotherapist, a clinical psychiatrist or a community residence staff member—whom they trust and to whom they can turn in times of trouble. The medication should be stabilized with provisions made for medical monitoring where appropriate. There should also be some ongoing periodic contact with the exresidents' families of origin, so that old pathological patterns will not reemerge without some provision for checking them. Finally, a continuing relationship with the residence, through an exresident program and personal ties to the house, is highly desirable. In sum, the program of the resident who is moving out should be intact and stable. This is another application of the principle that there should be no more than one significant life change at a time.

CONTROVERSIAL ADMINISTRATIVE ISSUES

It is not surprising that sheltered residential care is subject to a variety of serious controversial administrative issues, most often emanating from the community. Three legal areas will require careful resolution if community residential programs are to be enhanced—the issues of exclusionary zoning, building codes and licensing standards. First, the potential exclusion of community residences through local zoning ordinances is of vital importance to the development of community residential care.

This is a complicated legal field. The Mental Health Law Project in Washington, D.C., has been a national clearing house in relation to such issues. The reader should be aware of its publications summarizing all aspects of the law. They review types of local ordinances restricting community-based group homes and significant court decisions relating to them. Some of these are "interpretive," e.g., considering the term "family" in local zoning ordinances to include group homes. "These courts have held that because a group home functions as a family does, with residents living as a single unit, participating in housekeeping, cooking and other activities as a 'family' group, such a home fits within the definition of family." Other approaches of the courts have been to address whether there is existing state policy encouraging deinstitutionalization which preempts local ordinances which exclude group homes. A specific statute enacted by a state legislature intending to specifically override local law is an approach which could make the preemption argument far stronger.

The Mental Health Law Project's recent publication concludes:

> A review of the case law discloses conflicting decisions by courts on virtually every legal theory. Some of the best decisions, especially those turning on the definition of the term "family" in local ordinances, could easily be eliminated by more careful drafting of local ordinances by communities opposed to group homes. Further, before any of these cases get to court, months of delay have occurred. Not only is the delay attributable to the slow pace of the courts, but in most instances, complicated and time-consuming local procedures must be exhausted before a case can be filed. Many group homes will not have the resources to pay rent while a house remains empty. Because the success of a group home ultimately depends upon good relationships with the community and with its neighbors, litigation can be counter-productive. Attempts should be made before undertaking litigation to educate and to work politically with the local community. [Mental Health Law Project, 1980]

A second major administrative issue is building codes. It is vital that these codes permit the use of existing residences to allow true community integration. At the same time the occupants should be assured a safe environment. A successful resolution to this dilemma was achieved in Massachusetts where a unique fire safety system was developed that emphasized preserving life rather than the building. This system was based on three essential elements: 1) a fire detection alarm system; 2) two independent means of egress from each sleeping quarter; and 3) the certification of the capability of self-preservation of each occupant, assuring that egress was achievable within 2½ minutes of the alarm. This new system eliminated most of the structural changes required in stricter codes, which were not only expensive but also rendered homelike dwellings into institutionallike buildings. This system should be a model for the nation.

Adequate but fair licensing standards are essential if there is to be quality control on a statewide basis. At the same time, it is important that these programmatic standards set by governmental agencies not be so rigid as to interfere with program development, creativity and implementation. One critical issue is that the fear of potential provider abuse not be expressed by demanding more care than is required for the residence involved. For example, quality control that ignores the varying degrees of dependence of the residents could require excessive numbers of staff, which would make the program not only unmanageably expensive to operate, but would perpetuate the old system to relegating citizens to unnecessary dependence on professional helpers.

Furthermore, some states have tried to limit the size of community residences to no more than eight residents. For the mentally ill population, not only is such a small program impractical, causing very high per-person costs, but also, such smallness limits too severely the social network necessary to mobilize residents with poor ego and social skills. Experience has shown that fifteen to twenty persons per program has enhanced socialization.

The staffing of these programs with trained and effective workers is another important goal for the future. It is essential that community residential programs continue to be operated by people with a commitment to growth and rehabilitation. The spark of enthusiasm accompanying creativity and innovation should not be lost, for it fosters a lasting renewal of spirit that keeps the program vital and relevant to both the residents and the community. More and better staff will be needed in the future. Educational institutions must address this new field of community residential care in planning curricula in the human services. Staff from phased-out institutions as well as new students must be educated in the principles of community and residential care.

Inadequate funding and community opposition represent two additional roadblocks to these programs. We must pursue the slow process of educating the public and setting society's priorities to cope with these complex issues. Community residential programs are caught in the funding intricacies of a mental health delivery system in evolution. Innovative programmatic concepts and court orders insuring the constitutional rights of mental patients have not been matched by legislative appropriations. There are a multitude of state and federal funding programs involving, among others, Title XX, the Social Security Act, the Community Mental Health Center Act and HUD allocations which are both confusing and inadequate. All of this is in spite of the fact that a variety of investigators have shown that, from the view of cost effectiveness, there are distinct financial as well as clinical advantages to these community programs.

CONCLUSION

In conclusion, a successful community residence program engages almost all of the modalities discussed within this entire volume. These include the skillful implementation of the psychosocial therapies, the careful use and monitoring of the pharmacotherapies, and the awareness of the program's role within the larger context of the political, legal and economic arenas of society. Such a program is in a strategic position to foster the broadest growth of the people it serves. It can enhance the capacity for optimal adaptation in the resident's natural quest for a satisfied and dignified life within the community.

REFERENCES

Anthony, W. A. Efficacy of psychiatric rehabilitation. *Psychology Bull.* 78: 447–456 (1972).

Bachrach, L. L. A conceptual approach to deinstitutionalization. *Hosp. Comm. Psychiat.* 29: 573-578 (1978).

Beigel, A. The politics of mental health funding: Two views, a look at the issues. *Hosp. Comm. Psychiat.* 28: 194-196 (1977).

Beigel, A., Hollenbach, H., and Gurgevich, S. Practical issues in developing and operating a halfway house program. *Hosp. Comm. Psychiat.* 28: 601-607 (1977).

Budson, R. D. The psychiatric halfway house. *Psychiat. Ann.* 3(6): 64-83 (1973).

Budson, R. D. Legal dimensions of the psychiatric halfway house. *Comm. Ment. Health Journal.* 11(3): 316-324 (1975).

Budson, R. D. *The Psychiatric Halfway House: A Handbook of Theory and Practice*. Pittsburgh: University of Pittsburgh Press, 1978a.

Budson, R. D. Community residential care for the mentally ill in Massachusetts: Halfway houses and cooperative apartments, in *New Directions in Mental Health Care: Cooperative Apartments*, J. Goldmeier, F. V. Mannino, and M. F. Shore, eds. Monograph, NIMH, DHEW Pub. No. (ADM) 78-685, Adelphi, MD (1978b).

Budson, R. D., and Jolley, R. E. A crucial factor in community program success: The extended psychosocial kinship system. *Schiz. Bull.* 4: 609-621 (1978).

Burger, A. S., Kimelman, L., and Lurie, A. Congregate living for the mentally ill: Patients as tenants. *Hosp. Comm. Psychiat.* 29: 590-593 (1978).

Cannon, M. S. Selected characteristics of residents in psychiatric halfway houses. HSMA, NIMH Statistical Note 93, Rockville, MD, NIMH (1973).

Cannon, M. S. Halfway houses serving the mentally ill and alcoholics, United States, 1973. Mental Health Statistics, Series A, No. 16, Rockville, MD, NIMH (1975).

Carpenter, M. D. Residential placement for the chronic psychiatric patient: A review and evaluation of the literature. *Schiz. Bull.* 4: 384-398 (1978).

Chien, C., and Cole, J. O. Landlord supervised cooperative apartments: A new modality for community based treatment. *Am. J. Psychiat.* 130: 156-159 (1973).

Chouinard, E. Family homes for adults. *Soc. and Rehab. Record.* 2: 10-15 (1975).

Chu, F. D. and Trotter, S. *The Madness Establishment.* New York: Grossman, 1974.

Cumming, J., and Cumming, E. *Ego and Milieu.* New York: Atherton, 1963.

Dobson, W. R., and Patterson, T. W. A behavioral evaluation of geriatric patients living in nursing homes as compared to a hospitalized group. *Gerontol.* 1: 135-139 (1961).

Dubin, W. R., and Ciavarelli, B. A positive look at boarding homes. *Hosp. Comm. Psychiat.* 29: 593-596 (1978).

Epstein, L., and Simon, A. Alternatives to state hospitalization for the geriatric mentally ill. *Am. J. Psychiat.* 124: 955-961 (1968).

Fairweather, G. W., Sanders, D. H., and Maynard, H. Community life for the mentally ill: An alternative to institutional care. Aldine, Chicago (1969).

Fields, S. Asylum on the front porch: Foster communities for the mentally ill. *Innovations* 1: 3-10 (1974).

Fields, S. Rethinking rehabilitation: 1) Breaking through the boarding homes blues; 2) A vocation in Vermont; 3) No bedlam in Bethlehem. *Innovations* 2: 2-14 (1975).

Gaitz, C. M., and Baer, P. E. Placement of elderly psychiatric patients. *J. Am. Ger. Soc.* 19: 601-613 (1971).

Gibson, R. L., Marone, J., and Coutu, G. A rehabilitation program for chronically hospitalized patients. *Hosp. Comm. Psychiat.* 23: 381-383 (1972).

Glasscote, R. M., Gudeman, J. E., and Elpers, J. R. Halfway houses for the mentally ill. Washington, D.C., Joint Information Services of the APA and the NAMH (1971).

Goldmeier, J. Community residential facilities for former mental patients: A review. *Psychosoc. Rehab. J.* 1: 1-45 (Summer 1977).

Goldmeier, J., Mannino, F. V., and Shore, M. F., eds. *New Directions in Mental Health Care: Cooperative Apartments.* Monograph, NIMH, DHEW Pub. No. (ADM) 78-685, Adelphi, MD (1978).

Goldstein, S. E., and Rogers, L. Community liaison with a mental hospital. *J. Am. Ger. Soc.* 21: 538–545 (1973).

Gumrukeu, P. The efficacy of a psychiatric halfway house: A three-year study of a therapeutic residence. *Sociol. Quart.* 9: 374-386 (1968).

Gunderson, J., and Mosher, L. The cost of schizophrenia. *Am. J. Psychiat.* 132: 901-906 (1975).

Huessy, H. R. Spring Lake Ranch—The pioneer halfway house, in *Mental Health with Limited Resources*, H. R. Huessy, ed. New York: Grune & Stratton, 1966, pp. 63–72.

Jones, M. *The Therapeutic Community.* New York: Basic (1953).

Koltuv, M., and Neff, W. S. The comprehensive rehabilitation center: Its role and realm in psychiatric rehabilitation. *Comm. Ment. Health J.* 4: 251–259 (1968).

Kopolow, L. E., Brands, A., and Burton, J. Litigation and mental health services. Rockville, MD, NIMH, DHEW Pub. No. (ADM) 75-261 (1975).

Lamb, H. R. What array of residential programs is required to meet the full range of special needs. *Presentation of viewpoint in Community Living Arrangements for the Mentally Ill and Disabled: Issues and Options for Public Policy.* NIMH, Rockville, MD (1976).

Lamb, H. R. Board-and-care home wanderers. *Arch. Gen. Psychiat.* 37(2): 135–137 (1980).

Lamb, H. R., and Goertzel, V. Discharged mental patients—are they really in the community? *Arch. Gen. Psychiat.* 24: 29–43 (1971).

Lamb, H. R., and Goertzel, V. High expectations of long term ex-state hospital patients. *Am. J. Psychiat.* 129: 471-475 (1972).

Landy, D., and Greenblatt, M. *Halfway Houses.* Washington, D.C., U.S. Dept. of Health, Education and Welfare, Vocational Rehabilitation Administration (1965).

Linn, M. W., Klett, C. J., and Caffey, E. M., Jr. Foster home characteristics and psychiatric patient outcome. *Arch. Gen. Psychiat.* 37(2): 129–132 (1980).

Mannino, F. V., Ott, S., and Shore, M. F. Community residential facilities for former mental patients: An annotated bibliography. *Psychosoc. Rehab. J.* 1: 1–43 (Winter 1977).

McDonald, L., and Gregory, G. W. The Fort Logan Lodge: International community for chronic mental patients. NIMH Final Report, Grant No. 1 ROL MH15853-02, NIMH, Rockville, MD (1971).

Mental Health Law Project: Combatting exclusionary zoning. The right of handicapped people to live in the community. Washington, D.C. (1980).

Melick, C. F., and Eysaman, C. O. A study of former patients placed in private proprietary homes. *Hosp. Comm. Psychiat.* 29: 587–590 (1978).

Morrissey, J. R. The case for family care of the mentally ill. *Comm. Ment. Health J.* Monograph Series. 2: 1–64 (1967).

Murphy, H. B. M., and Datel, W. E. A cost-benefit analysis of community versus institutional living. *Hosp. Comm. Psychiat.* 27: 165–170 (1976).

Murphy, H. B. M., Pennee, B., and Luchins, D. Foster homes: The new back wards? *J. Canada's Mental Health.* 20: 1–17 (1972).

National Institute of Mental Health: Reference Data on Halfway Houses for the Mentally Ill and Alcoholics, United States. Superintendent of Documents, U.S. Govt. Prtg. Office, Washington, D.C. (1973).

Raush, H. L., and Raush, C. L. *The Halfway House Movement: A Search for Sanity*. New York: Appleton-Century-Crofts (1968).

Reich, R., and Siegel, L. The chronically mentally ill shuffle to oblivion. *Psychiat. Ann.* 3: 33-55 (1973).

Roberts, P. R. Human warehouses: A boarding home study. *Am. J. Pub. Health* 64: 276-282 (1974).

Rothwell, N. D., and Doniger, J. M. *The Psychiatric Halfway House: A Case Study*. Springfield, IL: Charles C. Thomas (1966).

Sandall, H., Hawley, T., and Gordon, G. L. The St. Louis community homes. *Am. J. Psychiat.* 32: 617-622 (1975).

Segal, S. P. Individual characteristics affecting the sheltered care needs of the mentally ill. *Health Soc. Work* 4: 41-58 (1979).

Shadoan, R. A. Making board and care homes therapeutic, in *Community Survival for Long-Term Patients*. H. R. Lamb, and Associates, eds. San Francisco: Jossey-Bass (1976), pp. 56-73.

Sharfstein, S., and Nafsiger, J. C. Community care: Costs and benefits for a chronic patient. *Hosp. Comm. Psychiat.* 27: 170-173 (1976).

Smith, B. J. A hospital's support system for chronic patients living in the community. *Hosp. Comm. Psychiat.* 15: 508-509 (1974).

Stanton, A. H., and Schwartz, M. S. *The Mental Hospital*. New York: Basic, (1954).

Test, M. A., and Stein, L. I. Special living arrangements: A model for decision making. *Hosp. Comm. Psychiat.* 28: 608-610 (1977).

Tunakan, B., and Schaefer, I. The community boardinghouse as a traditional residence during aftercare. *Cur. Psy. Ther.* 5: 235-239 (1965).

Van Putten, T., and Spar, J. E. The board-and-care home: Does it deserve a bad press? *Hosp. Comm. Psychiat.* 30: 461-465 (1979).

Wechsler, H. Halfway houses for former mental patients: A survey. *J. Soc. Issues* 16: 20-26 (1960).

Wechsler, H. Transitional residences for former mental patients: A survey of halfway houses and rehabilitation facilities. *Mental Hyg.* 45: 65-67 (1961).

Weinman, B., Sanders, R., and Kleiner, R. Community based treatment of the chronic psychotic. *Comm. Ment. Health J.* 6: 13-21 (1970).

Weisbrod, B. A., Test, M. A., and Stein, L. I. An alternative to mental hospital treatment: III. Economic benefit-cost analysis. *Arch. Gen. Psychiat.* (in press).

PART III

PHARMACOLOGIC TREATMENT PRINCIPLES

EDITOR'S COMMENTARY: PART III

A question that has concerned thoughtful practitioners is how to meaningfully relate different biological "explanations" of drug action to the fact that drug therapy occurs in a social context. A drug can interact with a receptor at the molecular level and modulate a physiological process, as well as produce a particular therapeutic effect. Drug action, therefore, can be described in several ways, reflecting different levels of biological organization. Previous chapters in this book have reviewed some of the social determinants of the therapeutic status of the chronic psychiatric patient. Such factors include the degree the person's dysfunction is exacerbated by psychosocial conditions (i.e., the social breakdown syndrome), the amount of support the person receives from the social and therapeutic systems in which he participates (i.e., day clubs, psychotherapy sessions, vocational training programs, etc.) and the extent to which the individual complies with the medication regimen, and their schedule. Another crucial variable which ultimately affects the clinical status of the patient is the precision with which the physician makes a host of related decisions. For example, should the person be medicated; does the benefit/risk ratio warrant prescribing the medication; what type medication should be used; what dose, and for how long; is the patient compliant and taking his medication; are there any serious early side effects; and when should the medication be stopped? Thus, the pharmacological therapy of the psychiatric patient operates in the social and biological matrix in which the medication both acts and is acted upon by the patient. The dilemma for the clinician is to understand which of these factors is operational at any one moment.

Integration of drug therapy into the overall management of the chronic psychiatric patient will require balancing:

- the objective of symptom reduction versus the occurrence of the adverse physical consequences of antipsychotic drug administration (e.g., tardive dyskinesia),
- the objective of facilitating function, free of drug administration, versus the hazard of psychotic relapse consequent to lack of this medication, and
- the objective of encouraging drug compliance versus the phenomena of patient self-adjustment of drug dosage with inadvertent benefit.

Each of these issues are addressed in the following chapters, sometimes implicitly, sometimes explicity. This information should help the practitioner develop alternative strategies to manage each of these dilemmas.

One of the essential barriers to the integration of pharmacotherapy into the psychological therapies is the nonspecific, or undesired side-effects of drugs. New developments in the biology of mental illness, however, hold promise of possible change in the design and development of neuroleptic agents (e.g., the neuropeptides; Ananth and Callman, 1979; Verhoeven, et al. 1979). Ultimately, it is hoped that what now could be deemed to be only palliative therapy may be replaced some day with pharmacological treatments which are more specific in relieving the target symptoms and free of all other undesired effects.

Readers of the three chapters of this section will be impressed by the progress that has been made in the chemotherapeutic management of the chronic psychiatric patient. Continued progress will require careful monitoring of the patient's functional status, balancing of the application of therapies—each of which have limited efficacy, and the development of alternative pharmacological agents that reflect new biological principles characteristic of the chronic psychiatric patient.

The reader should also note that patients retain the right to refuse treatment and that the very prescribing of medication in some instances has been legally characterized as unlawful chemical constraint. This is yet another reality of today's social context of medication.

REFERENCES

Ananth, J., and Callanan, T. S. Importance of endorphins in psychiatry. *Comprehensive Psychiatry* 20: 246-255 (1979).

Verhoeven, W. M. A., van Praag, H. A., van Ree, J. M., and deWied, D. Improvement of schizophrenic patients treated with [Des-Tyr[1]]- and -endorphin (DT&E) *Archives General Psychiatry* 36: 294-298, 1979.

CHAPTER 12

CLINICAL EXPERIENCES AND PRINCIPLES IN SELECTION OF MEDICATION

JONATHAN O. COLE, M.D.

This paper will review common problems encountered with chronic or relapsing patients and offer suggestions for optimizing their drug therapy. It will consider separately chronic schizophrenia, chronic or recurrent unipolar depression, recurrent bipolar manic-depressive illness and chronic anxiety.

CHRONIC SCHIZOPHRENIA

Most patients with recurrent schizophrenic psychoses requiring hospitalization are placed on long-term maintenance antipsychotic drug therapy. It is clear from present evidence that such patients are *less* likely to relapse and require rehospitalization if they are on an antipsychotic drug but are still prone to relapse unpredictably. Hogarty's studies suggest a relapse rate of 85% over a 2-year period if patients are in an aftercare program on placebo as against a 45% relapse rate on oral chlorpromazine.[1] Used in this way antipsychotic drugs are likely to be serving a prophylactic function; patients on placebo before they actually relapse are no sicker than patients on chlorpromazine. It is therefore unlikely that patients who are persistently somewhat psychotic even on maintenance antipsychotics will benefit strikingly from large increases in drug dosage or shifts to another and different antipsychotic. Occasional patients do benefit from such alterations but they appear rare. On the other side of this issue, many chronic schizophrenics become psychologically strongly attached to a particular drug; changing the medication against their will can sometimes initiate relapse.[2] Therefore, with chronic patients who are stable in the community and reliably take their medication, changes should only be made for a good clinical reason.

Some chronic patients are rather inert, passive and retarded and only function independently to a limited extent. While some of these patients are only showing the effects of chronic psychosis, others are either oversedated by their medication or are suffering from akinesia—forced inactivity secondary to a neurological drug side effect. If the problem is akinesia, it should respond to antiparkinsonian drugs. As Rifkin has pointed out, patients on high-dose depot fluphenazine are particularly apt to develop akinesia.[3] Akinesia is an important indication for not routinely stopping antiparkinsonian drugs in schizophrenic patients, even for those on them for more than 6 months, as DiMascio and others have recommended.[4] Thus patients being weaned off antiparkinsonian drugs, after a sensible period, should be watched for increased anergia, while anergic patients on antipsychotics but not on antiparkinsonian drugs should have a trial on added antiparkinsonian medication. Though any antiparkinsonian drug should work, Artane is perhaps a bit more stimulating than Cogentin and certainly less sedative than Benadryl. If this approach does not work and the patient is on one of the more sedative antipsychotics (e.g., chlorpromazine, thioridazine or loxapine), lowering dose or shifting to a high-potency drug (e.g., perphenazine, haloperidol, fluphenazine) should be tried. If medication is being given during the day, moving the whole dose to bedtime can also decrease day-time sedation.

In some chronic schizophrenics on maintenance antipsychotics, some degree of depression is present and interferes with functioning. In such cases the addition of a tricyclic antidepressant can often be helpful. Given that both antipsychotics and tricyclics both have anticholinergic side effects, probably desipramine as the least anticholinergic available tricyclic may be the drug of choice. Often lowish dosages (50–100 mg a day) work rather rapidly, perhaps because the antipsychotic slows tricyclic metabolism, leading to higher plasma levels at low doses.

Van Putten describes below (see pp. 383-393) two major reasons why chronic schizophrenics fail to continue to take prescribed antipsychotic medication in the community. One group is grandiose and happier when psychotic,[5] a problem not directly manageable by drug therapy except by some carefully monitored regimen such as depot fluphenazine coupled with a reliable social support system which assures that the patient gets the regular injection. The other group feels chronically miserable on medication because of akathisia, a muscular and sometimes psychic discomfort, often manifested by leg jiggling, inability to sit still or pacing, which may be confused with anxiety or agitation and therefore inappropriately treated.[6] Even when diagnosed accurately, akathisia's response to antiparkinsonian medications is often unsatisfactory. Benzodiazepines sometimes help in such situations. Uncontrolled observations have been based on diazepam use.[7,8] Clinical experience at McLean Hospital reveals some success with akathisia resistant to antiparkinsonian drugs by using lorazepam 1 to 2 mg b.i.d. to t.i.d.

The literature on differential response to antipsychotics—the right antipsychotic for each patient—has generally been disappointing. The patient's psychopathology and psychiatric history do not predict better response to one drug than to another. Nevertheless, occasionally a patient will do much better on a particular antipsychotic for unknown reasons; sometimes side-effect differences can explain the special effect. Once in a while depot fluphenazine is superior to oral medication, perhaps because this route of administration bypasses the gut and the liver where antipsychotics may be deactivated metabolically.

In the next few years perhaps plasma level determinations of antipsychotic drug concentrations will become really useful.[9,10] Or the measurement of dopamine-blocking activity level in plasma will prove a more usable general method that is applicable to all antipsychotic drugs.

In my experience molindone does appear to facilitate weight loss in schizophrenic patients who are becoming progressively more obese on other antipsychotics.[11]

The addition of lithium carbonate to antipsychotics in schizophrenics is controversial. Given lithium's recently discovered rare adverse effects on the kidney,[12] lithium should not be used for prolonged periods in schizophrenics in the pious hope that it may some day be vaguely helpful. On the other hand, schizoaffective-appearing patients with acute affective episodes and good adjustment between episodes may well be atypical manic-depressives and may respond well to lithium.[13,14] Occasionally, impulsively assaultive schizophrenics or even ordinary schizophrenics may also be helped by lithium.[15,16] Its use in such situations is certainly outside current FDA-approved indications.

CHRONIC AND RECURRENT DEPRESSIONS

Patients without a history of mania often show moderate to severe depression which may either be recurrent (unipolar) or chronic. In either group of patients, once they have responded to an antidepressant—either a tricyclic (TCA) or a monoamine oxidase inhibitor (MAOI)—the issue of prolonged maintenance therapy arises. Conventional wisdom, unsupported by real data, suggests that patients with single or infrequent depressions of brief duration (e.g., several months or less) should stay on the drug for 6 months after responding to it, perhaps at half the original therapeutic dose if side effects are bothersome. After 6 months the drug should be slowly tapered over a few weeks. Abrupt termination regularly causes unpleasant withdrawal effects, chiefly nausea, vomiting, restlessness and malaise.[17]

If the patient was steadily depressed for several years before an effective treatment was found, withdrawal at 6 months often may lead to a return of symptoms and prolonged maintenance treatment with the drug may be necessary. It is often necessary to keep such patients on medication until a particularly stable period in their life occurs, and then to try withdrawal again, sometimes successfully.

In patients who have frequent unipolar depressions, prolonged maintenance therapy is indicated with the drug that induced a remission in the last depression. On the average, imipramine is as effective as lithium carbonate in preventing future depressions, working well in 50–60% of cases.[18] If a tricyclic has worked in relieving the depression and is well tolerated as a maintenance treatment, there is no compelling reason for shifting to lithium with its more elaborate necessary serum monitoring and low risk of renal damage. To date there is no evidence that prolonged use of either TCAs or MAOIs leads to any chronic toxicity with use for months or years. The main problems with tricyclics are dry mouth, trouble urinating, blurred vision, sweating, tachycardia, hypotension, jitteryness or sedation, weight gain and impotence or frigidity and memory impairment and speech blockage. All of these except weight gain are most common early in therapy and tend to stay the same or ameliorate a bit if treatment continues. Thus, the problem is more one of finding an effective and well-tolerated antidepressant initially than of worrying about long-term consequences. It is my clinical impression that weight gain on TCAs is most common with amitriptyline and least common with desipramine.

With MAOIs, the problem side effects are hypotension, fatigue or insomnia or overstimulation, rare lack of orgasm in women or impotence in men, weight gain and, of course, the hypertensive crises with severe headache that follow ingestion of tyramine-containing foods or drugs which raise blood pressure.[19] Again, if a patient with a chronic or frequently recurring depression responds uniquely to an MAOI, maintenance therapy usually does not cause more side effects than short-term therapy, though the risk of hypertensive crisis remains and patients must be regularly reminded to observe the major dietary precautions.

In rare depressions which respond only to electroconvulsive therapy (ECT) and relapse in a few weeks after each course of therapy, maintenance ECT is believed to be effective by some practitioners.[20] No formal studies of its efficacy are available. Its potential for inducing organic brain changes is similarly unstudied.

Occasional depressions unresponsive to any other therapy will respond to stimulants (methylphenidate, d-amphetamine, magnesium pemoline) without developing either tolerance or abuse and may require such therapy for prolonged periods.

Some adult patients with symptoms resembling those seen in hyperkinetic children—restlessness, impulsivity, short attention span, irritability—are termed Adult Minimal Brain Dysfunction (MBD) and respond well to stimulants and, if clearly benefited, may need prolonged maintenance therapy.[21,22]

BIPOLAR AFFECTIVE DISORDER

Patients with either recurrent mania or both recurrent mania and depression are sometimes helped markedly by maintenance lithium therapy. Other patients may have the severity of their mood swings reduced but not abolished.[18] In some patients recurrent manic episodes occur because they unilaterally stop their lithium periodically and then relapse. If lithium alone does not work, maintenance antipsychotic therapy may work in some patients but has never been formally studied and carries a risk of tardive dyskinesia. Some patients (or their relatives) can learn to abort incipient mania by taking antipsychotics in low doses at the first sign of sleeplessness or racing thoughts.

Maintenance lithium therapy is said to be more effective at serum levels above 0.8 milliequivalents. Some patients require even higher levels (e.g., 1.2 meq), and some who can't tolerate higher dosages do well on levels as low as 0.4 meq.

Lithium therapy is not without its drawbacks. Tremor is common and can sometimes be controlled by propranolol. Acneform rash, weight gain, hair loss, hypothyroidism, fatigue and nausea are less common adverse effects.[23] Probably a quarter or more of patients on maintenance lithium develop some polyuria and polydipsia. In a few this reaches the severity of true diabetes insipidus with urine volumes of 8-10 litres a day. This can often be ameliorated by adding a thiazide diuretic. Since such diuretics reduce lithium excretion, the lithium dose must be markedly reduced and the serum level restabilized if a thiazine diuretic is added. There is also an unknown risk of pathological kidney changes and reduced renal clearance of creatinine and other substances on prolonged lithium therapy with or without added diuretic. Serious changes seem rare to date, but only a few preliminary surveys have been reported.[12]

The implication of the renal changes is that patients with unclear benefit from lithium should be tried off the drug to see if it is really providing enough benefit to match the low but real risk.

CHRONIC ANXIETY

Here the data is particularly weak. Essentially all studies of benzodiazepines and other antianxiety drugs in anxious patients cover only 4-6-week treatment periods. Since at least some patients become mildly physically or psychologically dependent on these drugs, and have trouble withdrawing themselves from them, and may well also have developed tolerance to their anxiety-relieving actions, such drugs should ideally be given only for 2–4-week periods and then tapered and reused sparingly or occasionally for the temporary relief of exacerbations in anxiety.[24]

Psychiatrists usually encounter these patients already on chronic maintenance benzodiazepine therapy and have to decide how hard to try to get patients off the drug. Dosages over 30 mg a day of diazepam or the equivalent in other benzodiazepines, or around 3,200 mg a day of meprobamate maintained for several months should be suspected of having caused some dependence, and the dose should be tapered slowly, perhaps 10–20% a week. It should also be remembered that diazepam and other benzodiazepines with a halflife over 30 hours may not cause severe withdrawal effects for about

4 days after the drug is abruptly stopped but can then cause agitation, convulsions and delirium.

In some patients with mixed anxiety and depression, TCAs are more effective and may cause fewer problems. Tybamate and hydroxyzine are nondependence-inducing antianxiety drugs which can sometimes replace benzodiazepines in relieving anxiety (but cannot prevent the severe withdrawal symptoms of physical dependence). Propranolol may also have a role, particularly in patients with autonomic symptoms of anxiety.[25] Low dosages of antipsychotics sometimes relieve chronic anxiety but have their own problems, mainly tardive dyskinesia.

GENERAL

The physical status of any patient on prolonged maintenance drug therapy should be medically evaluated yearly. In lithium patients, thyroid and renal function should be closely checked. In patients on antipsychotics, tardive dyskinesia should be watched for and cardiac status should be checked. Since the TCAs also alter cardiac function, usually in mild manner, and can aggravate narrow angle glaucoma, these areas should also be watched.

SUMMARY

The uses and problems attached to maintenance drug therapies for chronic psychiatric patients have been reviewed. The relative efficacies of antipsychotics in stabilizing chronic schizophrenics, tricyclics in recurrent and chronic depression and lithium in bipolar affective disorders are clear, and these medications are often quite useful.

REFERENCES

1. Hogarty, G., Goldberg, S. and Schoder, N. Drug and sociotherapy in the aftercare of schizophrenic patients: II. Two year relapse rates. *Arch. Gen. Psychiat.* 31: 603-608, 1974.
2. Gardos, G., Finnerty, R. J., Lilliscare, J. and Cole, J. O. Social functioning of chronic schizophrenics in the community under three drug conditions. Exhibit at Hosp. and Comm. Psychiat. Meeting. Denver, 1974.

3. Rifkin, A., Quitkin, F., Kane, J., Struve, F. and Klein, D. Are prophylactic antiparkinson drugs necessary? *Arch. of Gen. Psychiat.* 35: 483–489, 1978.
4. DiMascio, A., Demirgian, E. Antiparkinson drug overuse. *Psychosomatics.* 11: 596-601, 1970.
5. Van Putten, T., Crumpton, E. and Yale, C. Drug refusal in schizophrenics and the wish to be crazy. *Arch. Gen. Psychiat.* 33: 1442–1446, 1976.
6. Van Putten, T. Why do schizophrenics refuse to take their drugs? *Arch. of Gen. Psychiat.* 31: 67–72, 1975.
7. Donlon, P. The therapeutic use of diazepam for akathisia. *Psychosomatics.* 14: 222-225, 1973.
8. Gagrat, D., et al. Intravenous diazepam in the treatment of neuroleptic-induced acute dystonia and akathisia. *Amer. Journal Psychiat.* 135: 1232–1233, 1978.
9. Davis, J., Erickson, S. and DeKirmenjian, H. Plasma levels of antipsychotic drugs and clinical response. In: Lipton, M., DiMascio, A. and Killam, K. (Eds.). *Psychopharmacology: A Generation of Progress.* Raven Press, New York. pp. 905-916, 1978.
10. Baldessarini, R. Status of psychotropic drug blood level assays and other biochemical measurements in clinical practice. *Am. Journal of Psychiat.* 136: 1177-1180, 1979.
11. Gardos, G. and Cole, J. O. Weight reduction by molindone in schizophrenics. *Am. J. of Psychiat.* 134(3): 302–304, 1977.
12. Cole, J. Lithium and the kidney. *McLean Hospital Journal.* In Press, 1979.
13. Rapp, M. and Edwards, P. A high prevalence of affective disorders in a "schizophrenia" clinic. *Canadian Psychiatric Association Journal.* 22: 181–183, 1977.
14. Perris, C. Morbidity suppressive effect of lithium carbonate in cycloid psychosis. *Archives of Gen. Psychiat.* 35: 328–331, 1978.
15. Van Putten, T. and Sanders, D. Lithium in treatment failures. *Journal of Nervous and Mental Diseases.* 161: 255-264, 1975.
16. Small, J., Kellams, J., Milstein, V. and Moore, J. A placebo-controlled study of lithium combined with neuroleptics in chronic schizophrenic patients. *Amer. Journal of Psychiat.* 132: 1315-1317, 1975.
17. Shatan, C. Withdrawal symptoms after abrupt termination of imipramine. *Canadian Psychiatric Association Journal.* 11: Suppl. 5150-5158, 1966.
18. Davis, J. Overview: Maintenance therapy in psychiatry: II. Affective disorders. *American Journal of Psychiat.* 133: 1–12, 1976.
19. Ravaris, C., Robinson, D., Nies, A., Ives, J. and Bartlett, M. The use of MAOI antidepressants. *American Family Physician.* pp. 105–111, July, 1978.
20. Fink, M. Convulsive therapy: Theory and practice. Raven Press, New York, 1979.
21. Wood, D., Reimherr, F., and Wender, P. Diagnosis and treatment of minimal brain dysfunction in adults. *Archives of General Psychiat.* 33: 1453–1462, 1976.
22. Bellak, L. (Ed.) Psychiatric Aspects of Minimal Brain Dysfunction in Adults, Grune and Stratton, New York, 1979.
23. Altesman, R. and Cole, J. Lithium therapy: A practical review. *McLean Hospital Journal.* 3: 106–121, 1978.
24. Cole, J. Drug treatment of anxiety. *McLean Hospital Journal.* 3: 42–55, 1978.
25. Cole, J., Altesman, R. and Weingarten, C. Beta-blocking drugs in psychiatry. *McLean Hospital Journal.* 4: 40–68, 1979.

CHAPTER 13

CLINICAL PHARMACOLOGY AND SIDE EFFECTS OF ANTIPSYCHOTIC AND MOOD-STABILIZING DRUGS USED IN THE TREATMENT OF PSYCHIATRIC PATIENTS WITH CHRONIC OR RECURRENT DISORDERS

ROSS J. BALDESSARINI, M.D.

INTRODUCTION

The past two decades have produced almost revolutionary changes in the pattern of care of psychiatric patients. Important features of this revolution are a strikingly decreased prevalence of psychiatric hospitalization, the phasing out of many public mental institutions, the early return of psychotic patients to home and work, the development of open psychiatric units in general hospitals and an increased reliance on local community and outpatient treatment facilities, even for patients with severe psychotic illnesses such as schizophrenia and manic or depressive disorders, many of whom are treated effectively by physicians without specialized training in psychiatry. These changes almost certainly are the result of a complex interplay among new forms of medical treatment of psychiatric patients, administrative decisions, social and philosophic changes in medicine, and cultural and historical factors that are still poorly understood (1).

Among these factors, the introduction of effective and relatively safe new antipsychotic medications that are useful in schizophrenia, paranoid disorders, mania and some severe forms of depression, the availability of effective antidepressants, and the usefulness of antidepressants and lithium salts for the long-term prevention or amelioration of recurrent mood disorders (1), as well as the rise of the new discipline of psychopharmacology since the early 1950s have surely had an important effect. This era was opened by the introduction of reserpine, chlorpromazine (Thorazine) and the monoamine oxidase (MAO) inhibitors into the treatment of severely disturbed psychiatric patients in the early 1950s, and imipramine (Tofranil) in the late 1950s. The new psychopharmaceuticals lead to rapid control of psychotic or depressive symptoms and behavior and have profound preventive effects, both of a direct pharmacologic type and by preventing the untoward complications of prolonged institutionalization.

This chapter summarizes some aspects of the clinical use of antipsychotic drugs and emphasizes the important toxic reactions associated with these agents. Despite the problems of side effects and limited efficacy, it is important to emphasize at the outset that chemotherapy in psychiatry has had extremely beneficial direct effects on patient care and has also helped to draw psychiatry closer to medicine. The result has been the requirement for greater emphasis on careful differential diagnosis and substantial support for biologic approaches in psychiatry that complement still useful earlier psychosocial theories and therapies.

ANTIPSYCHOTIC AGENTS

Clinical Pharmacology of Antipsychotic Drugs

Antipsychotic agents include compounds proven effective in the management of a broad range of psychotic symptoms and particularly useful in the treatment of schizophrenia and mania. Nearly all produce neurological effects in animals and in patients. The evidence that this class of substances has real and selective antipsychotic effects in schizophrenia and other disorders marked by abnormalities of thought associations, perceptions and beliefs is now overwhelming (1). Although the antipsychotic drugs also calm excited, agitated or manic behavior, they are not merely a special kind of sedative and their older appellation "tranquilizers" is a misnomer. Some psychopharmacologists have been so struck by the regular association between antipsychotic effects and extrapyramidal motor effects that they have suggested the term *neuroleptic* (producing signs of neurological disorder) for this class of drugs. The preclinical screening of new agents in this class has depended almost entirely on the observation of motor effects in animals. Although this manner of developing new agents has had practical advantages, it may have retarded the search for agents that have antipsychotic effects without neurological side effects. The recent description of experimental agents that may have such desirable properties supports the conclusion that the more general and hopeful term *antipsychotic* is to be preferred while the search for drugs lacking neurological toxicity is pursued. The earliest antipsychotic drugs were the phenothiazines and the *Rauwolfia* alkaloids, notably reserpine (1952-53), although the usefulness of lithium salts for the management of excited or manic patients had been described earlier (1949). The first antipsychotic phenothiazine, chlorpromazine (Largactil), was developed in France (1952), and introduced into American medicine as Thorazine (1954).

At the present time, American practice accepts more than a dozen neuroleptic drugs of scientifically demonstrated clinical value for the treatment of psychoses (Table 1). These include the phenothiazines of low mg-potency (*not* efficacy)—with aliphatic or piperidine side-chains in their chemical structures—which have relatively greater tendency to induce sedation, hypotension and other autonomic side effects; the high-potency piperazine phenothiazines, which have relatively greater effects on extrapyramidal function; the *non*-phenothiazine tricyclic compounds (thioxanthenes and dibenzazepines); a butyrophenone; and its still experimental analogues, the orally, relatively long-acting diphenylbutylpiperidines; an indolone; and the now rarely used *Rauwolfia* alkaloids.

Despite the clinical availability of antipsychotic drugs for more than two decades, there is a striking lack of quantitative pharmacological information based on human studies, although a few general principles can be derived from studies in laboratory animals and from the available clinical literature. For example, a careful dose-response relationship has not been worked out for any antipsychotic drug in man. The best available information is derived from a reanalysis of published "success rates" (superior to placebo in overall group response) in studies comparing the antipsychotic effects of chlorpromazine with a placebo. These results suggest that the chance of a study's reporting success was about 60% when less than 300 mg of chlorpromazine was given per day, 80-90% at doses of 300-500 mg, and virtually 100% at doses of 500-800 mg or more. The dose-response relationship in man must be very broad as it is possible to obtain clinical estimates only of approximately minimally effective doses, whereas maximally effective doses are not known. Recommended doses are thus usually set above minimally effective doses, but as low as possible to avoid toxicity. In the attempt to

Table 1. Equivalent Doses of Commonly Used Antipsychotic Agents by Chemical Type

Generic Name	Trade Names[a]	Approximate Equivalent Daily Dose (mg)[b]
Phenothiazines		
Aliphatic		
Chlorpromazine	Thorazine, etc. (generic)	100
Triflupromazine	Vesprin	30
Piperidines		
Mesoridazine	Serentil	50
Piperacetazine	Quide	12
Thioridazine	Mellaril	95
Piperazines		
Acetophenazine	Tindal	20
Butaperazine	Repoise	12
Carphenazine	Proketazine	25
Fluphenazine	Prolixin, Permitil	2[c]
Perphenazine	Trilafon	10
Trifluoperazine	Stelazine	5
Thioxanthenes		
Aliphatic		
Chlorprothixene	Taractan	65
Piperazine		
Thiothixene	Navane	5
Dibenzazepines		
Loxapine	Loxitane, Daxolin	15
Clozapine	(Leponex, experimental)	60
Butyrophenones		
Haloperidol	Haldol, Serenace	2-3
Droperidol	Inapsine (for injection)	1-2[d]
Diphenylbutylpiperidines		
Pimozide	(Orap, experimental)	0.3-0.5
Penfluridol	(experimental)	2 (1-week dose)[c]
Fluspirilene	(experimental)	—
Indolones		
Molindone	Moban	10
Rauwolfia Alkaloids		
Reserpine	Serpasil, etc. (generic)	1-2

[a]Trade names in parentheses are not yet licensed in the U.S. The commercial preparations are available as soluble salts (most are hydrochlorides; Loxitane or Daxolin is a succinate; Repoise is a maleate). Other agents that are not commonly employed now or are less effective are not included, e.g., mepazine (Pacatal), promazine (Sparine), prochlorperazine (Compazine). While the tabulated drugs vary by over 100-fold in *potency*, they are very similar in their clinical *efficacy*.

Table 1. (continued)

[b]Data are summarized as averages from several sources, some of which vary greatly. These numbers are only an approximate guide, and dosage for each patient must be established by the clinical response. In switching from high doses of one agent to a dissimilar one, it is well to proceed gradually over several days to decrease the risk of side effects from the newly introduced drug.

[c]Injectable fluphenazine esters are used in doses of 25-100 mg every 1-4 weeks. Long-lasting diphenylbutylpiperidines can be used once weekly; penfluridol can be used as 2% of a *weekly* dose of chlorpromazine (i.e., 40 mg/week can replace 2100 mg/week of chlorpromazine).

[d]The only butyrophenone routinely used in the United States as an antipsychotic agent is haloperidol (Haldol). Another butyrophenone, droperidol (Inapsine) is an extremely potent neuroleptic, now used mainly as a preanesthetic or coanesthetic agent i.m. or i.v., although it has powerful antipsychotic-sedative effects that could be used in psychiatric emergencies too.

Adapted from Baldessarini, 1977 (1).

establish an ideal dose, there are two important clinical problems: the available methods have not provided quantitative evaluation of partial responses, and antipsychotic effects are essentially all-or-none phenomena and not clearly dose-related, except in the region of a "threshold" dose. A certain percentage of patients do not respond adequately even to doses equivalent to 1000 mg of chlorpromazine a day, although the occasional unresponsive patient may improve with a higher dose than usual, or with injected medication, or after a delay of several months. In recent studies that have compared ordinarily recommended doses (Table 1) of potent antipsychotic agents, such as fluphenazine and haloperidol, with doses more than an order of magnitude higher, it has not been possible to demonstrate consistently appreciable increases in group success rates, particularly when the comparison was extended for 2 to 3 months. The failure rate can also be reduced by the use of liquid oral preparations of antipsychotic drugs to avoid surreptitious disposal of pills. Unique metabolic characteristics of unresponsive patients might account for their failure to respond to antipsychotic medications, but these have not been described.

Animal studies do not permit estimations of dose-response relationships that allow meaningful predictions of clinical response, but they do reflect what is also known clinically, namely, that the therapeutic index (the ratio of a toxic dose to a dose that produces noticeable behavioral effects) for most of these agents is extremely high. It is also not possible to ascertain lethal doses, and it is almost impossible to commit suicide with these agents, unless medical assistance is unavailable or there are secondary complications of severe sedation. More than 10 grams of chlorpromazine has been ingested acutely by patients who survived.

In addition to the lack of lethality of the antipsychotic drugs, they are not particularly addicting. There is no craving for them on withdrawal, partly because they do not produce euphoria. The rebound excitation reported in animals after the abrupt discontinuation of very high prolonged doses of phenothiazines is virtually unknown clinically, with one important exception. Experimental use of ultrahigh doses (hundreds of mg/day) of powerful agents, such as fluphenazine, has been associated with a high risk of inducing acute dyskinesias (but not seizures) on withdrawal, if the high doses are suddenly terminated. This effect may be particularly likely to occur in children. There is, fortunately, little evidence of tolerance to the main effects of the antipsychotic drugs. There is, however, considerable evidence of tolerance to many of their side effects, including sedation, hypotension, anticholinergic effects, acute dystonic reactions, and even parkinsonism (a fact that challenges the routine use of antiparkinson medications beyond the period of risk in the first 2 or 3 months of treatment).

The metabolism of antipsychotic drugs has been best evaluated in the cases of chlorpromazine and haloperidol, although many generalizations apply equally well to other agents. The drugs are rapidly absorbed after oral administration and produce clinical effects within 30 to 60 minutes, and in 10 minutes or less after intramuscular injection. Anticholinergic agents, including antiparkinson drugs, can *decrease* intestinal absorption of antipsychotic drugs, possibly by slowing gut motility and allowing local bacterial inactivation to occur. However, it is not clear that such decreased absorption is clinically important, or even that it occurs at all to a significant extent. The antipsychotic agents are highly lipid-soluble and have a high affinity for membranes, including the surface of neurons. There is no impressively regional distribution of antipsychotic drugs in the central nervous system (CNS). The antipsychotic agents are known to be only partially excreted each day; a highly variable and unpredictable proportion is retained in lipid and connective-tissue pools, which saturate slowly and undergo slow turnover. Chlorpromazine can be found in the skin, cornea and lens after prolonged exposure to high doses. Metabolites of chlorpromazine have been detected in the urine many weeks and even months after discontinuation of treatment. These pharmacokinetic facts may contribute to the clinical observations that it takes several days or weeks for optimal antipsychotic action to evolve, whereas relapse after discontinuation of treatment is usually delayed for several weeks or months. Moreover, the slow elimination of antipsychotic agents suggests that it is reasonable eventually to administer the drugs only once a day, after tolerance to the acute side effects has been demonstrated, and to include periods without daily intake of drug during prolonged maintenance so as to mobilize stored drug.

The detoxification and inactivation of the antipsychotic drugs occurs largely through oxidation by hepatic microsomal enzymes. Oxidation converts these molecules to more polar, water-soluble metabolites and thus facilitates renal excretion. More than 100 metabolites of chlorpromazine alone have been identified. Most of these (about 80%) result from ring oxidation to form phenolic derivatives, some of which are pharmacologically active. The major metabolic change of butyrophenones is a form of oxidative dealkylation that splits the molecule to form inactive metabolites. Variable amounts of the metabolites are then excreted in bile and urine.

The complex metabolism of antipsychotic drugs, the bewildering array of active as well as inactive metabolites, and the enormous differences in metabolism of these drugs by individual patients are factors that have frustrated attempts to correlate blood drug levels with clinical responses, in contrast to the relative successes in this attempt with antidepressants and lithium (2). While chemical assays can typically detect only the parent drug and a few metabolites at best, the concept that antidopamine effects of the neuroleptics are a prominent if not crucial aspect of their action mechanisms (see section below on actions) has led to the development of a test-tube bioassay that can detect all circulating antidopamine metabolites. Thus, assays of the ability of serum from neuroleptic drug-treated patients to interfere with the binding of "neuroleptic-dopamine receptor" labeling agents such as [^{3}H]-spiroperidol to beef caudate nucleus membranes is such an approach (3). Nevertheless, this approach, too, has failed to provide clear guidelines to optimal blood levels of antipsychotic agents, although some progress is being made by the study of patients under better controlled circumstances that include use of fixed, moderate doses of one agent for acutely ill patients likely to improve rapidly.

Clinical Use of Antipsychotic Agents

There is now abundant evidence that the currently available antipsychotic drugs are effective in treating psychosis. Controlled therapeutic trials utilizing more than 300 mg/day of chlorpromazine or the equivalent (see Table 1) of other drugs have consistently demonstrated their efficacy, for the most part in patients within the schizophrenia spectrum of diagnoses. These results have led to the current impression that it is irresponsible not to treat relatively acute exacerbations of psychosis, including those occurring in chronic forms of schizophrenia, with adequate doses of antipsychotic medication, even though these drugs are rarely "curative." Moreover, it is important to emphasize that the neuroleptic agents are not selective for schizophrenia. In fact, the antipsychotic drugs are quite nonspecific in their effect on a number of severe psychiatric illnesses including schizophrenia, mania, agitated psychotic depression, paranoid disorders, involutional and senile psychoses, psychotic reactions to amphetamines, and even some aspects of organic dementia and acute brain syndromes. Moreover, the antipsychotic effects are most readily observed in acute and florid cases of psychotic excitement with considerable anxiety and agitation. It is possible that effects on thinking and social behavior are secondary to reduction of these aspects of psychotic affect. The main clinical consideration is that psychoses should not be treated with sedatives (except for rapid sedation in emergencies) or antianxiety agents, nor should antipsychotic agents ordinarily be used to treat anxiety. The target symptoms that consistently benefit from antipsychotic drugs include combativeness, tension, hyperactivity, hostility, negativism, hallucinations, acute delusions, insomnia, poor self-care, anorexia and sometimes seclusiveness, whereas improvement in insight, judgment, memory and orientation is less likely. In addition to acuteness and excitation, many other predictors of a favorable response to antipsychotic drugs include those features of psychotic illness generally associated with a favorable prognosis or with a favorable response to other forms of treatment. These include lack of an insidious, prolonged onset or a long chronic history; history of a relatively healthy premorbid adjustment and of social, educational and occupational accomplishment; current episode being the first psychotic breakdown; and prior favorable responses to similar medications or other medical treatments.

Because there are clear differences in the incidence of side effects with different classes of antipsychotic agents, the selection of a drug can rationally be made on the basis of predicted side effects. Whereas the *potency* (effect per mg) of antipsychotic agents can vary by more than 100-fold (Table 1), the overall clinical *efficacy*, as determined in controlled comparisons of many cases of psychosis, for most agents is remarkably similar provided that adequate doses were used—at least the equivalent of 300–400 mg of chlorpromazine a day. Similar data based on large numbers of systematic comparisons are unfortunately not available for forms of psychosis other than those called schizophrenia (which, in the past, has been a somewhat ambiguous term that included some acute or recurrent psychoses as well as chronic idiopathic disorders), although the same generalization appears clinically to be valid for most types of psychotic illness. There are a few notable exceptions to this rule, including promazine (Sparine), mepazine (Pacatal), and reserpine, all of which have failed to outperform a placebo in an appreciable number of clinical trials. Molindone, in a relatively small number of trials, has not been as consistently effective as other antipsychotic drugs, but its chemical dissimilarity to the phenothiazines is an advantage in cases of dangerous sensitivity reactions; the same advantage is offered by haloperidol and loxapine. Nearly every other antipsychotic agent currently in common use produced better results than placebo in at least 80–90% of comparisons. Among the many consistently effective antipsychotic agents, there is no evidence that one type is better than another for particular types of psychotic patients, nor is there a rational basis for combining antipsychotic agents—clinical folklore on these issues notwithstanding.

An important question is how long to pursue treatment with antipsychotic drugs. Although there is compelling evidence that antipsychotic drugs prevent recurrent exacerbations of schizophrenia (Table 2), in truly chronic, "poor-prognosis schizophrenia, the benefits of indefinite chemotherapy become increasingly difficult to demonstrate as the duration of illness and treatment increases, and in view of the risks involved: particularly the potentially irreversible neurological sequelae, notably tardive dyskinesia and more subtle

Table 2. Rate of Recurrence of Schizophrenia with and without Antipsychotic Agents

Treatment	N[a]	Relapsed	Percent Relapsed	Mean Relapse Rate ± SEM
Antipsychotic agent	1858	370	19.9	15.4 ± 0.6%[b]
Placebo	1337	698	52.2	55.7 ± 1.0%

Source: J. M. Davis, 1975, (4).
[a]N = 3195 patients in 22 controlled studies.
[b]When statistical analysis of the pooled data assumed that N = 22 studies, then $p<0.0001$ (a conservative method of computation); when it assumed that N = 3195 subjects, $p<10^{-80}$, using statistical methods explained in the source cited.

impairment of some higher cortical functions and psychomotor skills. Unfortunately, the best data refer only to relatively short periods of maintenance with the antipsychotic agents; they suggest that there is an appreciable relapse rate following recovery from an acute psychotic illness or an exacerbation of schizophrenia when active medication is discontinued immediately upon discharge from hospital. Relapse is unusual within the first few weeks after discontinuation of medication, most likely to occur between the second and twelfth months, and its risk may diminish after the second year (5). For this reason, the usual practice is to continue antipsychotic medications (or lithium, if indicated) for several months, even a year or longer, after the period of initial improvement from an episode of acute psychosis. Reasons for the slow or delayed emergence of relapse are obscure but may include the gradual clearance of medication accumulated in the initial weeks of treatment. In management of patients with chronic psychotic illnesses over many years, the conduct of a medication regimen requires considerable clinical judgment and a flexible response to the changing clinical needs of the patient. The safest guideline is to use the least medication for the shortest time necessary to obtain the desired results, with occasional attempts to reduce the dosage and to evaluate not only the continuing need for it, but also objective evidence of beneficial *response* to it, while examining specifically also for early signs of tardive dyskinesia.

General Toxicity and Side Effects of Antipsychotic Drugs (1)

The most important point to clarify in regard to the toxicity and side effects of the antipsychotic agents is that they are, in general, among the safest drugs available in medicine. This safety in no small measure accounts for their enormous popularity and widespread use. The overall incidence of important side effects is a few percent, although there are regularly occurring effects that are more annoying than dangerous. These include peculiar feelings of heaviness, sluggishness, weakness or faintness and a variety of mild, presumably anticholinergic effects, including dry mouth and blurred vision. Among the most common side effects characteristic of neuroleptic agents are those involving movements and posture, as will be discussed below, but there are a few other forms of toxicity that should also be emphasized.

The peripheral *anticholinergic actions* of most antipsychotic agents are modest and usually limited to annoying symptoms, such as dry mouth and blurred vision, although ileus and urinary retention can occur, particularly in older patients. Precipitating an acute attack of glaucoma with any agent having anticholinergic activity is always a worry, but even with antidepressant drugs this event is rare. A number of other *opthalmologic* problems occur with the antipsychotic agents. The most serious is an irreversible degenerative pigmentary retinopathy caused by large doses of thioridazine (above 900 mg/day). In addition, prolonged high doses of low-potency phenothiazines and thioxanthenes have also been associated with the deposit of drug substances and pigment in the cornea and lens, as well as in the skin. *Skin reactions* include photosensitivity early in treatment and later a blue-gray discoloration, usually associated with prolonged high doses of chlorpromazine. Maculopapular rashes occur on occasion, and there is some risk of contact dermatitis among those handling solutions of antipsychotic agents.

The risk of severe *cardiovascular* toxicity due to antipsychotic agents is not high. Although frank hypotension is not frequently encountered, orthostatic hypotension can be a problem, especially with the less potent phenothiazines and in elderly patients. The hypotensive effects of these agents are quite idiosyncratic and poorly correlated with doses. If severe hypotension does develop, it can usually be managed by bed rest, elastic stockings and elevation of the legs. If a vasoactive agent is required, the rational choice is a purely alpha-adrenergic pressor amine such as metaraminol (Aramine) to reverse the modest alpha-antagonistic effects of phenothiazines; beta-agonistic cardiac stimulants increase splanchnic pooling of blood and thus worsen the hypotension.

Other annoying side effects of antipsychotic agents include presumably peripheral *autonomic or hypothalamic effects* such as changes in appetite, weight gain, fluid retention, breast enlargement and engorgement (in males as well as females) and even galactorrhea, changes in libido and ejaculatory incompetence in males. These effects are most often associated with the less potent phenothiazines and particularly with thioridazine. The sustained prolactin-increasing action of most antipsychotic agents (mediated by the antagonism of hypothalamic dopamine at the anterior pituitary) and even small doses of reserpine as used to treat hypertension represents a theoretical risk in patients with an occult or identified carcinoma of the breast. However, there is at present no compelling evidence that antipsychotic agents have a tumor-inducing effect.

Although there has been a great deal of concern about jaundice and agranulocytosis due to antipsychotic agents, these problems are in fact encountered infrequently. The *jaundice* is almost always an allergic cholestatic type and is usually transient. Frank *agranulocytosis* is rare (incidence less than 0.01%), has a peak incidence within the first two months of treatment and is particularly observed in older females. Agranulocytosis has almost always been associated with low-potency phenothiazines or other low-potency antipsychotic agents such as clozapine and is virtually unknown with haloperidol, fluphenazine or thiothixine. Agranulocytosis is a potentially catastrophic and often rapidly developing medical emergency with a high mortality rate. It can rarely be predicted from occasional routine white blood cell counts and *must be suspected* and promptly evaluated in cases of malaise, fever or sore throat that occur *early* in the course of antipsychotic chemotherapy.

The safety of antipsychotic agents in *pregnancy and lactation* has not yet been established. These agents do pass the blood-placenta barrier as well as the blood-brain barrier, and they are to some extent secreted in human milk. They can induce a mild degree of sedation followed by motor excitement in the newborn. There is no evidence that they are responsible for an increased incidence of fetal malformations. Nevertheless, the current consensus is that the use of antipsychotic agents should be avoided as far as possible in pregnancy and lactation, and certainly in the first trimester of pregnancy. On the other hand, clinical judgment must be exercised when the indications for medication or psychiatric hospitalization during pregnancy are sufficiently compelling as to indicate cautious trials of the smallest effective divided doses for the shortest possible time.

Elderly patients treated with antipsychotic agents are particularly likely to be troubled by toxic effects of all types, and unwanted effects on the brain and behavior may be most striking.

Actions of Neuroleptic-Antipsychotic Drugs

Although the antipsychotic-neuroleptic drugs represent a wide variety of chemical structures, their pharmacology and spectrum of activity are remarkably similar (1). Thus, the antipsychotic agents in current use in this country all regularly produce a variety of presumably extrapyramidal disorders of the control of posture, muscle tone and movement. A crucial question is whether the almost routinely encountered neurologic ("neuroleptic") effects of the antipsychotic drugs are essential to their actions. The fact that several effectively antipsychotic drugs have relatively little tendency to induce acute neurologic reactions (dystonias, parkinsonism and restlessness) now strongly challenges the inevitability of the association of neurologic and antipsychotic effects. Such drugs include thioridazine (Mellaril), clozapine and its congeners, and possibly sulpiride (experimental agents), and their existence offers some hope that better antipsychotic agents with diminishing neurologic side effects can be developed.

Thioridazine does produce extrapyramidal effects, but appears to be among the least likely to do so of currently available agents. Unfortunately, it does produce other autonomc and metabolic side effects, and its maximum daily dose is limited to 800 mg/day due to reports of rare but potentially irreversible and sight-damaging retinal toxicity (retinitis pigmentosa). Clozapine is of great theoretical interest as its extrapyramidal side effect risk is extremely low, but its present status has been in doubt due to its association with agranulocytosis. Both of these agents are strongly anticholinergic; sulpiride is not. The uniqueness of sulpiride and other benzamide agents is somewhat uncertain as they appear to penetrate the CNS poorly, and at high, antipsychotically effective doses (about 1,000 mg/day), they can induce extrapyramidal effects.

An important fact (or artifact) is that the methods of screening new substances for potential antipsychotic utility have essentially involved seeking neurologic reactions in laboratory animals, because there are no satisfactory animal tests for schizophrenia. This impasse, coupled with current conservatism of the system for development and testing of new agents, particularly in the United States, has contributed to a repeated "rediscovery" of agents with very similar actions and limitations over the past 30 years.

In the past, a number of mechanisms had been proposed to explain the actions of the antipsychotic drugs. They differ from most other depressants of the CNS in several ways. Thus, they have limited ability to induce generalized sedative effects or coma until enormous overdoses are taken; in addition, tolerance to their antipsychotic effects is rare (and virtually unknown with 1–2 years of treatment) and addiction does not occur. Unlike sedatives, they have been reported to have greater ability to diminish conditional behavioral responses than to depress unconditional responses. They may have a selective ability to dampen the neurophysiologic effects of peripheral stimuli on the forebrain, while inhibiting to a much lesser extent the effects of stimulating electrodes placed in the brain-stem. In addition to these distinctions from sedatives, antipsychotic drugs have striking inhibitory effects on autonomic and motoric expressions of arousal and strong affect in animals, presumably mediated by actions in the limbic forebrain and hypothalamus. The cellular and biochemical events underlying these behavioral and physiologic actions, however, have remained obscure until recently.

It was proposed by European pharmacologists as long ago as the early 1960s that the neurologic, and possibly also the antipsychotic, effects may reflect the ability of antipsychotic drugs to interfere with synaptic transmission in the brain mediated by dopamine (6). This suggestion arose largely from the observation that among the biochemical consequences of giving an antipsychotic drug to an animal, there was a consistent increase in levels of the metabolites of dopamine, but variable effects on the metabolism of other neurotransmitters. The possible importance of dopamine was given strong support by early histochemical studies of the normal distribution of amine-containing neurons in the mammalian brain, which indicated a preferential distribution of dopamine fibers between midbrain and the basal ganglia (notably, the nigroneostriatal tract), and within the hypothalamus. More recently, anatomists have come to appreciate the existence of other dopamine projections from midbrain nuclei to forebrain regions that are associated with the limbic system and probably not the extrapyramidal motor system, as well as to deep temporal and mesial prefrontal cerebral cortical areas closely interlinked with the limbic system (Fig. 1). A somewhat simplistic, but attractive, concept has been that many extrapyramidal neurologic effects of the antipsychotic drugs may be mediated by antidopamine effects in the basal ganglia, and that some of their antipsychotic effects may be mediated by the antagonism of "dopaminergic" neuro-transmission in the limbic system, hypothalamus and cortex. The latter supposition has been given indirect general encouragement by repeated "natural experiments" that have associated psychotic mental phenomena with lesions of the temporal lobe and other portions of the limbic system.

In recent years, a large body of data has accumulated to support the theory that the antagonism of dopamine-mediated synaptic neurotransmission is an important action of antipsychotic-neuroleptic agents (Table 3). Thus, antipsychotic agents, but not their nonantipsychotic congeners, are reported to increase the rate of production of dopamine metabolites (notably, dihydroxyphenylacetic and homovanillic acids), the rate of conversion of tyrosine to dopamine and its metabolites, and the firing rate of presumably dopamine-containing neuronal cell bodies in midbrain. These effects have been interpreted as secondary or compensatory responses of

DOPAMINE PROJECTIONS: HUMAN BRAIN

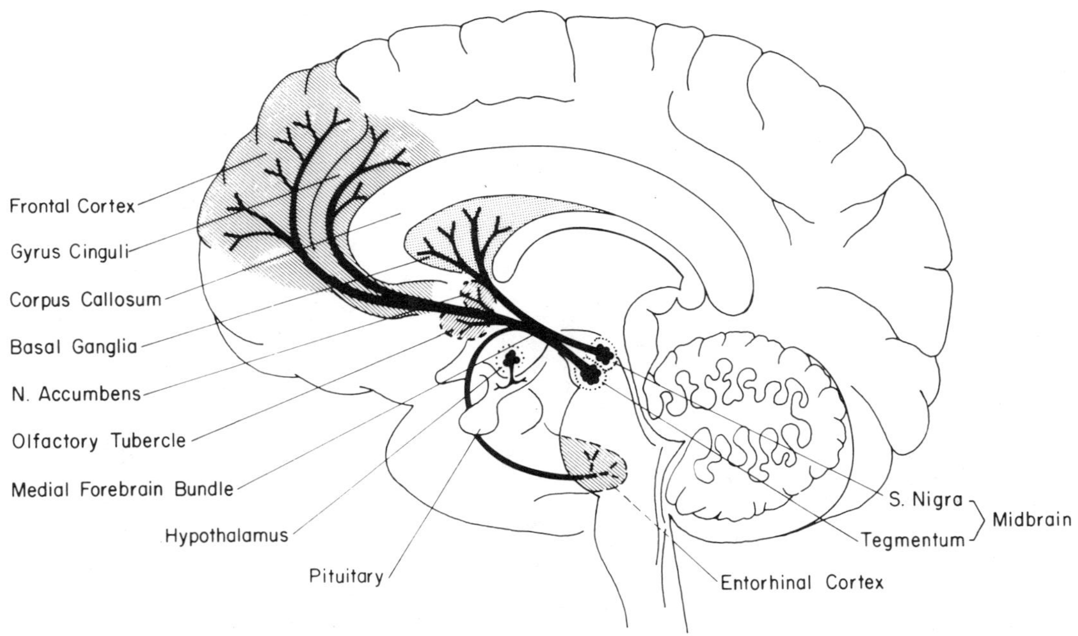

Figure 1. Dopamine-Containing Neurons in the Mammalian Brain. The major systems involving dopamine are: the *nigrostriatal* pathway from the zona compacta of the midbrain substantia nigra to the neostriatum (caudate and putamen); *mesolimbic* projections from midbrain tegmentum through the lateral hypothalamus to limbic structures, including the septal nuclei (e.g., nucleus accumbens septi) and olfactory tubercle; and related *mesocortical* projections, also arising in midbrain, and projecting particularly to prefrontal and temporal areas of the cerebral cortex; there is also a *tuberoinfundibular* dopamine-containing (TIDA) system within the hypothalamus. The scheme is based heavily on studies in rat, for which most information is available, although the dopamine systems in man are believed to be very similar.

Table 3. Effects of Neuroleptic Drugs on CNS Dopamine-Containing and Dopamine-Sensitive Neurons

1. Block DA receptors (as evidenced by antagonism of DA-sensitivity adenylate cyclase or of binding of ^{3}H-labeled drugs to DA receptor sites in brain, and by blockade of DA iontophoretically applied to single receptive cells).
2. May alter DA release (uncertain).
3. Block behavioral effects (hyperactivity and stereotyped movements) of dopamine agonists administered systemically or by local intracerebral injection (esp. in caudate nucleus and limbic areas).
4. Block behavioral effects (self-stimulation) mediated by electrodes placed in DA-rich brain pathways (extrapyramidal and limbic).
5. Increase DA cell firing rate in midbrain.
6. Increase turnover of DA in forebrain (HVA increases; conversion of tyrosine to DA increases).
7. TIDA—neuroendocrine effects (e.g., PL increases, and PL decrease in response to DA agonists is blocked).

Abbreviations: DA: dopamine
HVA: homovanillic acid
PL: prolactin
TIDA: tuberoinfundibular hypothalamic DA system

plastic and adaptive neuronal systems attempting to maintain homeostasis in the face of what is assumed to be a primary interruption of synaptic transmission at the dopamine terminals in the caudate nucleus, septal nuclei and cerebral cortex. Figure 2 shows the metabolic arrangements at such synapses.

Evidence that a crucial primary event may be the blockade of postsynaptic dopamine receptor sites includes the ability of small doses of antipsychotic agents to block behavioral or endocrine effects of dopamine agonists. Examples are stereotyped gnawing behavior in the rat induced by the direct dopamine agonist, apomorphine, possibly acting at the caudate nucleus; the locomotor excitement induced by the injection of dopamine into the nucleus accumbens septi of the limbic system; or the prolactin-decreasing response to apomorphine or L-dihydroxyphenylalanine (L-dopa) believed to be mediated by dopamine receptor in the anterior pituitary. Such "tests" have been proposed as screening methods to detect even more agents of the kinds already available. More direct evidence of a receptor blockade has been provided by the antagonism of a dopamine-sensitive adenylate cyclase (an enzyme that mediates the action of many hormones) in homogenates of caudate or limbic tissue, and the interference with electrophysiological responses to dopamine locally applied to receptive cells in the caudate nucleus—a blockade overcome by presumed circumvention

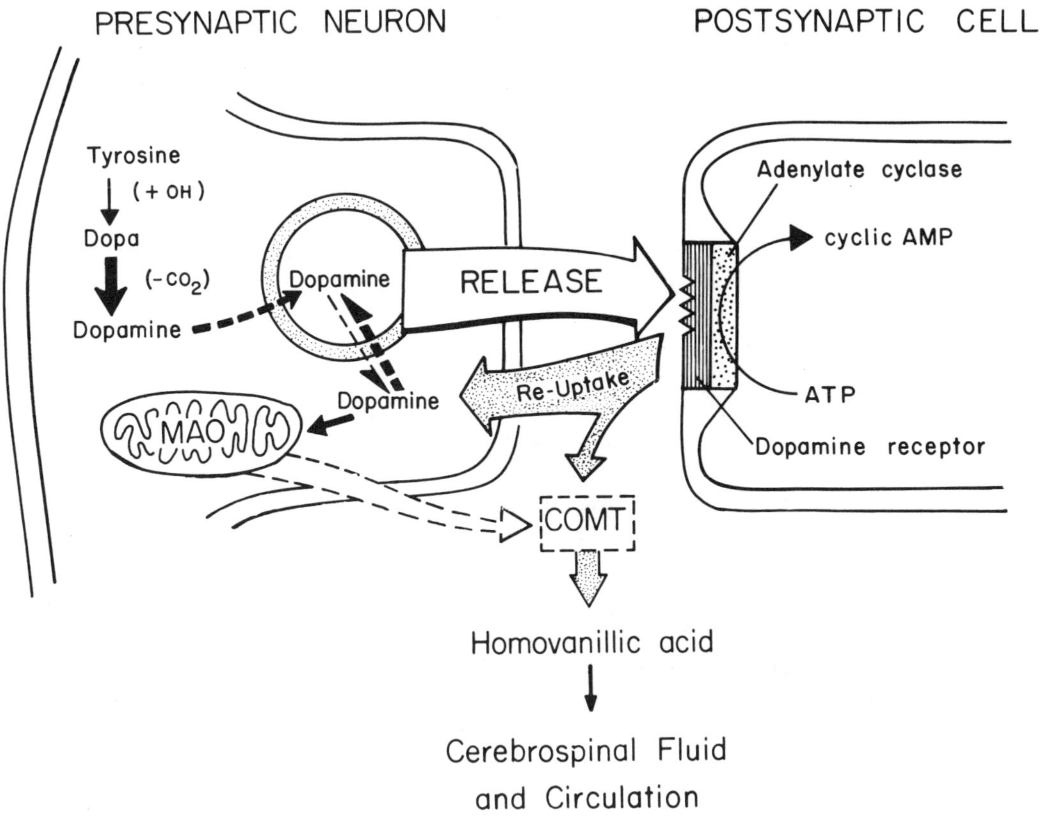

Figure 2. Metabolism at a Dopamine Synapse in the Brain. Dopamine is formed from tyrosine by hydroxylation (the rate-limiting step) to dihydroxyphenylalanine (dopa), which is rapidly decarboxylated. Dopamine is stored in presynaptic vesicles (shaded circle), from which release occurs into the synpatic cleft by neuronal depolarization in the presence of calcium. The released amine has a postsynaptic effect, possibly mediated by a recognition molecule (receptor) associated with adenylate cyclase. Neurotransmitter is inactivated largely by efficient high-affinity reuptake into the presynaptic terminals; excess dopamine that is not stored can be metabolized by monoamine oxidase (MAO) in the mitochondria and catechol-*O*-methyltransferase (COMT), largely extra-neuronal, to produce homovanillic acid from dihydroxyphenylacetic acid, an intermediary metabolite; the metabolites are removed in the cerebrospinal fluid and venous circulation via the choroid plexus.

of the receptor sites on the cell surfaces (Fig. 2) by analogues of cyclic-AMP (the product of adenylate cyclase and ATP) (7). A more recent development is the application of "radioligand" binding assays using homogenates of mammalian caudate nucleus and low concentrations (nanomolar or 10^{-9} M) of intensely radioactive [^{3}H]-labeled neuroleptic drugs (haloperidol or spiroperidol). Pharmacologic evidence supports the suggestion that the binding of these ligands to brain tissue represents an interaction with a dopamine "receptor" site. Correlations between the potency of antipsychotic drugs of all types to interfere with the binding of such ligands, and estimates of their potency to block the effects of dopamine agonists in animals or to produce clinical benefits in psychotic patients (6,8) are impressive. Chemical analogues or isomers of the antipsychotic drugs that are clinically inactive lack this ligand-binding antagonistic effect. It is particularly interesting that two antipsychotic agents (thioridazine and clozapine) with relatively weak acute neurologic side effects seem to have antidopamine effects in the ligand-binding assays that correlate closely with their clinical potencies (6,8). Although their relative lack of extrapyramidal toxicity has been explained by a countervening antimuscarinic (antiparkinsonism?) action of these two drugs, this explanation is not satisfactory for a similar drug, sulpiride (7). Analogous approaches have led to the suggestion that hypotensive and sedative effects of the less potent phenothiazines may correspond to their relatively strong antagonistic effects at central and vascular alpha-noradrenergic receptors (9).

Although these findings together strongly support the theory that antipsychotic agents interfere with the actions of dopamine as a synaptic neurotransmitter in the brain, they do not prove the antidopamine effects are either necessary or sufficient for antipsychotic efficacy. They strongly suggest, however, that some of the extrapyramidal neurologic effects of this class of agents may be produced by antagonism of dopamine, largely on the basis of analogy to the demonstrated loss of dopamine in the caudate nucleus, and the beneficial responses to its precursor L-dopa, in idiopathic Parkinsonism.

Neurologic Side Effects of Antipsychotic Drugs

The common and sometimes troublesome neurologic side effects of antipsychotic drugs represent a unique constellation of syndromes not associated with other psychotropic agents. These reactions can be subdivided into several categories, as are outlined in Table 4. Other classes of psychotropic drugs, including sedatives (e.g., barbiturates), tranquilizer-antianxiety agents (e.g., benzodiazepines such as diazepam

[Valium]), and even tricyclic antidepressants and lithium salts, are more likely to express toxic effects in the CNS, especially on overdosage, with generalized depressant effects, toxic delirium, and eventually coma and death. The antidepressants are also likely to produce atropinelike signs and symptoms on acute overdose, which are discussed below. The monoamine oxidase (MAO) inhibitor antidepressant agents (also used to treat certain anxious-phobic reactions) as well as the classical stimulants (notably, amphetamines) are more likely to produce toxic states of excitement, hypertension and eventually collapse on acute overdosage.

Thus, for the antipsychotic agents, CNS toxicity is expressed in several characteristic syndromes. Except for parkinsonism, the pathophysiology of these reactions is still poorly understood, although it is suspected that effects on dopamine-mediated systems in the basal ganglia are involved (Table 4). These syndromes are as follows.

Acute dystonias typically occur within the first few days of orally administered treatment although they occasionally follow each dose of long-acting injections of fluphenazine esters. They involve hyperkinesias of the musculature of the neck, mouth and tongue and may include opisthotonos or oculogyric crises. The main problem with this syndrome is to recognize it and not to ascribe it to a seizure disorder, tetany or tetanus, or "hysteria." Treatment by injection of an antiparkinson agent is usually dramatically effective; diphenhydramine (Benadryl, 25 or 50 mg given intramuscularly or 25 mg intravenously) and benztropine mesylate (Cogentin, 2 mg given intravenously) are currently popular choices. If dystonic reactions recur frequently, calcium metabolism should be evaluated. The pathophysiology of these reactions remains obscure, in part because so many different classes of drugs (including stimulants, sedatives, anticholinergics, antihistamines, etc.) have been reported to be therapeutically useful. One interesting lead is that the maximum time of risk of dystonias is when blood levels of a neuroleptic are at a maximum rate of decline some hours after an acute dose (10).

Drug-induced parkinsonism is similar to other forms of the disease, except that tremor is typically less prominent. The clinical pharmacology of drug-induced parkinsonism as well as the clinical signs of the disorder are strikingly similar to the idiopathic forms of the illness, which is almost certainly due, at least in part, to a deficiency of dopamine in the basal ganglia. Thus, it is likely that neuroleptic-induced parkinsonism is due to the pharmacologic blockade of dopamine-mediated neurotransmission. The onset of the syndrome is usually after the first week of treatment, but within the first month. There appears to be some "tolerance" to this effect, as the signs

Table 4. Neurological Side Effects of Neuroleptic-Antipsychotic Drugs

Reaction	Features	Onset (Max. Risk)	Proposed Mechanism	Treatment
Acute dystonia	Spasm of muscles of tongue, face, neck, back; may mimic seizures; *not* hysteria	1–5 d	Unknown	Antiparkinson agents are diagnostic and curative (i.m. or i.v., then p.o.)
Parkinsonism	Bradykinesia, rigidity, variable tremor, mask-facies, shuffling gait	5–30 d	DA-blockade	Antiparkinsonism agents help (p.o.)
Akathisia	Motor restlessness; *not* anxiety or agitation	5–60 d	Unknown	Reduce dose or change drug; antiparkinsonism agents or benzodiazepines may help
Tardive Dyskinesia	Oral-facial dyskinesia; choreoathetosis	mos.–yrs. (worse on withdrawal)	DA-excess?	Prevention best; treatment unsatisfactory, but often spontaneously disappear gradually
"Rabbit" Syndrome	Perioral tremor (late Parkinson variant?)	mos.–yrs.	Unknown	Antiparkinsonism agents may help

usually fade away over 2 or 3 months, with a decreasing requirement for antiparkinson medications. Antipsychotic agents with higher milligram potency induce dystonic reactions and parkinsonism with greater frequency than less potent agents, while the latter tend more often to induce sedation and autonomic effects.

Severe akinetic, catatonic reactions and mutism, sometimes with hyperthermia and other signs of autonomic instability, have also been associated with relatively high doses of potent antipsychotics, such as the piperazine phenothiazines and thioxanthenes and the butyrophenones. This reaction is usually termed the "neuroleptic malignant" syndrome. While the temptation is to suspect worsening functional psychosis and give even higher doses of the offending agent, improvement usually follows reduction in its dosage. The antiparkinson agents, including anticholinergics or amantadine (Symmetrel), may also help.

There are now a variety of agents used for the treatment of idiopathic as well as drug-induced parkinsonism. Those used in psychotic patients (L-dopa is too likely to produce agitation for routine use in such patients) are listed in Table 5. Most of these drugs (except amantadine [Symmetrel]) are strongly antimuscarinic (atropinelike),

Table 5. Equivalent Doses of Antiparkinsonism Agents

Generic Name	Trade Names	Usual Dose Range (mg/day)
Amantadine	Symmetrel	100–300
Benztropine	Cogentin	1–6
Biperiden	Akineton	2–6
Diphenhydramine	Benadryl	25–100
Ethopropazine	Parsidol	5–0
Orphenadrine	Disipal, Norlex	300
Procyclidine	Kemadrin	6–20
Trihexyphenidyl	Artane, etc. (generic)	5–15

These agents are commonly prescribed orally three times a day to provide the total daily adult doses stated above. Benztropine (2 mg) and diphenhydramine (25–50 mg) are commonly used intramuscularly or intravenously to reverse acute dystonic reactions to antipsychotic agents. Amantadine has recently been used to treat drug-induced parkinsonism and catatonia; it is relatively expensive and may lose effectiveness in a few weeks; overdoses may respond to physostigmine. Diphenhydramine and orphenadrine are antihistaminic and anticholinergic; ethopropazine is strongly anticholinergic phenothiazine; the other agents are atropinelike. Most are available as soluble hydrochlorides.

From Baldessarini, 1977 (1).

so that they can induce the syndrome of anticholinergic poisoning: restless agitation, confusion, disorientation, perhaps seizures and hyperthermia, dry and sometimes flushed skin, tachycardia, sluggish and at least moderately dilated pupils, decreased bowel sounds and often acute urinary retention. These effects are probably due to peripheral and central anticholinergic actions of these potent muscarinic blocking agents (11). This syndrome is best managed by removal of the offending agent and the use of physostigmine (eserine, Antilirium)—the only available centrally (CNS) as well as peripherally active reversible anticholinesterase agent (11). It can be seen from Table 6 that the antiparkinsonism and tricyclic antidepressant drugs are among the most potent centrally active anticholinergic agents used in medicine. The potential to induce CNS toxicity is only one of the problems associated with antiparkinsonism agents that indicates caution in their use with psychotic patients being treated with neuroleptics, or especially with antidepressant agents (Table 7). While the antiparkinsonism agents are sometimes given prophylactically to avoid acute extrapyramidal effects of antipsychotic agents, this practice is often unnecessary. Furthermore, sound practice requires the attempt to withdraw these drugs after several weeks, and certainly within 4-12 weeks after the onset of an acute extrapyramidal reaction, due to "tolerance" developing within that time for acute dystonias and even parkinsonism (see Table 4).

Akathisia—motor restlessness, fidgeting, pacing, "restless legs," and the drive to move about—is a common motor symptom complex that typically follows the time course of parkinsonism. This syndrome, like other extrapyramidal reactions, should not be mistaken for increasing psychotic anxiety or agitation or treated by increasing the dose of an antipsychotic drug. It can sometimes be managed by reducing the dose or changing to a different chemical class of antipsychotic agents. Antiparkinsonism drugs may have a beneficial effect, as may anxiolytic agents with muscle-relaxing properties, such as diazepam (Valium) or lorazepam (Ativan). Unfortunately, many cases respond poorly to treatment, and a clinical decision must be made to weigh the distress of the akathisia against the need for antipsychotic medication. This reaction may persist or reoccur indefinitely, even though it is usually said to have its peak incidence within the first two months of treatment (see Table 4). Tolerance to akathisia seems less likely than to dystonic and parkinsonism reactions. The pathophysiologic basis of akathisia is unknown, although antidopamine effects are suspected.

Table 6. Antimuscarinic Effect of CNS Agents: Rank-order of Potencies

Agent	Potency
Scopolamine	+++++
Atropine	+++++
Trihexyphenidyl (Artane)	++++
Benztropine (Cogentin)	++++
Amitriptyline (Elavil, etc.)	++++
Doxepin (Sinequan)	+++
Imipramine (Tofranil, etc.)	+++
Nortriptyline (Aventyl)	++
Protriptyline (Vivactil)	++
Desipramine (Norpramin, etc.)	+
Clozapine (Leponex)	++++
Thioridazine (Mellaril)	+++
Chlorpromazine (Thorazine, etc.)	+
Triflupromazine (Vesprin)	+
Fluphenazine (Prolixin)	+
Acetophenazine (Tindal)	+
Perphenazine (Trilafon)	+
Haloperidol (Haldol)	±
Trifluoperazine (Stelazine)	±
Iproniazid (Marplan)	0
Nialamid (Niamid)	0
Phenelzine (Nardil)	0
Trazodone	0

Rankings (strength from 0 to 5+) are based on data for the half-maximally effective concentrations (EC_{50}) of drugs which compete for the binding to tissue of the labeled test agent, ^{3}H-QNB—an avid and selective muscarinic antagonist (^{3}H-3-quinuclidinylbenzilate)—as estimated in rat brain homogenates by Snyder, Yamamura and Greenberg, 1974 (12) and 1977 (13). Additional data were from Richelson and Divenetz-Romero (1977) (18), on the potency of the test drugs in blocking the formation of cyclic guanosine-3′,5′-cyclic-monophosphate (cyclic-GMP) by carbamylcholine (a stable acetylcholine analogue), using cultured mouse neuroblastoma cells. The two methods are compared by the rank-order of potencies, disregarding the absolute values obtained which were usually, but not always, similar.

Tardive dyskinesia (late and persistent dyskinesia) is the late-developing extrapyramidal syndrome that has led to a reappraisal of the value of uninterrupted and indefinitely prolonged antipsychotic therapy (7,14). The syndrome consists of involuntary or semivoluntary movements of a choreiform (ticlike) nature, sometimes with an

Table 7. Potential Problems with Prolonged Use of Antiparkinson Agents

1.	Complicates regimen for doctor and patient.
2.	Unpleasant anticholinergic side effects.
3.	Risk of delirium, especially in elderly and with other drugs.
4.	Need decreases over 1-3 mos. (tolerance to drug-induced parkinsonism).
5.	Habituation and abuse occur.
6.	May decrease GI absorption of antipsychotics.
7.	Possibly reduced efficacy of antipsychotics (not proven).
8.	Possible contribution to risk of tardive dyskinesia (dubious).

athetotic or dystonic component. These classically affect the tongue, facial and neck muscles but often also affect the extremities and muscles that control posture and sometimes those used in breathing. Early signs of tardive dyskinesia are movements of the tongue or extremities. Oral-lingual-masticatory movements are common, especially in older patients; it is usual to find abnormalities of posture and at least subtle choreiform movements of the fingers as well, especially in younger patients.

The movements in tardive dyskinesia are much less voluntary and purposeful and more classically choreoathetotic than the stereotyped mannerisms and posturing that occur in schizophrenia. They usually become worse temporarily if the antipsychotic agent is withdrawn, and can be suppressed, at least temporarily, by readministering a neuroleptic drug or an amine-depleting agent. The "differential pharmacology" or pattern of drug responses that indicate worsening or improvement of tardive dyskinesia (Table 8) strongly suggests that this syndome may represent a functional *overactivity* of central *dopamine* mechanisms, possibly arising in compensation for prolonged blockade of dopaminergic synaptic transmission by an antipsychotic drug (7). Since the syndrome may be irreversible or persist for many months even after withdrawal of antipsychotic agents, it seems probable that other irreversible neurotoxic effects on central neurons also occur. Although painless, the syndrome can be embarrassing and distressing, especially in relatively well-functioning outpatients; in some cases it is as disabling as the impaired movement control of Huntington's chorea.

At the present time the conclusion seems inescapable that an important and relatively selective action of the antipsychotic-neuroleptic drugs is to block the actions of dopamine as a neurotransmitter in various regions of the CNS. Acute extrapyramidal and sustained neuroendocrine side effects of these agents are almost certainly, in part at least, reflections of this action in the basal ganglia and hypothalamus

Table 8. The Differential Pharmacology of Tardive Dyskinesia

Agents that may partially suppress tardive dyskinesia
- Dopamine antagonists
  - Apomorphine (in low dose)
  - Butyrophenones
  - Clozapine
  - Papaverine (mechanism uncertain)
  - Phenothiazines
  - Pimozide
- Amine-depleting agents
  - Reserpine
  - Tetrabenazine
- Blockers of catecholamine synthesis
  - Alpha-methyldopa
  - Alpha-methyltyrosine
- Blockers of catecholamine release
  - Lithium salts
- Cholinergic agents
  - Deanol (mechanism uncertain)
  - Physostigmine
  - Choline and Lecithin
- "GABA agonists"
  - Valproate (mechanism uncertain)
  - Baclofen (mechanism uncertain)
  - Benzodiazepines

Agents with variable, negligible or uncertain effects
- Alpha-methyldopa
- Amantadine
- Antihistamines
- Barbiturates
- Benzodiazepines
- Methylphenidate
- Penicillamine
- Physostigmine
- Pyridoxine (B_6)
- Tryptophan

Agents that worsen tardive dyskinesia
- Anticholinergic agents
  - Antiparkinsonism agents (e.g., benztropine)
- Dopamine agonists
  - Amphetamines
  - L-DOPA

  - Phenytoin

Some drugs appear in more than one category, reflecting ambiguity in the literature. Note that while apomorphine is usually classed as a dopamine-agonist, it actually has complex mixed actions, may antagonize DA at low doses and has clear antidyskinetic effects.

Adapted from Baldessarini & Tarsy, 1979 (7).

or pituitary, respectively. Antipsychotic effects may further in part reflect antidopamine effects in the limbic or cortical portions of the forebrain, although this hypothesis remains highly tentative. There is also excellent evidence that prolonged exposure to antidopamine drugs can lead to a variety of secondary or partially compensatory adjustments in the physiology and biochemistry of dopamine neurons and other cells with which they interact in the animal or human CNS. Among these adjustments, some tend to increase the effectiveness of dopamine as a neurotransmitter, particularly in the basal ganglia. These effects may help to explain the clinical observation that the risk of acute clinical extrapyramidal reactions diminishes in time, as the risk of tardive dyskinesia increases. Another crucial source of support for a "dopamine supersensitivity" hypothesis in tardive dyskinesia is the now considerable amount of clinical pharmacologic evidence to suggest that a functional overactivity of extrapyramidal mechanisms mediated by dopamine is an important aspect of the pathophysiology of tardive dyskinesia. An explanation for the prolonged and even irreversible course of some cases of tardive dyskinesia awaits further research, especially as it suggests that irreversible neurotoxic or degenerative effects of neuroleptic agents may occur.

While the precise pathophysiology of tardive dyskinesia remains uncertain, the study of neurological, behavioral and endocrinological effects of the neuroleptic agents on the CNS has contributed to an improved understanding of their actions, at least equal to that of many other drugs used in medicine. Moreover, insights arising from studies of the antidopamine effects of the antipsychotic drugs in various brain regions promise to lead the way to a more rational basis for developing new, less neurotoxic, but effectively antipsychotic agents.

A thorough neurologic examination of patients with tardive dyskinesia includes a vigorous attempt to exclude other forms of choreiform disease, such as Huntington's disease, rheumatic chorea, hyperthyroidism, Wilson's disease, and other rare toxic or degenerative dyskinetic syndromes as well as heavy metal poisoning (Table 9). The prevalence of the syndrome has varied widely among several epidemiologic studies (5 to 50%), largely as a reflection of differences in diagnostic criteria, but has averaged between 10 and 15% of patients chronically maintained on antipsychotic medication for several years. It is unusual to develop the syndrome in less than a few months, and there is growing evidence that if antipsychotic agents are withdrawn early, the signs of tardive dyskinesia may fade away spontaneously within several months, especially in younger patients.

Table 9. Differential Diagnoses to Consider in Evaluating Tardive Dyskinesia

- Neuroleptic withdrawal or transient dyskinesias
- Late and persistent "classical" tardive dyskinesia itself
- Stereotyped movements of schizophrenia
- Spontaneous oral dyskinesias of senility
- Oral dyskinesias related to dental conditions or prostheses
- Torsion dystonia and oromandibular dystonia with blepharospasm
- Huntington's disease
- Gilles de la Tourette's syndrome
- Wilson's disease (hepato-cerebral-lenticular degeneration due to abnormal copper metabolism), manganism and other heavy metal intoxications
- Fahr's syndrome with calcification of the basal ganglia
- Postanoxic or postencephalic extrapyramidal syndromes
- Rheumatic chorea ("St. Vitus' Dance" or Sydenham's Chorea)
- Drug intoxications (L-dopa, amphetamines, less commonly anticholinergics, antidepressants, lithium, phenytoin)
- CNS complications of systemic metabolic disorders (e.g., hepatic or renal failure, hyperthyroidism, hypoparathyroidism, hypoglycemia, vasculitides)

The treatment of tardive dyskinesia is highly unsatisfactory (see Table 8). Antiparkinsonism agents usually worsen the condition. The most effective short-term treatment is to suppress the manifestations with potent antipsychotic or amine-depleting (e.g., reserpine) agents. This approach may require increasing doses of the suppressing agent, may eventually fail, and in principle seems irrational, since it could contribute further to the underlying problem (although evidence is lacking that continued suppression of the symptoms results in their eventual worsening). The best means of dealing with the problem, as the search for "cleaner" or "nonneuroleptic" antipsychotic agents continues, is to seek to avoid it by the thoughtful and conservative use of antipsychotic agents in effective but not excessive doses, and only as indicated by *objectively discernible and clinically responsive* signs of psychotic thought, mood or behavior disorders. Suggested guidelines for dealing with this problem are presented in Table 10.

It is also well to realize that in the present era of the use of increasingly large doses of the more potent neuroleptic agents, sudden discontinuation of such treatment can lead to choreoathetotic reactions. These have been called "*withdrawal dyskinesias*" (15), are usually transient (several days to weeks), may occur early or late in treatment and may or may not reflect pathophysiologic mechanisms similar to those that underlie the tardive dyskinesias. They may be particularly likely to occur in children.

"*Rabbit*" *Syndrome*—perioral tremor—is another reaction associated with neuroleptic drugs that usually occurs late in therapy. This

Table 10. Suggested Guidelines for the Avoidance and Management of Tardive Dyskinesia

1. Consider the indications for prolonged and sustained antipsychotic-neuroleptic drug therapy carefully; the indications (chronic psychosis) should be serious, and there should be objective evidence of clinical benefit.
2. Seek alternative therapies for cases of neurosis, mood disorders and character disorders.
3. Advise patients and their families about the risks and benefits and arrive at a mutual decision when the use of neuroleptic agents exceeds one year. Note this discussion and agreement in the clinical record.
4. Examine the patient regularly and specifically for early signs of choreoathetosis and oral-lingual dyskinesia. Consider alternative neurologic diagnoses (See Table 9).
5. Reevaluate the continuing indications for neuroleptic treatment (need and response) at least every 6-12 months and attempt to reduce the dose.
6. Lower the dose; change to a less potent agent; or ideally stop treatment altogether at the earliest sign of dyskinesia and try to await spontaneous remission over many weeks or months for as long as the psychiatric status permits.
7. Attempt to treat the dyskinesia with benign agents first (diazepam, deanol, choline or lecithin in high doses, possibly lithium; stay alert to new experimental therapies as they are developed), if only to bide for time and offer hope. Suppress symptoms by reinstitution of neuroleptics only as an extreme measure for extraordinarily severe disabling dyskinesias, using the lowest doses that are feasible.

timing has led to its (probably erroneous) association with the tardive dyskinesias. It may represent an atypical and localized variant of parkinsonism since the rate of the mouth movements is similar to more typical parkinsonian limb tremors, and the reaction sometimes responds favorably to treatment with antiparkinson agents (16) and withdrawal of the neuroleptic agent.

In addition to these more specific neuroleptic-induced neurologic syndromes, other effects of antipsychotic drugs on the CNS have also been described. They include the following.

Seizures: There is some evidence that neuroleptic drugs, and perhaps especially low-potency phenothiazines, slightly increase the incidence of seizures in epileptic patients, while the piperazines and haloperidol may have somewhat less tendency to do this. As yet, there are few helpful data to guide the clinician in the selection of a specific agent least likely to have this effect. Usually a clinical judgment is required to balance the patient's need for antipsychotic medication with his need for anticonvulsants, and the dosage of the latter may need to be increased.

"Hypothalamic crises": Antipsychotic agents, and particularly chlorpromazine, have also been associated with severe reactions that are marked mainly by hyperthermia, but that may also include sweating, drooling, tachycardia, dyspnea, seizures and unstable blood pressure. Similar rare reactions have been ascribed to the tricyclic antidepressants. This syndrome is probably indistinguishable from the "malignant neuroleptic" syndrome mentioned above.

Acute intoxication: In contrast to most other central nervous system depressants, the antipsychotic agents' lethality on acute overdose and their potential for inducing deep and prolonged coma and respiratory depression are limited. That is, they have a very high therapeutic index (ratio of toxic or lethal dose to effective dose). The lethal doses (LD_{50}) for most of these agents are not known. Patients have survived ingestions of many grams, and it is virtually impossible to commit suicide by taking an overdose of an antipsychotic agent (17). On the other hand, it is essential to consider the possibility of more lethal and treatable forms of acute intoxication, since ingestions are often mixed. For example, the patient may also have taken alcohol, barbiturates or agents with important central anticholinergic activity, such as the tricyclic antidepressants and antiparkinsonism drugs as well as some antipsychotic agents, such as thioridazine. Dialysis can be used to remove barbiturates, but it is not useful in removing antipsychotic or antidepressant medications because of their strong binding to protein and lipids. The reversible anticholinesterase agent physostigmine (eserine or Antilirium) can be administered for the central anticholinergic syndrome (11). Attempts to induce vomiting after overdoses of antipsychotic agents may be unsuccessful, owing to their antiemetic effects. One indication of the antipsychotic agents' limited toxicity and addiction potential is the fact that large quantities of these drugs can be prescribed with relative impunity, even for patients with impaired judgment or little impulse control.

In conclusion, the antipsychotic agents have had a strong impact on modern psychiatry. Their influence on medical practice has been compared to the impact of the antibiotics, in terms of numbers of patients affected, quantity of research effort generated and changes in patterns of care delivery introduced. The currently available antipsychotic agents virtually all carry some risk of inducing early or late neurological toxic effects. Most of these can be managed with antiparkinsonism agents or by thoughtful and conservative use of the available neuroleptics as we await the development of more selectively antipsychotic chemicals.

DRUGS USED TO STABILIZE MOOD

Clinical Pharmacology of Mood-Altering Drugs (1,19)

Since the 1950s, the treatment of depression and manic-depressive disorders has been advanced dramatically with the introduction of several effective and safe medications that are widely used by primary care physicians as well as by psychiatrists. These agents include the tricyclic antidepressant drugs (such as imipramine) and the now less commonly employed monoamine oxidase (MAO) inhibitors. Antidepressants are impressively effective in the treatment of the more serious, recurrent depressions or isolated depressive illnesses ("unipolar" mood disorders); lithium salts are now well established as an effective treatment for acute manic illnesses and for recurrent mood disorders marked by manic and depressive phases ("bipolar" affective disorders). While they are not specifically mood-altering agents, the antipsychotic drugs are also effective in the treatment of mania and can be helpful adjuncts to antidepressant treatment or electroconvulsive therapy (ECT) in the treatment of severely agitated or psychotic depressed patients.

Although the present discussion centers on drugs, it should be realized that ECT still has an important role in the treatment of serious depression, even though it has acquired a mixed reputation due to its relative inconvenience and sometimes overly zealous applications in the past. Nevertheless, in many controlled comparisons between adequate doses of the best antidepressant drugs and ECT, the latter more venerable treatment has emerged as the most effective treatment modality for severe depression yet devised. In some very serious forms of depression, characterized by refusal to eat or drink and suicidal behavior, ECT is rapidly effective and can sometimes be lifesaving.

Imipramine and similar chemicals had been known since the 1940s to have antihistaminic and sedative properties, as well as considerable anticholinergic activity. Because many of these properties and the structure of imipramine were superficially similar to those of the phenothiazines, which were introduced into psychiatry for the treatment of psychoses in the early 1950s, a prediction was made that imipramine might have antipsychotic properties. In one of the initial clinical trials of the new drug, Kuhn in Switzerland found in 1957–58 that it had little antipsychotic efficacy but seemed to have mood-elevating and behavior-activating properties. Since that time, imipramine and other structurally related "tricyclic" or "heterocyclic" agents have been repeatedly demonstrated by controlled comparisons with a placebo or a stimulant to be effective in several types of depression. Although these clinical effects have not always been easily demonstrated, and despite the considerable toxicity and side effects of this class of drugs, these agents have become by far the most popular and common medical treatment for depressions of all kinds, and particularly severe depression.

Inhibitors of the enzyme monoamine oxidase (MAO) are historically important, as they had a major impact on the medical treatment of depression and on the biologic theories that attempt to relate brain metabolism to psychiatric illness (1,20). In 1952 the first useful antidepressant, iproniazid (Marsilid), was introduced in the U.S., and its inhibitory effects on MAO were described. A few years later, the ability of reserpine to deplete serotonin and norepinephrine in the mammalian brain while inducing behavioral "depression" was noted. Speculation then began that a functional deficiency of brain amines may underlie depression and that MAO inhibitors and other antidepressants act by reversing this deficiency. After that time, the MAO inhibitors had fallen into a position of very limited use until recently. The tricyclic agents were consistently superior as antidepressants until recent studies of higher doses of MAO inhibitors demonstrated their efficacy in depression and several other conditions (such as hysteroid dysphoria and panic disorder). The imipramine-like tricyclic agents also do not have the complex effects of the MAO inhibitors on interaction with certain foodstuffs and many drugs. The MAO inhibitors are severely toxic on acute overdosage and can induce dangerous interactions with other drugs, chemicals, hormones or metabolic conditions. Although the likelihood of inducing serious drug reactions with an MAO inhibitor is small, the reactions can be severe and potentially fatal when they do occur. Thus, the dangers of toxicity, the inconvenience of restrictions required for the safe use of MAO inhibitors have resulted in their relatively infrequent use in this country and somewhat undeservedly poor reputation. The only commonly used MAO inhibitors are phenelzine (Nardil) and tranylcypromine (Parnate); isocarboxazid (Marplan) is also available but less commonly used. The complex and highly specialized nature of the use, pharmacology and toxicology of this class of agents as well as the classical stimulants is beyond the scope of the present chapter, and the interested reader is referred elsewhere for further information (1,19,21). It is important to emphasize that when used in adequate doses (e.g., more than 45 mg/day, and up to 75 or even 90 mg/day of phenelzine), that MAO inhibitors are effective antidepressants worthy of consideration if a vigorous trial of a tricyclic agent is not successful.

Although antipsychotic drugs are used in the treatment of mania, *the lithium ion* is a unique agent with considerable selectivity in the treatment of this serious psychiatric illness (22). Lithium is greatly inferior to the antipsychotic agents in the treatment of other forms of psychosis, and particularly in schizophrenia. It may have beneficial effects on certain acute psychoses, sometimes called "acute schizophrenic reactions," in which an affective or mood disturbance is very prominent, and many of which may represent atypical forms of mania (23). Lithium salts also have a unique place in the long-term maintenance of patients with a variety of severe, recurrent mood disorders. The differential effectiveness of antipsychotic agents and lithium salts has led to a much needed reawakening of interest in the careful diagnostic differentiation of acute psychoses and to a reconsideration of the tendency in American medicine to use the term "schizophrenia" inappropriately, almost as a synonym for "psychosis" (23).

In 1949 Cade in Australia noted interesting behavioral aspects of lithium salts in animals and gave lithium to psychiatric patients, reporting striking anecdotes of favorable responses among severely disturbed manic patients. This report led to an intense investigation of the biology and clinical actions of lithium salts in Europe in the 1950s and 1960s. The results of several studies led to the early acceptance of lithium in European practice as a highly effective and safe treatment for manic-depressive illness, both for the treatment of acute mania and for reducing the frequency and severity of recurrent mania and depression. Lithium salts were not accepted into American practice until 1970. Reasons included strong scepticism among American physicians about the safety of lithium salts, after several cases of severe intoxication and even death were reported in 1949-50 among patients using large, uncontrolled amounts of lithium chloride as a salt substitute while on a sodium-restricted regimen for cardiac or renal failure. It is now known that sodium restriction and diuresis markedly increase the retention and toxicity of the lithium ion and that lithium salts cannot be used safely in gram quantities without careful monitoring of blood levels. In addition, lithium has a very narrow margin of safety (a low therapeutic index). Another factor contributing to a slow development of lithium therapy was the lack of commercial interest in this inexpensive, unpatentable mineral, and consequently the lack of industrial support to demonstrate the efficacy and safety of its use. Before lithium was accepted in American psychiatric practice, an overwhelming amount of evidence accumulated to support its usefulness and safety.

Heterocyclic antidepressants (Table 11) are rapidly absorbed after oral administration. Although several of them, including imipramine and amitriptyline, are available in injectable form, injection probably does not appreciably increase their speed of action or efficacy. Their elimination is multiphasic. About half is rapidly eliminated—two thirds in the urine and one third in the feces—within 2 or 3 days, but the fraction that remains more firmly bound to plasma and tissue protein undergoes slower excretion over several days. A practical consequence of the strong affinity of the antidepressant drugs for tissue and plasma proteins is that it is not possible to remove these agents by any known dialysis technique with sufficient speed to be of clinical benefit in the management of acute overdosage. The heterocyclic antidepressants, like the antipsychotic agents, are metabolized mainly by oxidation by hepatic microsomal enzymes. The activity of these enzymes is determined genetically, is poorly developed in infants, is diminished in the elderly and is enhanced or diminished by many drugs. These drug-metabolizing reactions include ring hydroxylation and oxidation of the terminal amino nitrogen of the side-chain, sometimes yielding active metabolic products such as the *N*-demethylated forms of imipramine and amitryptyline that are themselves used clinically (Table 10). The oxidized products are more polar, more water soluble and thus more readily excreted.

There have been attempts to utilize information about the pharmacokinetics and metabolism of the heterocyclic antidepressants to improve their clinical effects. An important application of pharmacokinetics has been the evaluation of blood levels of heterocyclic antidepressants, particularly in attempts to explain clinically unsatisfactory results (2). There are clear, and presumably genetically determined, individual abilities to metabolize and excrete these agents; "steady-state" plasma concentrations (determined at approximately 12 hours following the last daily dose after several weeks of treatment) vary among individuals by more than 20-fold. There are almost certainly minimally effective blood levels of all tricyclic antidepressants below which a therapeutic response is unlikely, and there may be optimal blood levels of some antidepressants (notably nortriptyline), as diminished effectiveness may correlate with either very low or very high blood levels of drug. There are also suggestions that patients who produce unusually high or low blood levels of one antidepressant are likely to do so with others. In Europe, these various clinical correlations are considered sufficiently useful that blood levels of antidepressants are monitored almost routinely in some

Table 11. Equivalent Doses of Antidepressants[a]

Generic Name	Trade Names	Dose Range (mg/day)
Heterocyclics		
Amitriptyline	Elavil, etc., generic	50–300
Amoxapine[c]	Ascendin	200–300
Desipramine[d]	Norpramin, Pertofrane	75–200
Doxepin	Adapin, Sinequan	75–300
Imipramine	Tofranil, etc., generic	50–300
Maprotiline	Ludiomil	100–150
Nortriptyline[d]	Aventyl	50–150[b]
Protriptyline	Vivactil	15–60
Trazodone	Desyrel	150–250
Trimipramine	Surmontil	75–150
MAO Inhibitors		
Isocarboxazid	Marplan	10–60
Phenelzine	Nardil	15–60
Tranylcypromine	Parnate	20–30

[a]Although the ratio of a severely toxic or lethal dose to a typical daily dose (approximate therapeutic index) may be as high as 10 to 30, 5–10 days' supply is a safer amount to dispense. Doses above 250 mg of imipramine or the equivalent of other agents are best reserved for inpatients. Daily doses are initially divided into 2 or 3 portions, but total doses of 150 mg or less can later be given at bedtime for convenience. Amitriptyline is available in combination with perphenazine (Etrafon, Triavil) and with chlordiazepoxide (Limbitrol). Most commercial preparations are soluble hydrochlorides. Imipramine is also available as the slower-acting pamoate (Tofranil-PM), which can be given in the same daily dose as the hydrochloride, in 1 or 2 portions, but is more expensive and probably not safer than giving the hydrochloride twice a day or at bedtime. The usually effective dose is 150–200 mg of imipramine hydrochloride (or the equivalent of another agent) achieved over several days; smaller doses are used in children and elderly patients. In changing agents, it is wise to make the conversion gradually over several days to avoid intoxication. Another new benzodiazepine, alprazolam (Xanax) may have antipanic and antidepressant activity at higher doses than are currently recommended for anxiety.

[b]Recent studies suggest that optimal blood levels of nortriptyline are most commonly attained at doses of 100–150 mg/day, although the manufacturer's current upper limit of recommended dosage is only 100 mg/day.

[c]Amoxapine (nor-loxapine) may also have neuroleptic activity.

[d]Note that these N-demethylated agents are also formed as active metabolites of their "parent" compounds, imipramine and amitriptyline, respectively, and so probably contribute to the clinical action of the latter drugs.

centers, and interest is growing in the United States in the application of these methods, at least to patients who respond poorly to routine treatment with antidepressants. More and more hospital and commercial laboratories now perform such assays of antidepressant

Table 12. Suggested Therapeutic Blood Levels of Heterocyclic Antidepressants (ng/ml)[a]

II° Amines	
Nortriptyline (Aventyl)	50–150 (window)
Protriptyline (Vivactyl)	100–200 (window)
Desipramine (Norpramin, Pertofrane)	100–300 (window?)
Maprotiline	200–500
III° Amines (Plus active II° amine metabolites)	
Imipramine (Tofranil, etc.)	150–300 (linear)
Amitriptyline (Elavil, etc.)	100–250 (linear)
Doxepin (Sinequan)	100–200 (linear?)

[a]These assays are currently performed on plasma or serum with powerful and selective gas chromatrographic methods. Results are usually expressed as nano (n)g/ml (10^{-6} mg/ml). Values reported are not firmly established, vary somewhat among laboratories and represent approximate averages of the currently available data. Toxicity can be expected at levels 2–3 times above the recommended upper limits (or over 500 ng/ml, with serious toxicity to be expected above 1000–2000 ng/ml). It has been suggested that the demethylated agents desipramine and nortriptyline have optimal levels or a "therapeutic window," while their parent compounds imipramine and amitriptyline usually have better clinical response in approximately direct proportion to blood levels up to toxic levels. Assays of this kind tend to be expensive at the present time ($15 to $50/assay) and are used judiciously, and most commonly in cases that respond unsatisfactorily.

blood levels, as well as levels of platelet MAO activity as a way to monitor the action of MAO inhibitors, the efficacy of which is best at levels of inhibition above 85% (21). An attempt to provide a rough guide to optimal suggested blood levels from the complex and still evolving research on this question is provided in Table 12.

The mechanisms of action of the heterocyclic antidepressant agents remain poorly understood, although the leading hypothesis (19,20) can be recapitulated as follows. It suggests that nearly all of them (trazodone is an exception) block the uptake of amines acting in the brain as synaptic neurotransmitters or as local neurohormones, and thus potentiate norepinephrine and perhaps serotonin (5-hydroxytryptamine), while their muscarinic receptor-blocking effects antagonize acetylcholine. The catecholamines are believed to have an important role in central mechanisms underlying sympathetic autonomic effects, drive states, appetive behavior, arousal and the like; these are sometimes called "ergotropic" actions. Effects of the antidepressants on indoleamines, including serotonin, and on acetylcholine may also contribute to antidepressant and other actions of the tricyclic drugs. The latter amines are centrally quieting, parasympathetic or "trophotropic" neurohumors. Accordingly, the more sedating heterocyclic antidepressants, including amitriptyline, clomipramine (experimental) and a number of other tricyclic *di*-methylated amines, may have relatively potent uptake-blocking and function-potentiating effects on serotonin as well as norepinephrine, while the less sedating *de*methylated tricyclic agents such as desipramine and nortriptyline, as well as the demethylated metabolite of clomipramine, exert preferential potentiating effects on norepinephrine. The reason for the delay of several days to 3 weeks for the antidepressant clinical effects of these agents to appear is still uncertain. Furthermore, this delay presents a problem for the amine hypotheses, inasmuch as the amine-potentiating actions of the drugs are immediate. The clinical delay might reflect the saturation of certain tissue pools, possibly at a crucial site on neuronal membranes. It has also been suggested that changes in postsynaptic beta-adrenergic receptors (decreases) for norepinephrine in the brain may evolve over several weeks, and even more interesting, that decreased sensitivity of *pre*synaptic (α_2 adrenergic) receptors may lead to increased release of this transmitter into the synapse (24).

Lithium is usually administered as 300-mg tablets or capsules of the dibasic carbonate salt Li_2CO_3 (as the generic substance or as the commercially available preparations Eskalith, Lithane or Lithonate, or the more slowly released Lithobid). Other salts of lithium can also be used and the citrate (as a liquid preparation) is now commercially available. Long-acting preparations of lithium salts are being tested in Europe for once-a-day administration. Lithium is readily absorbed after oral administration; injectable forms are not used. It is easily measured by techniques used to assay sodium and potassium. Unlike sodium and potassium ions, lithium lacks a strongly preferential distribution across cell membranes, and tends to distribute evenly throughout the total body water space. There is some lag in penetration into the cerebrospinal fluid, but there is no absolute barrier to entry into the brain; equilibration between blood and brain is nearly complete within 24 hours. The metabolism of lithium ion is almost entirely by renal excretion. As with sodium, 70–80% of the lithium ions, which readily pass into the glomerular filtrate, are reabsorbed in the proximal renal tubules; although there is further absorption of sodium distally (10–20%), there is almost no absorption of lithium in the distal renal tubules. Because the proximal reabsorption of these two ions is competitive, sodium diuresis and a deficiency of sodium tend to increase the retention of lithium, and hence to increase its toxicity. The renal excretion of lithium is maximal within a few hours and then proceeds more slowly over several days. The average half-life of lithium in the body varies with age, from about

12 hours in young adults to as long as 36 hours in elderly patients. The relatively short half-life requires dividing the daily dose into two to four portions for safety and to diminish the peaks and troughs of tissue levels (which may also be diminished by slowly released preparations such as Lithobid). An important feature of the renal excretion of the lithium ion is that its rate of removal cannot be increased by the administration of most diuretic agents; similarly additional sodium input has little effect on the excretion of lithium, while sodium deficiency has a large effect. These physiologic facts therefore have important implications for the medical management of toxic overdoses of lithium salts.

The mechanisms of action of lithium ion in affective disorders are still not clearly established, although several interesting aspects of its effects have been elucidated. Much attention has been directed to the effects of lithium on electrolyte balance across cell membranes, including those of neurons. In addition, lithium at clinical concentrations can antagonize synaptic transmission mediated by catecholamines (see Fig. 2); it inhibits the release of norepinephrine and dopamine and weakly increases the uptake and decreases retention of catecholamine neurotransmitters in presynaptic nerve terminals. Lithium ion may also interfere with the ability of several hormones, including the antidiuretic hormone (ADH) and thyroid stimulating hormone (TSH), to stimulate adenylate cyclase, which is believed to be an important component of the receptor mechanisms of many hormones, including the catecholamines. There is also recent evidence that lithium may minimize the changes in catecholamine receptor sensitivity that follow altered transmitter availability (25). All of this information accords well with the popular hypothesis that in mania catecholamines may be functionally overactive in the brain, but it does not help to explain the reported mood-normalizing actions of the ion in recurrent depressive illnesses.

Clinical Use of Mood-Altering Agents (1,19,22)

Treatment of depression is made difficult by the diversity of conditions subsumed under the generic term "depression," and by the inconsistency with which clinicians and investigators categorize depressions. Regardless of the scheme of categorization, it is generally agreed that depressions vary in severity. The more severe or "major" forms include those formerly referred to as "endogenous," "manic-depressive," "retarded," "involutional," "agitated," "psychotic" or "vital," depending on the clinical form of the illness and the patient's history. In contrast, the less severe forms are said to be "minor," "reactive," "neurotic," "situational" or "anxious" depressions. Also currently popular is the distinction between *primary* affective (mood) disorders (no other obvious psychiatric or medical illness associated) and *secondary* affective disorders associated with a predisposing medical disease or treatment (e.g., cancer, endocrine disorder, other chronic metabolic disorders or infections, use of antihypertensive agents, addictions), or other psychiatric illness (such as schizophrenia, a character disorder or alcoholism). Moreover, manic-depressive disorders are sometimes designated "bipolar disorders." In these, hypomania or mania alternates with depression, either spontaneously or as the evident result of provocation by antidepressants or ECT; such provocation is sometimes called the "switch process." Another class of pure recurrent depressions ("unipolar depressive illnesses") has traditionally also been considered to exist, but this group is less likely to represent a biologically distinct syndrome than are the bipolar manic-depressive illnesses. Finally, it has recently been suggested that a subtype of recurrent depressions may include episodes of subclinical mild euphorias or periods of increased energy below the level of hypomania. Depressions of this type are sometimes called "bipolar type II" manic-depressive disorders in contrast to those with clear-cut episodes of spontaneous or treatment-related mania or hypomania, which are designated "type I" bipolar disorders.

Although the prognosis for the less severe depressions is better, efficacy of medical treatments has been more clearly demonstrated for the more serious depressions with more pronounced "biologic" symptoms such as anorexia, insomnia, loss of drive and sexual interest and diurnal change. Patients with the lesser depressive illnesses tend to recover more rapidly or even spontaneously and respond to psychotherapy, sedatives, antianxiety medications and stimulants or to nonspecific treatments, including placebos, about as well as to antidepressants. The best performance of the drugs has been documented in trials that attempted to exclude the less severe depressions, used adequate daily doses of medication (more than 125 mg imipramine or the equivalent of another agent; see Table 10) and continued for at least a month. In controlled trials with a mixture of depressive syndromes of varying severity, overall improvement rates with heterocyclic antidepressants have been about 70% in contrast to about 40% with placebo; thus, only an additional 30% of patients with significant depressive illnesses respond to the active medication. A few who respond poorly to a heterocyclic agent respond satisfactorily to an MAO inhibitor, and about half of those who respond poorly to a tricyclic agent respond to ECT. ECT has consistently outperformed MAO inhibitors or heterocyclic antidepressants, but the overall gain is only on the order of 10–20%. Among the specific antidepressants, there are more similarities than differences in overall effectiveness (1,26,27). The heterocyclic antidepressants have performed better than MAO inhibitors, with the exception of tranylcypromine (Parnate), and high doses (>45 mg/day) of phenelzine (Nardil).

While differences in the overall efficacy of the various tricyclic antidepressants are not easy to document, subtleties based on the relative chances of various side effects or drug interactions call for some judgment and the selection of a specific agent on the basis of sound pharmacologic principles and clinical observations, as are reviewed elsewhere in greater detail (1,19). An example of how to make clinical use of the differences in action and side effects is provided by amitriptyline (Elavil). Its relative prominent and early sedative effects are often useful early in therapy of depression with insomnia. The demethylated antidepressants, and especially protriptyline (Vivactil) are much less sedating. Another important differentiating characteristic of the tricyclics are their anticholinergic side effects. Amitriptyline has more potent anticholinergic activity than other tricyclic antidepressants, and desipramine about the least, with other agents clustering between them (see Table 6). This consideration suggests that desipramine may be a more rational choice for elderly patients at high risk of anticholinergic brain syndrome or of cardiac toxicity. Although its greater safety (as well as that of doxepin [Sinequan]) does not have strong clinical support, some suggestive data have been reported (28).

It has been suggested that biochemical tests of the excretion of amine metabolites might lead to a more rational selection of a specific antidepressant in a specific case. However, this approach has not yet been reduced to practice. Since antidepressant blood level assays are expensive and not always readily available, it may be simplest to rely first on drugs such as imipramine and amitriptyline, where a poor response is probably best managed by *increasing* the dose to increase the blood level, whereas (without blood assays) it is impossible to guess whether to increase or decrease the close of the demethylated agents due to their complex and possibly biphasic relationship between blood level and efficacy (see Table 12).

It is most important to appreciate the fact that the *most common cause of poor response* to an antidepressant is inadequate treatment: the use of doses below the equivalent of 150 mg/day imipramine is common, but even this dose is often barely adequate. The half-lives

Table 13. Rate of Relapse of Unipolar Depression with Tricyclic Antidepressants or Placebo

Treatment	N[a]	Relapsed	Percent Relapsed	Mean Relapse Rate ± SEM (Percent)
Antidepressant[b]	162	44	27.2	28.1 ± 8.9[c]
Placebo	202	107	53.0	59.7 ± 9.4

Source: J. M. Davis, 1976 (29).
[a]N = number of patients in controlled studies, a total of 364 patients.
[b]Tricyclic antidepressants included imipramine or amitriptyline. Placebo included inert tablet or diazepam.
[c]$p < 2 \times 10^{-8}$, comparing results for antidepressant vs. placebo, using pooled data.

of the tricyclic agents are long enough that it is reasonable to use the bulk of a day's dose at bedtime, both for convenience and to combat insomnia. Furthermore, it is best to prescribe preparations of heterocyclics with the highest unit strength (mg/tablet or capsule), as this is usually the least expensive. When large doses of an antidepressant are used (above the equivalent of 150 mg/day imipramine), it is probably safer to use divided doses to minimize anticholinergic and potential cardiotoxic actions of the drugs, as well as nightmares that occasionally follow large doses at bedtime, especially in children, who may be less able to metabolize these drugs. The clinically "equivalent doses" of antidepressant agents summarized in Table 11 have been established on the assumption that the *doses are attained gradually*. Thus, to avoid toxic reactions, it is best to avoid switching immediately from equivalent doses of one agent to another, and to allow several days for a gradual transition. Because of the potentially severe toxicity and limited margin of safety of all antidepressant agents, it is unwise to dispense more than a week's supply to a depressed and possibly suicidal outpatient. It is important to remember that the risk of suicide may increase with initial improvement, since activity usually increases before mood elevation. It is also likely that inadequate treatment contributes to the risk of suicide.

After appreciable clinical improvement of a severe depressive illness has been achieved with heterocyclic antidepressant agent, it is usual to continue the treatment at approximately 150 mg/day imipramine or its equivalent for several months, and perhaps up to a year for severe illness or in patients with a history of frequently recurrent depression (29). Discontinuing treatment too early is often associated with relapse, but even doses as low as 75–100 mg in this

Table 14. Rate of Recurrence of Affective Illness with Lithium or Placebo

Treatment	N[a]	Relapsed	Percent Relapsed	Mean Relapse Rate ± SEM (Percent)
Lithium salt	329	117	35.6	31.9 ± 7.2[b]
Placebo	330	262	79.4	74.6 ± 6.6

Source: J. M. Davis, 1976 (29).
[a]N = 659 patients in 9 controlled studies.
[b]Statistical analysis of the pooled data results in $p<0.001$ if N assumed to be 9 studies (a conservative method), and $p<10^{-80}$ if N assumed to be 659 subjects, as explained in the reference cited.

phase of treatment are questionably effective in preventing relapses. A similar regimen should be followed by patients treated initially with ECT. This approach has evolved from clinical experience and many reports of relapse after partial treatment of depressions. The exact duration of the treatment depends on the individual patient's response, ability to resume normal responsibilities, premorbid personality, ongoing stresses and life situation, and the duration, rate of recurrence and response to treatment of prior depressions. There is encouraging evidence that the sustained use of antidepressant agents in unipolar depressive illness may be nearly as useful as lithium is in preventing or diminishing bipolar or unipolar illnesses (29; Table 13), although the efficacy and safety of indefinitely prolonged antidepressant therapy are not fully established. The usefulness of indefinitely continued treatment in outpatients with "chronic characterologic depressions" (sometimes misdiagnosed when depression is simply inadequately treated) is not clear, although this is occasionally done when the medication seems to be effective by clinical observation of individual patients.

Despite the proven efficacy of *lithium carbonate* in acute episodes of hypomania and mania, and its well-demonstrated preventive effects in recurrent mood disorders, and especially in bipolar manic-depressive illness (1,19,22,29), a recent estimate for the United States is that only about 50,000 patients are receiving this agent, while perhaps a million or more Americans with severe recurrent mood disorders could be so treated. A large number of controlled studies demonstrate the efficacy of lithium carbonate in hypomania and acute mania, with improvement typically of 70–80% of patients in 10–14 days. A summary of some of the evidence for a preventive or "prophylactic" effect of prolonged lithium treatment is presented in Table 14. The

Table 15. Principles of the Use of Lithium Ion

Indications
- Acute hypomanic and manic episodes
- Recurrent manias, bipolar illness and perhaps depressions

Acute Treatment
- Slow action as plasma Li+ reaches 1.1-1.3 mEq/L
- Usually add antipsychotic agent during early phase of treatment
- Monitor serum level frequently and watch closely for toxic signs
- Expect toxicity at 2-3, and lethality above 5-7 mEq/L

"Maintenance" Treatment
- May add antidepressants, ECT or antipsychotics as needed
- Plasma levels 0.75-1.0 mEq/L
- Monitor serum levels infrequently
- Li+ retention and toxicity increased if Na+ decreased: with sweating, diarrhea, diuresis (including postpartum diuresis); and on resolution of mania
- Watch skin, thyroid, renal function

prophylactic effect of lithium seems to occur in the depressive as well as the manic phases of bipolar disorders, although it sometimes provides only a partial protective effect by reducing the severity or frequency of attacks of mood disorders. The initial indication for which lithium carbonate was licensed was the treatment of mania itself, although at present prolonged use of lithium for the prevention of recurrent mania and bipolar mood disorders is already a widely accepted practice. The evidence for utility of lithium salts in the treatment of "unipolar" recurrent depressive disease is also encouraging, but not yet sufficient to establish this use of lithium as a routine clinical practice. The evidence for usefulness of lithium as a primary treatment for depressive illnesses is weak and inconsistent.

Due to the low therapeutic index (margin of safety) for lithium salts, careful monitoring of patients receiving lithium for the treatment of acute or recurrent mood disorders is required. Indeed, the dose given is frankly irrelevant as one attends *only to the blood level* and clinical responses in establishing and monitoring the treatment regimen. The safe clinical management of lithium treatment is outlined in Table 15 (21).

Side Effects and Toxicity of Antidepressant Drugs (1,19)

Important toxic effects occur in perhaps 5% of patients treated with *heterocyclic antidepressants*; of these, more than 10% represent cerebral intoxication, and the incidence of nervous system toxicity is much higher in patients over age 50.

Anticholinergic actions

The most common toxic side effects of the heterocyclic antidepressants are extensions of their adrenergic and anticholinergic pharmacologic activities. These include anticholinergic actions leading to dry mouth, sweating and opthalmic changes, which are variable but usually include mild mydriasis and often some degree of cycloplegia with blurred near vision because of impaired accommodation. These problems are more annoying than dangerous and can usually be managed by simple means such as the use of sugar-free candy or mild mouthwashes to offset reduced salivation and reading lenses to compensate for reduced near vision. Cholinergic eyedrops and cholinergic mouthwashes or systemic medications have been tried for these various symptoms but are usually not very helpful. Moreover, some degree of tolerance to the side effects normally develops. The overuse of ordinary candy for dry mouth can lead to monilial infections and dental caries. Patients may also complain of a vile taste or epigastric distress and "indigestion" while taking antidepressants. Grossly excessive water intake secondary to dry mouth on rare occasions can lead to water intoxication due to significant hyponatremia, particularly in confused patients. Water intoxication also occurs infrequently with the use of antipsychotic drugs; it is not yet clear whether this is due to endocrine effects of antidepressant or antipsychotic agents, such as an inappropriate increase in the release of antidiuretic hormone (ADH).

Among more serious aspects of the anticholinergic actions of antidepressants is the induction of glaucoma, especially acute "closed-angle" glaucoma in the elderly that requires miotic eyedrops and careful opthalmologic supervision. Serious antivagal effects of this highly anticholinergic class of agents include paralytic ileus and urinary retention; thus extra caution is required in elderly patients and men with prostatism, and urgent medical intervention is necessary when these conditions develop. Treatment entails eliminating or reducing the dose of antidepressant and giving cholinergic smooth-muscle stimulants such as bethanechol (Urecholine), 2.5 or 5.0 mg subcutaneously as needed. When severe inhibition of gastrointestinal or urinary function occurs with even small doses of antidepressants, it may be necessary to change the treatment to ECT or an MAO inhibitor. Among the heterocyclic agents, desipramine (Norpramin, Pertofrane) has the least peripheral and CNS antimuscarinic activity in animal tissues, while amitriptyline (Elavil) is the most potently anticholinergic (see Table 6). Amitriptyline has 5% the potency of atropine, but is given in doses more than 100 times greater than is atropine!

Systemic reactions

Various skin reactions have been described. An allergic-obstructive type of jaundice occasionally occurs early in the course of treatment. Purpura has been reported in a few cases. Agranulocytosis is rare. There may be a tendency to gain weight, and there are occasional hypoglycemic effects of the tricyclic agents.

Cardiac toxicity

This is a serious consequence of the anticholinergic and direct quinidinelike properties of the tricyclic antidepressants. Palpitations, tachycardia and arrhythmias are not unusual and are to be expected in acute overdosage. Electrocardiographic changes include tachycardia, prolongation of the Q-T interval and flattening of the T waves. The myocardium is often directly depressed; decreased strength of contraction creates some risk of syncope. Faintness due to postural hypotension also is not unusual, although the underlying mechanisms are not clear. Steroids such as cortisone, as well as dihydroergotamine (10 mg/day), have been reported to counteract postural hypotension resulting from administration of tricyclic antidepressants or MAO inhibitors when more conservative management did not suffice. Because there is an increased risk of malignant ventricular arrhythmias, cardiac arrest, left ventricular enlargement, myocardial damage and congestive heart failure with the tricyclic antidepressants, they are used in lower doses and with great caution in elderly patients at risk for myocardial infarction and stroke, and avoided soon after myocardial infarction. Amitriptyline may be particularly cardiotoxic, although this impression derives mainly from studies in animals and clinical experiences with acute overdoses. The potential clinical usefulness of the quinidinelike effects of these agents as a primary treatment for tachyarrhythmias is currently under investigation.

An important consideration in choosing the treatment for serious depression in elderly or infirm patients is that, with its modern modifications, ECT is probably as safe as the antidepressant drugs, if not safer. Mortality rates with both the tricyclic agents and ECT are low, and even lower than in untreated or undertreated depression (in which death is due to natural causes as well as suicide—the lifetime risk of which is about 15% in primary depression). The incidence of serious morbidity and mortality with the antidepressant drugs is probably even higher than with ECT if overdoses are included: certainly the total morbidity rate with the drugs is considerable, especially if minor as well as more serious toxic effects and overdosages are all taken into account.

Central nervous system effects

These include mild dizziness and lightheadedness, insomnia and restlessness or fatigue and somnolence. Fine and occasionally gross resting tremors are common and may respond to diazepam (Valium). Extrapyramidal syndromes are rare, possibly as a reflection of the powerful anticholinergic action of these drugs. The latter action is sufficient to produce antiparkinsonism effects, which are occasionally encountered when antidepressants are combined with parkinsonism-producing antipsychotic agents, or when they are given to depressed patients with Parkinson's disease. Tricyclic antidepressants must be used with caution by patients receiving anticholinergic antiparkinson medications or L-dopa, due to the risk of combined toxicity. They would be expected to worsen choreas, including Huntington's chorea and tardive dyskinesia, as antiparkinsonism drugs often do. There is some risk of provoking or worsening agitation and psychosis in patients with psychotic or unstable characterologic conditions in addition to depression, and large doses or acute overdoses of heterocyclic antidepressants can induce a toxic organic psychosis resembling that due to atropine poisoning (see Table 16). This toxic state is not always easy to diagnose in severely depressed patients who are already agitated and psychotic. Seizures and the worsening of epilepsy have also been associated with the antidepressants. Large doses of tricyclics at bedtime may produce nightmares. Withdrawal reactions have been reported to follow the abrupt discontinuation of high doses of tricyclic antidepressants (rare unless doses exceed 300 mg/day imipramine or its equivalent); they include restlessness, anxiety and akathisia (motor restlessness) but almost never seizures. Thus, it is best to discontinue unusually high doses *slowly*.

Acute overdosage

The agents used in the treatment of mood disorders (heterocyclic antidepressants, MAO inhibitors and lithium salts) are highly toxic in acute overdosage, and unfortunately must be given to patients at increased risk of attempting suicide. The heterocyclic antidepressants are an increasingly common choice in suicide attempts by increasingly younger persons. Acute doses above 1000 mg are almost always very toxic, but doses as low as a few hundred milligrams, especially of amitriptyline, have been severely toxic in adults as well as children. Acute doses in excess of 2000 mg can be fatal. The monomethylated (*de*methylated) derivatives may be slightly less toxic than the *di*methylated parent compounds. Because of the relatively low therapeutic index, or margin of safety, of all tricyclic antidepressants, it is unwise to dispense more than a week's supply, and certainly never more than 1000 mg of imipramine or the equivalent of another agent (see Table 11).

After an acute overdose, it is impossible to remove these agents by dialysis; forced diuresis also adds little and may contribute to cardiac failure. Although attempts to increase the dialysis of antidepressants by the use of oils, resins or charcoal have not been successful, activated charcoal is sometimes introduced into the gut during gastric lavage (preferably after tracheal intubation) in an attempt to bind and inactivate any remaining unabsorbed drugs. Since overdoses often involve several drugs and may include antipsychotic drugs, which are antiemetic, lavage may be preferable to induced emesis, unless the patient is alert and no agent with antiemetic effects has also been ingested.

Severe central nervous system depression and coma (rarely lasting more than 24 hours) can result from large doses of the antidepressants, but it is common to see signs of anticholinergic poisoning early, with restless agitation, confusion and disorientation, perhaps seizures and hyperthermia, dry, sometimes flushed skin, tachycardia, sluggish and at least moderately dilated pupils, decreased bowel sounds, and often acute urinary retention (Table 16). These effects are probably due to CNS and systemic anticholinergic and antivagal actions of these potent muscarinic blocking agents. The cardiac toxicity can be particularly dangerous and includes severe depression of myocardial conduction, with various forms of heart block, atrial fibrillation and more malignant ventricular arrhythmias or cardiac arrest. Widening of the QRS complex in excess of 75 (or, more clearly, 100) msec has been reported to correlate well with toxic plasma levels of imipramine antidepressants. A peculiarity of heterocyclic poisoning is that the risk of cardiac arrhythmias continues at least several days, and possibly up to a week or more after the initial brain syndrome has cleared considerably. Many of the agents commonly employed to manage ventricular arrhythmias can lead to further conduction blockade and cardiac depression. Electrical defibrillation, conversion and cardiac pacing may be necessary, and all patients with moderate to severe heterocyclic poisoning should ideally be managed in a medical intensive care unit, with constant cardiac monitoring and immediately available difribrillating and resuscitation

Table 16. Anticholinergic and Cholinergic Excess Syndromes

ANTICHOLINERGIC SYNDROME

Causes

Acute overdose or excessive prescription of medications with antimuscarinic properties, especially in combination: heterocyclic antidepressants, most antiparkinsonism agents, some antipsychotics (especially thioridazine), many proprietary sedative-hypnotics, many antispasmodic preparations, several plants (e.g., Jimson weed, some mushrooms).

Neuropsychiatric Signs

Anxiety, agitation: restless, purposeless overactivity; delirium, disorientation; impairment of immediate and recent memory; dysarthria; hallucinations; myoclonus; seizures.

Systemic Signs

Tachycardia and arrhythmias; large, sluggish pupils, scleral injection; flushed, warm, dry skin; increased temperature; decreased mucosal secretions; urinary retention; reduced bowel motility.

Treatment

Adults: initial or test dose, 1–2 mg physostigmine salicylate, intramuscularly or slowly intravenously; repeat as needed after at least 15–30 minutes.

Children: 0.5–1.0 mg physostigmine salicylate, as for adults (Neostigmine, pyridostigmine, etc., do not enter the CNS)

Note: In cases of severe (and especially mixed) overdoses with *coma*, and *unstable vital functions*, the first responsibility is to support respiratory and cardiovascular function; physostigmine's role is not clear and may even make such situations worse.

PHYSOSTIGMINE-INDUCED CHOLINERGIC EXCESS

Neuropsychiatric Signs

Confusion, seizures, nausea and vomiting, myoclonus, hallucinations, often after a period of initial CNS improvement when physostigmine is given to treat the anticholinergic syndrome.

Systemic Signs

Bradycardia, miosis, increased mucosal secretions, copious bronchial secretions, dyspnea, tears, sweating, diarrhea, abdominal colic, biliary colic, urinary frequency or urgency.

Treatment or Prevention

Atropine sulfate (acts in CNS as well as systemically, and so may reinstate previous anticholinergic delirium): 0.5 mg/mg of physostigmine, intramuscularly or subcutaneously.

Glycopyrrolate (Robinul) (no CNS action): 0.1–0.2 mg/mg of physostigmine, intramuscularly.

Methscopolamine bromide (Pamine) (no CNS action): 0.5 mg/mg of physostigmine, intramuscularly (methscopolamine and methylatropine, a similar agent, may not be readily available).

equipment. It is also wise to continue cardiac monitoring for several days after the initial recovery of consciousness and orientation, perhaps up to 7-10 days in severe poisoning. Whereas many cardiac drugs, including digitalis and quinidine, are contraindicated or dangerous, both the cardiac and central nervous system manifestations of anticholinergic poisoning can be successfully treated with reversible anticholinesterase agents. Neostigmine (Prostigmin) and prydiostigmine (Mestinon) have been successfully used in the management of the cardiac effects of a number of atropinelike agents, including tricyclic antidepressants and antiparkinsonism agents. However, these anticholinesterase drugs are charged quaternary ammonium compounds that penetrate the blood-brain barrier poorly, and only physostigmine (eserine, Antilirium) has both central and peripheral cholinergic activity. Physostigmine therefore represents the treatment of choice in the management of intoxications of *mild to moderate severity* with agents possessing significant anticholinergic activity (11). The principles of its use are outlined in Table 16. There is at least one recent report that prolonged coma due to an antidepressant, without prominent anticholinergic signs, was helped by large doses of physostigmine, although this experimental therapy and the role of this agent in severe cases of coma induced by drug overdosage are not yet established as effective or safe.

Other aspects of the pharmacology of the heterocyclics should also be appreciated in the management of their overdoses. For example, the ability of these compounds to potentiate directly sympathomimetic amines such as norepinephrine complicates the use of such pressor substances in managing the hypotension and shock of antidepressant poisoning. Furthermore, the tricyclic agents potentiate and prolong the actions of barbiturates, probably through competition for hepatic microsomal enzymes, which are particularly important in inactivating the shorter-acting barbiturates. Although small doses of very short-acting barbiturates have been advocated for the control of seizures associated with tricyclic poisoning, diazepam (Valium) or other benzodiazepines are probably safer anticonvulsants in this situation and are less likely to induce respiratory depression.

Drug interactions

Antidepressant agents have many interactions with other drugs. They increase the CNS depression caused by alcohol, barbiturates and some minor tranquilizers as well as antipsychotic agents and anticonvulsants. The barbiturates and glutehimide (Doriden) much more than the benzodiazepines also induce hepatic microsomal enzymes required for the metabolism of the tricyclic agents, and thus may decrease the efficacy of the heterocyclics. The seizure threshold may be lowered, so that increased doses of anticonvulsants may be required. The effect of any anticholinergic agent (including antiparkinson drugs [see Table 6]) will be increased additively by the antimuscarinic activity of the tricyclic antidepressants, and this combination creates a risk of toxic confusional brain syndrome, agitation and sometimes hyperpyrexia. Antipsychotic agents are contraindicated in cases of toxic agitation produced by overdoses of tricyclic antidepressants because of their own moderate anticholinergic actions.

A difficult combination to manage satisfactorily is depression and hypertension. Antihypertensive agents, possibly because of their central antiadrenergic properties, are sometimes associated with depression. This association may occur unpredictably at any point in the treatment of hypertension; it is most common in patients with a prior history of depression. It has most frequently been reported with reserpine and other *Rauwolfia* alkaloids, and occasionally with alpha-methyldopa (Aldomet). Guanethidine (Ismelin) is one of the few antihypertensive agents with little CNS activity and is not likely to induce or worsen depression, although, surprisingly, sporadic anecdotal reports of its association with depression exist. Owing to blockade by heterocyclics of guanethidine uptake into postganglionic sympathetic nerve fibers, the treatment of hypertension with guanethidine in patients who are also depressed is usually rendered unsuccessful by the addition of any of the currently available tricyclic antidepressants (and to some extent the antipsychotic phenothiazines as well, but less so haloperidol [Haldol] or molindone [Moban]). Although doxepin (Sinequan) has been claimed to have this effect much less than the other antidepressants, the claim is at best only partially valid for small doses of the antidepressant (less than 150 mg/day for brief periods of time (less than three weeks). The antihypertensive effects of a number of other agents, including reserpine and the *Veratrum* alkaloids, can also be diminished by the tricyclic antidepressants. It is safe to use diuretics with tricyclic antidepressants for the management of hypertension in depressed patients, although there is at least one report that moderate degrees of hyponatremia have depressant effects. It is also possible to treat hypertension with large doses of a beta-adrenergic blocking agent such as propranolol (Inderal) combined with the vascular smooth-muscle relaxant hydralazine (Apresoline); but high doses of the former can produce central sedative effects and may induce depression, and hydralazine has occasionally induced toxic psychoses. However, this combination of antihypertensive agents with heterocyclic antidepressants has evidently not yet been evaluated. Moreover, newer beta-blocking agents that are more selective for peripheral sites may avoid central depressant effects associated with propranolol. One other approach to the management of depression with hypertension might be to take advantage of the hypotensive effects of MAO inhibitors, and particularly the nonhydrazine pargyline (Eutonyl), which was initially withdrawn as an antidepressant because of its hypotensive effects and later relicensed as an antihypertensive agent. However, this use of pargyline has not yet been adequately evaluated; moreover, it must be used *alone* to avoid the risk of certain potentially severe toxic interactions of an MAO inhibitor with a tricyclic antidepressant, such as hypertension, seizures and hyperthermia.

Pregnancy and lactation

The safety of antidepressant drugs in these conditions and guidelines for optimal blood levels during pregnancy (when drug metabolism may *increase*) are not established. The tricyclic antidepressants pass the placental barrier and can be secreted at low levels in human milk. In severe pre- and postpartum depression, ECT can safely be used. There have been rare reports of neonatal distress in infants born to mothers given antidepressants: these reactions included muscle spasms, myoclonus, tachycardia, congestive heart failure and respiratory distress. Preliminary reports of some limb deformities in infants associated with prenatal exposure to imipramine and its congeners have not been supported in further extensive epidemiological investigations.

Elderly patients

Because of their decreased ability to metabolize drugs of all types, and probably as an expression of decreased functional "resilience" of the central nervous system, elderly patients treated with heterocyclic antidepressants are particularly likely to experience toxic side effects. Delirium and agitation are common, partly as an expression of the central anticholinergic syndrome, which should be suspected if there are signs of peripheral vagal and ciliary blockade, and evaluated pharmacologically with a small test dose of physostigmine (see Table 16). If this syndrome develops, antipsychotic agents are avoided, and either management is conservative (to allow time for elimination of the offending agent), or treatment is begun with small doses of physostigmine, or in uncertain cases with a benzodiazepine. Hypotension, cardiac arrhythmias and glaucoma are also particularly likely to occur in elderly patients. One other commonly encountered situation is the simultaneous use of anticoagulants and tricyclic antidepressants, which may compete for the same metabolic pathways, possibly increasing anticoagulant activity and the risk of bleeding, although recent studies have concluded that this effect is minor and unlikely to be clinically important.

The *MAO inhibitors* can present a complex variety of potentially serious problems, including parenchymal liver damage, *hypo*tension by themselves or profound *hyper*tension when given with sympathomimetic-amine-containing foods or drugs. In addition, they interact strongly to potentiate or alter the actions of many other classes of drugs. Due to the relative infrequency of long-term MAO inhibitor therapy for psychiatric patients treated in the community, and to the specialized nature of these complex toxicologic problems, the interested reader is referred again to more specialized sources (1,19, 21,30,34).

Side Effects and Toxicity of Lithium Salts

The most common problem associated with the use of lithium salts are mild or occasionally distressing nausea, vomiting and diarrhea, usually when doses are rapidly increased. Effects on the nervous system may also occur, including lightheadedness and some confusion, but typically the subjective effects of lithium are minimal, and patients rarely complain of feeling "medicated" or mentally dull. A fine resting tremor is common and is usually of no particular importance, although a clear increase in the tremor or appearance of unsteady handwriting can be an important early clue to incipient intoxication. More severe tremor not associated with acute intoxication occurs occasionally and in some cases has been reported to respond favorably to propranolol (Inderal).

Intoxication

The most important early means of detecting serious intoxication with lithium salts are the clinical signs, and blood assays should only be considered as secondary and confirmatory. When signs of intoxication are observed, the intake of lithium should be decreased or stopped without waiting for results of the blood lithium assay. Early signs of intoxication include increasing tremor, weakness, ataxia, giddiness, drowsiness or excitement, slurred dysphasic speech, blurred vision and tinnitus. More severe intoxication produces increased neuromuscular irritability, increased deep tendon reflexes and nystagmus; increasing confusion, lethargy and stupor may lead to coma, sometimes with generalized seizures. With ordinary doses of lithium, extrapyramidal reactions are rare, but choreoathetosis or other bizarre dyskinesias can occur with severe intoxication. The electroencephalogram (EEG) ordinarily reveals generalized slowing, with a prominent 4-6 Hz (cycles/second) activity, even without toxic levels of lithium. Toxicity can be expected at blood levels of 2-4 mEq/L, and levels much above 5 mEq/L may be fatal. In acute overdoses of lithium, the usual causes of death are the secondary complications of coma, including pneumonia and shock. A small number of cases of uncertain significance have been reported, which raise the question of whether the combination of lithium in high doses with haloperidol may produce severe forms of irreversible and even fatal CNS intoxication, although this combination has been safely used for many years throughout the world and continues to be used. It is particularly important to watch for subtle features of an organic mental syndrome (delirium) in elderly patients receiving prolonged lithium treatment, even if blood lithium levels are in a nominally "therapeutic" range.

In the medical management of acute intoxication with lithium, it is important to discontinue lithium treatment immediately. Usually, gastric lavage, the support of vital functions and electrolyte balance and careful nursing care in a specialized medical toxicology unit while the spontaneous elimination of lithium occurs are sufficient treatment. An important implication of the renal excretion of the lithium ion is that its rate of removal cannot be increased by the administration of most saluretic drugs; the thiazide diuretics or spironolactone, by preferential removal of sodium, may even increase the retention and toxicity of lithium. There is little evidence that intravenously administered solutions of sodium chloride appreciably increase the removal of lithium, but the management of lithium intoxication should include normal availability of sodium; the administration of sodium bicarbonate is also helpful. Fluid loading, solute-induced diuresis, as with mannitol, and theophylline can all contribute to some increased renal excretion of lithium in cases of intoxication, and dialysis techniques are very effective in serious overdosage. The use of lithium in patients with salt restriction or sodium wasting requires extra caution in monitoring blood levels of lithium and avoiding intoxication.

Cardiovascular problems

These are unusual in patients given controlled quantities of lithium salts. Hypotension and arrhythmias are rare, although ECG changes can occur. At doses that are likely to be encountered clinically, the most typical changes are similar to those associated with *hypo*akalemia, even though blood levels of potassium are almost always normal. These changes include flattening and even inversion of the T waves; the effects are dose-dependent and reversible. In experimental animals extraordinarily high concentrations of lithium (above 10 mEq/L, levels unlikely to be encountered clinically) have been reported to produce changes resembling those of hyperkalemia: high, peaked T waves; T-wave inversions; depressed S-T segment; widened QRS complex; and evidence of atrioventricular dissociation and conduction blockade. Depressed or absent P waves, atrial fibrillation and standstill with independent ventricular responses also occur.

Renal damage

Severe renal tubular damage due to lithium has been a concern, mainly because pathologic changes in the kidney of uncertain significance were reported in early instances of gross overdosage when lithium chloride was given to patients with preexisting circulatory and renal disease. Similarly, reports of renal tubular damage in the rat are hard to relate to the clinical use of lithium in psychiatry, inasmuch as these studies have used toxic doses of lithium salts. A more likely clinical problem is a form of nephrogenic diabetes insipidus manifested by the intake of many liters of water per day and the output of huge quantities of very dilute urine. This syndrome is now believed to result from the ability of lithium ion to interfere with the activity of antidiuretic hormone (ADH) on the renal tubules, either by preventing its access to the appropriate membrane site or by blocking the response of an ADH-sensitive adenylate cyclase. This syndrome is usually managed conservatively by reducing or completely discontinuing the intake of lithium as soon as possible, and it is almost always reversible. It often responds paradoxically to thiazide diuretics, as do other forms of nephrogenic diabetes insipidus, and when there are compelling indications to continue the use of lithium, this treatment might be considered, but will require a reduction in the dose of lithium.

Recently the question of possibly significant long-term kidney-damaging effects of lithium salts was raised again in a series of reports of small numbers of patients who had renal biopsies examined histopathologically. These examinations indicated some degenerative changes and scarring of the nephron that could reasonably be suspected as being due to response to lithium for at least several months (see 31,32). While there has been some evidence of mild impairment of maximal renal concentrating ability, there is other evidence against gross persistent polyuria and impaired average concentrating ability and against obvious abnormalities of blood urea or creatinine levels and of clinical urinalysis in such patients even after many years of lithium therapy (e.g., 31,32). While this potentially important problem receives further investigation, some clinical guidelines for the management of patients given lithium for prolonged periods, with special regard to their renal status, are offered in Table 17.

Goiter

Another metabolic abnormality is the development of benign diffuse nontoxic goiter in patients receiving ordinary doses of lithium salts for prolonged periods. The patients almost always remain euthyroid or only slightly hypothyroid, although there may be an increase in the circulating levels of thyroid-stimulating hormone (TSH). There is experimental evidence for the ability of lithium to

Table 17. Suggested Guidelines to the Clinical Management of Lithium Therapy

1. Consider the indications for lithium maintenance therapy carefully. While lithium is the treatment of choice for the "prophylaxis" of bipolar mood disorders (mania and depression), antidepressants are, on the average, as effective as lithium in decreasing recurrence of unipolar depressions.
2. Advise patients of the knowns and unknowns concerning lithium use; discuss potential risks and benefits, and arrive at a joint decision. Note this discussion and agreement in the clinical record.
3. Prior to initiating lithium therapy, inquire about any history of kidney-related illnesses or symptoms. Obtain a baseline serum BUN and creatinine and a routine urinalysis. Ask the patient to estimate his normal daily fluid intake and output.
4. During lithium treatment, again inquire about fluid balance. Patients who produce three to four liters of urine per day are more likely to show renal changes. Therefore, patients with polyuria and polydipsia, as well as those with increases in serum BUN or creatinine should be studied further with tests of 24-hour creatinine clearance and of renal concentrating capacity.
5. In all patients taking lithium, regularly assess the efficacy of continued maintenance therapy. If lithium is not clearly effective, consider other types of treatment.

These suggestions are adapted from Gelenberg, 1978 (33).

interfere with thyroid metabolism at several points, including the iodination and release of iodinated tyrosine, and some evidence of its interference with the actions of thyroxine on target tissues, much as it seems to impair the actions of ADH. There is no serious danger from the goiter, such as the development of thyroid carcinoma, but judgment must be exercised in deciding whether to continue the treatment with lithium. Rarely will significant functional hypothyroidism or frank myxedema occur, and in many cases treatment with thyroxine leads to regression of the goiter and permits maintenance of a euthyroid status while lithium therapy is pursued. (Lithium has even been suggested as treatment for hyperthyroidism and excesses of ADH.)

Skin reactions

Other toxic effects of lithium include the occasional development of localized edema, eruptions (especially a reversible, but potentially recurrent, form of folliculitis that resembles keratosis pilaris) or even ulcerations of the skin. An antihistaminic agent may be helpful for the rashes, and for the rare skin ulcers, topical steroids are useful. Thinning and loss of hair may also occur.

Other reactions

Hepatic and bone marrow toxicity are rarely associated with lithium therapy. Although it is not unusual to observe a mild *elevation* of the peripheral leukocyte count, the significance of this is uncertain. Lithium has been reported to worsen myasthenia gravis in rare instances.

Use in pregnancy and lactation

A great deal of concern surrounds the use of lithium in pregnancy and lactation partly because studies in classical embryology revealed grossly teratogenic effects of very high concentrations, and more recent evidence in experimental animals indicates that very high doses of lithium are associated with fetal wastage and anomalies of the central nervous system. There are also reports of uncertain significance that lithium can alter the metabolism of the rat testis, as well as the motility of human sperm. Together with other alterations in fluid and electrolyte metabolism in pregnancy, there is an increased clearance of lithium; with the diuresis after delivery there may be an increased retention of lithium and consequently an increased risk of intoxication. Fetal distress may occur when lithium is used near term, and there may be hypotonia, listlessness, lethargy, cyanosis, decreased suck response and startle reflex in the newborn infants of mothers taking lithium. In nursing mothers, breast milk lithium concentration is about 50% of the mother's blood level, leading to the calculation that the daily dose of a newborn on a per-kg body weight basis is about 10% of an adult dose. A small number of reports have associated human fetal anomalies (especially cardiovascular malformations) with the use of lithium in pregnancy, and suggest that the rate of such occurrence may be increased over that expected in the general population, and that cardiovascular anomalies as a fraction of all anomalies are in striking excess over the ratio presented by the general population. A reasonable position at the present time is that there is enough circumstantial evidence about the potential fetal toxicity of lithium to urge avoidance of its use in the early months of pregnancy, to advise caution and discontinuation of lithium before term, and to permit the use of lithium in pregnancy only for the most urgent indications.

In conclusion, the antidepressants and lithium have been shown to be of impressive utility not only in the management of some acute mood disorders and their recurrences, but also in the partial protection against recurrences, in long-term treatment of outpatients with manic-depressive (bipolar) and so-called unipolar disorders. Unfortunately, they are relatively toxic substances on acute overdosage, so that they require great caution with impulsive, unreliable or suicidal patients, and should usually be dispensed in limited quantities that reflect their known margin of safety (ratio of lethal to effective daily dose). Strong anticholinergic effects are typical of many heterocyclic antidepressants and these can be demonstrated and treated rapidly with physostigmine. Lithium had been judged safe when blood levels are closely controlled, although recent reports of possible renal changes following prolonged exposure to lithium are currently raising questions about the risk:benefit ratio similar to those being faced with the problem of neuroleptic drug-induced tardive dyskinesia.

SUMMARY

The antipsychotic drugs have provided an effective and relatively safe treatment of psychiatric patients with schizophrenia, paranoid illnesses, manic-depressive conditions and other illnesses marked by psychotic features. These agents are sometimes called "neuroleptic" as virtually all produce signs of extrapyramidal neurological disorders in addition to their antipsychotic actions—in part, evidently, as an artifact of the means of screening potential new agents. These agents have a strong and selective antagonistic action on synaptic mechanisms in the brain mediated by dopamine as a neurotransmitter. This antidopamine action almost certainly contributes importantly to the parkinsonism effect (basal ganglia), and the prolactin-elevating (pituitary) effect of these drugs; in addition, their antipsychotic actions may be mediated by antidopamine effects, possibly in cortical, limbic and other forebrain centers. The specific neurological side effects of these drugs include acute dystonias, parkinsonism, motor restlessness and late oral dyskinesias and choreoathetosis. The treatment of the acute reactions is usually effected by the use of anticholinergic agents; the treatment of the later dyskinesias is unsatisfactory, and they are to be avoided by judicious use of antipsychotic drugs for long-term treatment.

The modern medical treatment of mood disorders includes the use of antidepressant drugs and lithium salts, and ECT still has a place. In contrast to the largely antiadrenergic antipsychotic agents, the imipramine-like heterocyclic antidepressants, though analogues of the phenothiazines, potentiate the actions of norepinephrine; they also have strong antimuscarinic effects. The latter actions contribute to their annoying and more serious atropinelike effects on the eye, salivary glands, heart, gut, bladder and central nervous system. It is unfortunate that the drugs used for patients at increased risk of suicide are so toxic and potentially lethal. While antidepressant effects of the heterocyclic antidepressants have been demonstrated in controlled clinical trials among outpatients as well as inpatients, their efficacy is more impressive in the more severe forms of depression. For milder forms of the syndrome, their effects are not much better than those of antianxiety agents, a placebo or other nonspecific treatments, nor are they impressively better than psychotherapy. Even in serious depressions, the antidepressant drugs are usually not effective for a week or more after treatment is begun, and the rate of relapse is high unless patients are maintained on the medications for at least several months. In recurrent or so-called "unipolar" depressions, antidepressants are sometimes continued indefinitely. In severe cases of depression, more consistent and more rapid effects are obtained with ECT, which should still be used in the treatment of many very severe depressions, with acutely suicidal patients and when the antidepressant drugs fail to work within a month or so, as happens in as many as 30% of severe depressions. The antipsychotic agents and ECT are also useful in the treatment of agitated and psychotic forms of depression. The MAO inhibitors are now of renewed interest since they have been shown to be effective in depression at high doses and effective in panic disorder, obsessive-compulsive neurosis, and other neurotic dysphoric states. These useful effects are also found with many heterocyclic antidepressants, which are less encumbered by the complex and potentially dangerous interactions between MAO inhibitors with many other drugs and with tyramine-rich foods. Stimulants have little if any place in the treatment of serious depressive illnesses. Owing to the limited efficacy, slowness and toxicity of the currently available agents, the search for better antidepressants is being pursued. There has been little fundamentally new in the treatment of depression since the introduction of ECT in the 1930s and the MAO inhibitors and imipramine in the 1950s, although applications of biochemical measurements to evaluate blood levels of antidepressants show promise of optimizing existing treatments for individual patients, and the recent introduction of new antidepressants with uncertain mechanisms of action (such as trazodone) as well as experimentation with still others (such as bupropion, zimelidine, fluoxetine, iprindole, mianserin) with actions unlike those of imipramine are promising developments.

Lithium ion provides a useful and specific form of medical therapy for manic and hypomanic episodes. Its clinical actions may be delayed for a week or more, so the use of an antipsychotic agent may be required in the initial period to control the behavior of very disturbed patients. The main limitations of lithium are its narrow therapeutic index and requirement for close medical supervision. The most promising aspect of the use of lithium is its partial prophylactic effect in reducing the frequency and severity of manic and depressive attacks in manic-depressive illness. It is also being tried experimentally in other recurrent or cyclic disorders of mood or behavior. Possible problems in the long-term use of lithium are goiter and renal effects.

Overall, the record of the use of antipsychotic and mood-stabilizing agents for long-term psychiatric patients has been impressive. The present chapter has emphasized some of the side effects and problems sometimes encountered in short- or long-term use of these drugs. Nevertheless, it is important to point out that treatment of psychiatric patients with the chemical agents introduced in the 1950s and an understanding of the actions of these drugs have contributed in a most important way to the revolutionary changes in the pattern of care delivery as well as in modern psychiatric theory. Such treatment has helped greatly to reduce the need for prolonged institutional care and to maintain even patients with severe chronic or recurrent mental disorders in the community. The conduct of long-term maintenance or preventive chemotherapy for psychiatric patients with optimal efficacy and safety is one of the most important challenges of present-day clinical psychopharmacology.

REFERENCES

1. Baldessarini, R. J. *Chemotherapy in Psychiatry.* Cambridge, Mass.: Harvard University Press, 1977, 201 pp.
2. Cooper, T. B., Simpson, G. M., and Lee, J. H. Thymoleptic and neuroleptic drug plasma levels in psychiatry: current status. *Intl. Rev. Neurobiol.* 19: 269–309 (1976).
3. Creese, I., Snyder, S. H. A simple and sensitive radioreceptor assay for antischizophrenic drugs in blood. *Nature* 270: 180–182 (1977).
4. Davis, J. M. Overview: Maintenance therapy in psychiatry: I. Schizophrenia. *Am. J. Psychiatry* 132: 1239–1245 (1975).
5. Hogarty, G., and Ulrich, R. F. Temporal effects of drug and placebo in delaying relapse in schizophrenic outpatients. *Arch. Gen. Psychiatry* 34: 297–301 (1977).
6. Baldessarini, R. J. Drugs and the treatment of psychiatric disorders. Chapter 19 in *Goodman and Gilman's The Pharmacological Basis of Therapeutics*, Sixth Edition, A. G. Gilman, L. S. Goodman, and A. Gilman (eds.), New York, MacMillan Co., 1980, pp. 391–447.
7. Baldessarini, R. J., and Tarsy, D. Pathophysiology of tardive dyskinesia. *Int. Rev. Neurobiol.* 21: 1–45 (1979).
8. Creese, I., and Snyder, S. H. Behavioral and biochemical properties of the dopamine receptor, in *Psychopharmacology: A Generation of Progress*, M. A. Lipton, A. DiMascio, and K. F. Killam, eds. New York: Raven Press, 1978, pp. 377–388.
9. Snyder, S. H., U'Prichard, D. C., and Greenberg, D. A. Neurotransmitter receptor binding in the brain, in *Psychopharmacology: A Generation of Progress*, M. A. Lipton, A. DiMascio, and K. F. Killam, eds. New York: Raven Press, 1978, pp. 361–370.

10. Garver, D. L., Davis, J. M., Dekirmenjian, H., Jones, F. D., Casper, R., and Haraszti, J. Pharmacokinetics of red blood cell phenothiazine and clinical effects: acute dystonic reactions. *Arch. Gen. Psychiatry* 33: 862-866 (1976).
11. Granacher, R. P., and Baldessarini, R. J.: Physostigmine: its use in acute anticholinergic syndrome with antidepressant and antiparkinson drugs. *Arch. Gen. Psychiatry* 32: 375-380 (1975).
12. Snyder, S. H., Greenberg, D., and Yamamura, H. I. Antischizophrenic drugs and brain cholinergic receptors: Affinity for muscarinic sites predicts extrapyramidal effects. *Arch. Gen. Psychiatry* 31: 58-61 (1974).
13. Snyder, S. H., and Yamamura, H. Antidepressants and the muscarinic acetylcholine receptor. *Arch. Gen. Psychiatry* 34: 236-239 (1977).
14. Baldessarini, R. J., and Tarsy, D. Tardive dyskinesia, in *Psychopharmacology: A Generation of Progress,* M. A. Lipton, A. DeMascio, and K. F. Killam, eds. New York: Raven Press, 1978, pp. 993-1004.
15. Jacobson, G., Baldessarini, R. J., and Manschreck, T. Tardive and withdrawal dyskinesia associated with haloperidol. *Am. J. Psychiatry* 131: 910-913 (1974).
16. Jus, K., Jus, A., Gautier, J., Villeneuve, A., Pires, P., Pineau, R., and Villeneuve, R. Studies of the actions of certain pharmacological agents on tardive dyskinesia and on the rabbit syndrome. *Int. J. Clin. Pharmacol.* 9: 138-145 (1974).
17. Davis, J. M., Bartlett, E., and Termini, B. A. Overdosage of psychotropic drugs: A review. *Dis. Nerv. Syst.* 29: 157-164 (1968).
18. Richelson, E., and Divenetz-Romero, S. Blockade of psychotropic drugs of the muscarinic acetylcholine receptor in cultured nerve cells. *Biol. Psychiatry* 12: 771-785 (1977).
19. Baldessarini, R. J. Mood drugs. *Disease-a-Month* 24(2): 1-65 (1977).
20. Baldessarini, R. J. The basis of amine hypotheses in affective disorders. *Arch. Gen. Psychiatry* 32: 1087-1093, (1975).
21. Robinson, D. S., Nies, A., Ravaris, C. L., Ives, J. O., and Bartlett, D. Clinical pharmacology of phenelzine. *Arch. Gen. Psychiatry* 35: 629-635 (1978).
22. Baldessarini, R. J., and Lipinski, J. F., Jr. Lithium salts: 1970-1975. *Ann. Intern. Med.* 83: 527-533 (1975).
23. Pope, H. G., Jr., and Lipinski, J. F., Jr. Diagnosis in schizophrenia and manic-depressive illness. *Arch. Gen. Psych.* 35: 811-828 (1978).
24. Crews, F. T., and Smith, C. B. Presynaptic alpha-receptor subsensitivity after long-term antidepressant treatment. *Science* 202: 323-324 (1978).
25. Pert, A., Rosenblatt, J. E., Sivit, C., Pert, C. B., and Bunney, W. B., Jr. Long-term treatment with lithium prevents the development of dopamine receptor supersensitivity. *Science* 201: 171-173 (1978).
26. Appleton, W. S., and Davis, J. M. *Practical Clinical Psychopharmacology.* Second Edition, Baltimore: Williams and Wilkins, 1980, 173 pp.
27. Morris, J. B., and Beck, A. T. The efficacy of antidepressant drugs. *Arch. Gen. Psychiatry* 30: 667-674 (1974).
28. Blackwell, B., Stefopoulos, A., Enders, P., Kuzma, R., and Adolphe, A. Anticholinergic activity of two tricyclic antidepressants. *Am. J. Psychiatry* 135: 722-724 (1978).

29. Davis, J. M. Overview: Maintenance therapy in psychiatry. II. Affective disorders, *Am. J. Psychiatry* 133: 1–13 (1976).
30. Atkinson, R. M., and Ditman, K. S. Tranylcypromine—a review. *Clin. Pharmacol. Ther.* 6: 631–655 (1965).
31. Burrows, G. D., Davies, B., and Kinkaid-Smith, P. Unique tubular lesions after lithium. *Lancet* 1: 1310 (1978).
32. Cattell, W. R., Coppen, A., Bailey, J., and Rama Rao, V. A. Impairment of renal-concentrating capacity by lithium. *Lancet* 2: 44–45 (1978).
33. Gelenberg, A. J. Lithium and the kidney. *Mass. Gen. Hosp. Biol. Ther. Psychiatry Newsletter* 1: 25–28 (1978).
34. Baldessarini, R. J. *Biomedical Aspects of Depression*, Washington, D.C.: APA Press Inc., 1982 (in press).

CHAPTER 14

THE CLINICAL MANAGEMENT OF NONCOMPLIANCE

THEODORE VAN PUTTEN, M.D.

The value of antipsychotic drugs in the maintenance therapy of chronic relapsing schizophrenia is now well established. The problem is that at least 40% of unselected outpatients will not take their prescribed tablets reliably (Van Putten 1974). The long-acting injectable depot neuroleptics are an advance over the oral medication, but the patient still has to return to the clinic for his next injection. In the British experience, some 20% of patients on depot medications do not return (Johnson and Freeman 1973; Johnson 1976).

CAUSES OF DRUG DEFAULTING

Drug refusal cannot be managed well unless one can unravel its causes. In our experience it is useful to distinguish between deliberate and nondeliberate drug defaulting.

Nondeliberate Drug Defaulting

A sizable percentage of schizophrenics lack the motivation or drive to travel to an aftercare clinic. Given that some aftercare centers have "excessively compulsive and long-winded intake procedures," which serve as "endogenous defense mechanisms," (Raynes and Warren 1971), we cannot blame them. Kline and King (1973) also suggest that uncooperative patients, who fail to take medication, are often "pushed out" or "eased out" of treatment by subtle staff pressures.

Reduced motivation in schizophrenics to comply with maintenance antipsychotic medications extends to other medications as well. Ferebee (1964) reported that isoniazid reduced the incidence of tuberculosis by 80% in general patient populations, but by only 18% in schizophrenics with tuberculosis who adhered less readily to treatment.

In Great Britain, where a visiting nurse will administer a long-acting depot medication, depot fluphenazines (Prolixin) can decrease the outpatient drug default rate from as much as 50% to as little as 20%, depending on the vigor of the followup (Johnson and Freeman 1973). This suggests that some 30% of discharged patients are non-deliberate drug defaulters who would be compliant if they were reminded and if the taking of medicine were made easier for them.

Not taking maintenance medication may be different from the patient's perspective. Stopping maintenance medication does not result in immediate and disruptive consequences, such as in diabetes; rather, the patient may feel better as mild or subclinical side effects wear off. Also, many schizophrenics have no great investment in staying well, particularly when relapse means trading a stay in a caring hospital for a lonely hotel room and a welfare check.

Deliberate Drug Refusal

These patients purposively stop maintenance medication and often have a history of doing so. Nonjudgmental interviewing with some awareness of what to look for will usually disclose the reason. Not infrequently, deliberate drug refusers insist on telling us their reasons.

The British experience, in which maintenance depot fluphenazine is routinely administered, and dropouts to clinic are followed up with vigor, indicates that at least 20% of unselected patients stop their injections deliberately (Johnson and Freeman 1973; Johnson 1976).

Dysphoric Responders

Every clinician has encountered schizophrenic patients who, although clearly psychotic, refuse treatment with an antipsychotic drug claiming that it makes them feel worse, that they are "allergic" to these medications, that the drug effect is unbearable.

Such patients with a dysphoric response to an antipsychotic drug describe an effect somewhat akin to that experienced by normal persons given the same drug. Belmaker and Wald (1977) administered haloperidol, 5 mg intravenously, to themselves and described the effect as follows:

> . . . a marked slowing of thinking and movement developed along with profound inner restlessness. Neither subject could continue work, and each left work for over 36 hours. Each subject complained of a paralysis of volition, a lack of physical and psychic energy. The subjects felt unable to read, telephone or perform household tasks of their own will, but could perform these tasks if demanded to do so. There was no sleepiness or sedation; on the contrary, both subjects complained of severe anxiety.

When drug-free schizophrenic patients who signed consent were given a test dose, of either chlorpromazine (2.2. mg per kilogram or 1 mg/lb of body weight) or thiothixene (0.22 mg or 0.1 mg/lb), some 20% had a dysphoric response (Van Putten and May 1978; Van Putten et al. 1979). Some examples were: "It makes everything slower," "makes me feel down," "takes away motivation," "can't think straight," "makes me uptight," and one likened it to a "bad acid trip." Indeed, some dysphoric responders, although cooperative and calm to start with, became acutely panicked and objectively more disorganized several hours after the first dose.

Such an early dysphoric response was a powerful predictor of either immediate or eventual drug refusal, no matter how understanding the therapist. Further, even when we could persuade the patient to continue taking the medication, an early dysphoric response to chlorpromazine tended to augur a poor outcome—at least at conventional dosage levels (Van Putten and May 1978; Van Putten et al. 1979).

The rote—or coercive—insistence that a patient with a history of dysphoric response take antipsychotic medication like everyone else is likely to be viewed by the dysphoric responder as an assault on his personality. Some feel wronged by the drug and the doctor or institution that prescribed it. It is, we think, persons like these who develop adversary relationships with staff, and even become spokesmen in the various consumer movements that equate antipsychotic drugs with "psychiatric assault" and "chemical straightjacketing."

The mechanisms of dysphoric response to antipsychotic drugs is unclear. Dysphoric responders did experience significantly more extrapyramidal symptoms (EPS)—notably akathisia—during the 24 hours after a test dose (Van Putten et al. 1979), and it is our clinical experience that a dysphoric response can often be terminated by the administration of trihexyphenidyl (Artane). Since patients who view the medication as helpful (syntonic responders) also experience EPS, much may depend, as Sarwer Foner (1961, 1963) has suggested, on the meaning and significance a drug side effect has for a patient. Another view is that antipsychotic medication interferes with a psychotic equilibrium, however maladaptive (Nevins 1977).

It seems plausible that the stubborn drug refusal of some psychotic patients is rooted in the "Sauce Bearnaise Phenomenon." To quote Seligman (1972, p. 8): "Sauce Bearnaise . . . used to be my favorite sauce. It now tastes awful to me. This happened several years ago, when I felt the effects of the stomach flu about six hours after eating filet mignon with Sauce Bearnaise. I became violently ill and spent most of the night vomiting. The next time I had Sauce Bearnaise, I couldn't bear the taste of it." Such "interoceptive conditioning" (Barofsky 1976), with a somatically based dysphoric response as the paired event, may explain the stubborn drug refusal of some patients. Further, interoceptive conditioning can probably occur regardless of whether the subject is aware of the association of events. Or he might forget. As a result, patients may offer more "constructed" than "real" explanations for their noncompliance behavior.

Side Effects

Intolerance of side effects—particularly subtle extrapyramidal side effects (EPS) which can be mistaken for the vicissitudes of schizophrenia—prompt many a schizophrenic to stop his maintenance pills or injection. It is often not the side effects per se, but an interaction between a bothersome side effect and little investment in staying well or having little awareness of illness in the first place.

Akathisia

Akathisia is an emotional state and "refers not to any type of pattern of movement, but rather to a subjective need or desire to move" (Crane and Naranjo 1971). This urge to move is always accompanied by affective distress and, objectively, may be manifested by restless pacing, inability to sit still and continuous alterations in posture. With the subtler akathisias,* the patient may not use the word "restless" and complain instead of "jitteriness," inability to feel "comfortable," "impatient," "irritability," the feeling of being "keyed up" or "wired," or of being a "bundle of nerves" (Van Putten 1975). Many experience a vague sense of dread, and most will not tolerate an akathisia for very long. In our experience, patients who claim to be "allergic" to antipsychotic drugs often mean that they were tormented by an akathisia. Hodge (1959) stated that akathisia "may appear like an anxiety state . . . in which real anxiety can be neither recognized nor verbalized," and Kalinowsky (1958) remarked that akathisia can be "more difficult to endure than any of the symptoms for which (the patient) was originally treated." Other characteristics are that akathisia is nearly always experienced as ego-alien, that the inner agitation and restlessness are difficult to articulate, that the patient feels better when moving about, and that once the patient has gained relief from an antiparkinson drug, he will seek relief from the next episode. The subtler akathisias often go unrecognized by the physician—but not the patient! Even a mild akathisia can preclude sitting through the dinner hour, a movie, a therapy session, or a sedentary job.

The Subclinical Akinesias

In its grosser form, akinesia is a component of the "zombie" reaction. Clearly, such easily observable akinetic manifestations as slowed movement, shuffling gait, absence of spontaneous muscular movement and lifeless appearance are not desirable on a maintenance basis. A double-blind procedure in which patient received biperiden, 5 mg intramuscularly, alternating with placebo (or vice versa) and, in later trials, an oral test dose of 4 mg of trihexyphenidyl (Artane) alternating with placebo has enabled us to confirm subtler or subclinical akinesias. Objectively, these milder akinesias, as noted by

**In order for a particular emotional state to be scored as akathisia, the following test had to be passed: disappearance or marked improvement after intramuscular administration of 5 mg biperiden (Akineton), and no improvement after a placebo injection (double blind).*

Rifkin, Quitkin and Klein, are evident mostly as a "behavioral state of diminished spontaneity characterized by few gestures, unspontaneous speech and, particularly, apathy and difficulty with initiating usual activities" (Rifkin et al. 1975, p. 672).

Subjectively, these patients feel "blah," "listless," "tired," "old." Like parkinsonian patients, they may complain of vague joint pains and speak of having "no interest," "life" or "ambition." Some speak of having no feelings at all. Only about half of the patients with a mild akinesia complain of this subjective state: the remainder seem to accept it, and it does appear that both the doctor and patient can get "used to" a mild akinesia, particularly since akinesia is insidious. Further, it is not always easy to distinguish between a mild akinesia and blunted affect, schizophrenic apathy, institutionalization or its equivalent in community neglect, or nondrug-related psychomotor retardation. It is therefore helpful to know that there is a high association between akinesia and both objectively rated sedative effect ($r = + 0.71$) and ratings of subjectively experienced sedative effect ($r = + 0.70$) (Van Putten and May 1978).* Thus, an akinesia is not likely if the patient does not look or feel at least somewhat drowsy.

These invisible EPS contribute to drug defaulting. In one study (Van Putten 1974) of 85 chronic schizophrenics, who had been followed both as inpatient and outpatient for at least 2 years, we found a high association between subtle EPS (notably akathisia and akinesia) at usual maintenance dose and drug defaulting. Association, of course, does not mean cause, but our experiences are that few will tolerate an akathisia for long. Dyskinesias (abnormal involuntary movements), although they can be quite grotesque to the observer, are usually not a factor in drug defaulting as the patient tends not to be aware of them. About half uncomplainingly become accustomed to an akinetic lethargy or reduction of drive. Even so, a mild akinesia can have far-reaching consequences. One chronic schizophrenic lady, competitively employed as a maid, requested disability because she felt "too old and tired"; the addition of antiparkinson medication solved the problem. If such subtle side effects are not detected, many a schizophrenic will stop his maintenance medication. In such an instance, the patient will indeed feel better; the side effects will go away and relapse may not occur until 2 to 3 months later.

**Rated at 9 AM, 12 hours after H.S. dose.*

The role of other side effects in drug defaulting has not been studied. Sexual side effects (particularly erective impotence) are—when they occur—often attributed to medication. There is agreement that antipsychotic medication can be responsible for erective impotence and certainly retrograde ejaculation ("white urine").

Preference for a Schizophrenic Existence

Of course, intolerance of side effects is only a part of the noncompliance problem. Poor motivation, lack of insight, social isolation or just not caring (Blackwell 1976) all contribute. It may even be that some schizophrenics stop their medications because they prefer a schizophrenic existence.

In another study (Van Putten et al. 1976), we compared the extremes of drug compliance in chronic schizophrenics: habitual drug refusers who invariably refused to return for their injection after discharge, and drug-complier patients who habitually came in for their refills or injections of antipsychotic medication.

The drug refusers experienced the resurgence of a psychosis characterized by grandiose delusions and the relative absence of such dysphoric affects as anxiety and depression. The habitual compliers, in contrast, developed decompensations characterized by such dysphoric affects as depression and anxiety, virtual absence of grandiosity and some awareness of illness. A discriminant function analysis revealed grandiosity to be the most powerful discriminating variable between the two groups. Goldstein (1978), in a sample of 107 unselected acute schizophrenics treated with depot fluphenazine, also found grandiosity to be the most powerful predictor of noncompliance. We interpret these findings to mean that some schizophrenics, particularly those with nongratifying circumstances, prefer their grandiose delusions to a relative drug-induced normality.

Attitudes

It is particularly disturbing when a schizophrenic patient stubbornly refuses to take maintenance medication on his own, even though his illness is quite drug sensitive and there are no drug side effects. Some of these patients leave the hospital each time "promising" to take maintenance medication, much like a well-intended alcoholic promises sobriety. Some are younger schizophrenics who equate antipsychotic medication with irrational parental authority. For others, the tablet (or even the injection) can come to symbolize incurable mental illness. Still others, particularly those in whom the medication is only modestly effective to start with, never develop any useful awareness of illness. "Perceived severity" and "perceived susceptibility," two attitudes predictive of compliance in general medical prophylaxis (Sackett and Haynes 1976), are, of course, not applicable in those without awareness of illness. Many of these patients require institutional control of medication and, if they do ever take medication on their own, it certainly will not be out of any personal conviction that it is helpful. Some may acknowledge that they are better now than before medication, but they attribute this to "will" or some voluntary effort on their part, despite repeated demonstrations that the medication is the necessary ingredient in such improvement. In still others, the habitual drug refusal is unfathomable. The patients may agree to maintenance medication, but each time they stop taking maintenance medication—usually shortly after leaving hospital. When closely questioned, these patients often provide shallow-sounding reasons for their behavior.

CLINICAL MANAGEMENT OF NONCOMPLIANCE

A history of noncompliance should be identified as a core problem. Much can be learned from the taking of a detailed drug history: "What medications have you taken and how did each agree with you?"

If the patient has not been returning for his next supply of tablets or his injection because of lack of motivation or just not caring, telephone reminders and injections of depot fluphenazines by visiting nurses can—in the British experience—reduce the noncompliance rate from as much as 50% to as low as 20% (Johnson and Freeman 1973).

Improving drug compliance in nondeliberate drug defaulting requires effort of a very ordinary type—making phone calls, giving patients appointment cards, serving coffee and, if need be, making a house visit. Further, the effort—as in general medical compliance—must be continuing if it is to be effective. Moreover, there is little glamour in working with chronic schizophrenics. The typical poverty of speech, underactivity, social withdrawal, lack of motivation, stereotyped conversations and general lack of social intelligence in many of these patients are very wearing. I have never known a mental health worker who could work effectively with chronic schizophrenics 40 hours a week.

In all the compliance literature—psychiatric as well as medical—compliance is much improved if a spouse or significant other assumes a supervisory role (Blackwell 1976). At times, the history of noncompliance is such that a patient may need placement in a setting (board and care home) where medication is supervised; some patients will quite willingly take medication as long as it is given to them, but they will not take it on their own.

The management of *deliberate* noncompliance—particularly habitual drug refusal—requires expert assessment. Too often, an adversary relationship develops between a patient who believes that drugs have harmed him and a staff member who regards this as delusional thinking. At times, the adversary positions become so intense that the patient is given a larger than usual dose of depot fluphenazine (Prolixin). Even the rote administration of a usual dose (1 cc) of fluphenazine decanoate to a patient with a history of dysphoric response is likely to result in severe dysphoria, and a hardening of psychiatric mistrust.

Patients with a history of dysphoric responses to antipsychotic medications need to have their subjective reaction to medication acknowledged, and even then, they usually require considerable persuasion before they are willing to risk a trial with a new medication—or a lower dose of the same one. The effort is worthwhile because some dysphoric responders do have good short-term outcomes—both objectively and subjectively—on very low doses of antipsychotic drug (e.g., 5 mg of haloperidol, 5 mg of thiothixene [Van Putten et al. 1979]). Such patients can, in our experience, often be maintained on ultralow doses: e.g., 25 mg of thioridazine, 1/5 cc of fluphenazine decanoate per month, 1 or 2 mg of haloperidol. Since dysphoric responses, in our experience, are often extrapyramidally based, we believe that such patients should be given a prophylactic antiparkinson drug. Further, when any patient develops a dysphoric response to medication, one should search for subtle EPS and, when in doubt, we recommend a concomitant trial of antiparkinson drug. The faddish withholding of antiparkinson drug is not supported by rigorous data; indeed, the reappearance or development of subtle EPS (notably akinesia), when antiparkinson drugs are stopped in double-blind fashion, indicates that considerable numbers of patients would be deprived of a useful treatment by the withholding of antiparkinson drug (Rifkin et al. 1978).

Not only do dysphoric responders seem to require ultralow dose maintenance, but the indications are that most schizophrenics can get along with less maintenance medication than is commonly prescribed. Mean dosages in double-blind studies of the efficacy of maintenance antipsychotic drug treatment tend to be below 400 mg of chlorpromazine (CPZ) or equivalent per day. Leff and Wing (1971) used a mean of 157.1 mg of CPZ or equivalent in outpatients with illness of moderate severity. In the recent study of Hogarty et al. (1974), "drug survivors" were maintained on 270 ± 140 mg/day. Troshinsky (1962) studied 43 chronic schizophrenics who had been maintained for over 2 years in the community on a mean daily CPZ dose of 225 mg, and the better-adjusted discharged patients of Hargeaves et al. (1977) were maintained on 408 mg/day of CPZ. The recently completed study by Goldstein et al. (1978) shows that many young schizophrenics can be maintained on surprisingly small doses of fluphenazine (Prolixin) decanoate, 6 mg every two weeks, as long as they receive supportive family therapy. Experienced clinicians (e.g., Ban 1977) find that patients can be maintained on 50–200 mg of chlorpromazine (Thorazine) or its equivalent. The point is that patients can be effectively maintained on dosages commonly considered "placebo" or "homeopathic."

Maintenance at a lower dose—with fewer side effects—may have far-reaching consequences. Falloon et al. (1978), in a double-blind comparison of oral pimozide and injected fluphenazine, found at one-year followup, that the patients on oral drugs were significantly less impaired than those on the injected preparations, in respect to sociability, leisure interests, and function as a housewife and parent. This benefit in social behavior was found to be correlated with reduced extrapyramidal symptoms, particularly rigidity, which impairs expressive behavior and nonverbal communication. In Rifkin and coworker (1978), as well as in our experience, the milder akinesias are manifest at times only as diminished social interest or diminished interest in any activity. Some respond to akinesia with depression, and it is our belief that some "postpsychotic depressions" are primarily a toxic drug effect (Van Putten and May 1978). Goldstein et al. (1978) compared fluphenazine decanoate 25 with only 6 mg in young, newly admitted schizophrenic patients and found that the higher dose (which is the customary dose in many clinics) did protect more against relapse, but at a price. The men on the higher dose experienced significantly more anxious-depression. Thus, lower maintenance doses, although somewhat more risky, may result in improved social adjustment and less dysphoria.

When the drug defaulting is primarily attitudinal, the therapist resorts to persuasion. The patient—after a period of hospitalization—may correctly state that he is now well (that is, free of psychotic symptoms), "not nervous," or as well as he ever was, so why should he continue with maintenance medication. Certainly medication cannot be helpful in securing employment, straightening out an impossible family situation, etc. If the patient has had two or more psychotic episodes, he should be told that future relapses are a virtual certainty and that the purpose of low dose maintenance medication is prophylactic—that is, "to keep you well." At least those with a foothold in life will readily agree that psychotic relapses are too disruptive, that it becomes more and more difficult to reengage, to find a new job, etc. Those who equate the medication with irrational parental authority or societal control must be persuaded to take it for their own sake. When these patients rationalize their peculiarities or symptoms as inevitable or "normal" reactions to the environment, this may be impossible. No matter how persuasive the physician, many will promise to take the medication only when they "need it"—according to their own self-identified needs. This approach is usually doomed to failure as loss of awareness of illness is often one of the earliest symptoms of relapse.

REFERENCES

Ban, T. A., and Lehmann, H. E. Myths, theories and treatment of schizophrenia. *Dis. Nerv. Syst.* 38: 665–671 (1977).

Barofsky, I. Behavioral therapeutics and the management of therapeutic regimens, in *Compliance with Therapeutic Regimens.* D. L. Sackett and R. B. Haynes, eds. Baltimore: The Johns Hopkins University Press, 1976, pp. 100–109.

Belmaker, R. H., and Wald, D. Haloperidol in normals. *British J. Psychiatry* 131: 222–223 (1977).

Blackwell, B. Treatment adherence. *Br. J. Psychiatry* 129: 513–531 (1976).

Crane, G. E., and Naranjo, E. R. Motor disorders induced by neuroleptics. *Arch. Gen. Psychiatry* 24: 179–184 (1971).

Falloon, I., Watt, D. C., and Shepherd, M. The social outcome of patients in a trial of long-term continuation therapy in schizophrenia: pimozide vs. fluphenazine. *Psychological Medicine* 8: 265–274 (1978).

Ferebee, S. H. The schizophrenic and oral medication. *Lancet* 2: 147 (1964).

Goldstein, M. J., Rodnick, E. H., Evans, J. R., May, P. R. A., and Steinberg, M. Drug and family therapy in the aftercare treatment of acute schizophrenia. *Arch. Gen. Psychiatry* 35: 1169–1177 (1978).

Goldstein, M. J. Personal Communication. See above study.

Hargreaves, W. A., Glick, I. D., Drues, J. Showstack, J. A., and Feigenbaum, E. Short vs. long hospitalization: a prospective controlled study. *Arch. Gen. Psychiatry* 34: 305-311 (1977).

Hodge, J. R. Akathisia: The syndrome of motor restlessness. *Am. J. Psychiatry* 116: 337-338 (1959).

Hogarty, G. E., Goldberg, S. C., Schooler, N. R., Ulrich, R. F., and The Collaborative Study Group. Drug and sociotherapy in the aftercare of schizophrenic patients. II. Two-year relapse rates. *Arch. Gen. Psychiatry* 31: 603-608 (1974).

Johnson, D. A. W. The expectation of outcome from maintenance therapy in chronic schizophrenic patients. *British J. Psychiatry* 128: 246-250 (1976).

Johnson, D. A. W., and Freeman, H. Drug defaulting by patients on long-acting phenothiazines. *Psychol. Med.* 3: 115-119 (1973).

Kalinowsky, L. B. Appraisal of the "Tranquilizers" and their influence on other somatic treatments in psychiatry. *Am. J. Psychiatry* 115: 294-300 (1958).

Kline, J., and King, M. Treatment dropouts from a community mental health center. *Community Mental Health J.* 9: 354-360 (1973).

Leff, J. P., and Wing, J. K. Trial of maintenance therapy in schizophrenia. *Br. Med. J.* 3: 559-604 (1971).

Nevins, D. B. Adverse response to neuroleptics in schizophrenia. *International J. Psychoanalytic Psychotherapy* 6: 227-241 (1977).

Raynes, A. E., and Warren, G. Some characteristics of "drop-outs" at first contact with a psychiatric clinic. *Community Mental Health J.* 7: 144-150 (1971).

Rifkin, A., Quitkin, F., and Klein, D. F. Akinesia: A poorly recognized drug-induced extrapyramidal behavioral disorder. *Arch. Gen. Psychiatry* 32: 672-674 (1975).

Rifkin, A., Quitkin, F., Kane, J., Struve, F., and Klein, D. F. Are prophylactic antiparkinson drugs necessary? *Arch. Gen. Psychiatry* 35: 483-489 (April 1978).

Sackett, D. L., and Haynes, R. B., eds. *Compliance With Therapeutic Regimens.* Baltimore: Johns Hopkins University Press, 1976.

Sarwer-Foner, G. J. Some comments on the psychodynamic aspects of the extrapyramidal reactions. *Rev. Can. Biol. Extrapyramidal Sys. & Neuroleptics* 20: 527-533 (1961).

Sarwer-Foner, G. J. On the mechanisms of action of neuroleptic drugs: a theoretical psychodynamic explanation. *Recent Advances in Biological Psychiat.* 6: 217-232 (1963).

Seligman, M. E. P. Preface, in *Biological Boundaries in Learning,* M. E. P. Seligman and I. L. Hager, eds. Appleton-Century-Crofts, 1972, p. 8.

Troshinsky, C. H. Maintenance phenothiazine in aftercare of schizophrenic patients. *Pa. Psychiatr. Q.* 2: 11-15 (1962).

Van Putten, T. Why do schizophrenic patients refuse to take their drugs? *Arch. Gen. Psychiatry* 31: 67-72 (1974).

Van Putten, T. The many faces of akathisia. *Compr. Psychiatry* 16: 43-47 (1975).

Van Putten, T., Crumpton, E., and Yale, C. Drug refusal in schizophrenia and the wish to be crazy. *Arch. Gen. Psychiatry* 33: 1443-1446 (1976).

Van Putten, T., and May, P. R. A. Subjective response as a predictor of outcome in pharmacotherapy: The consumer has a point. *Arch. Gen. Psychiatry* 35: 477-488 (1978).

Van Putten, T., and May, P. R. A. "Akinetic depression" in schizophrenia. *Arch. Gen. Psychiatry* 35: 1101-1107 (1978).

Van Putten, T., May, P. R. A., Wittman, L. A., and Marder, S. R. Subjective response to antipsychotic drugs. *Arch. Gen. Psychiat.* 38: 187-190 (1981).

PART IV

SELECTED APPLICATIONS OF TREATMENT PRINCIPLES

EDITOR'S COMMENTARY: PART IV

The previous chapters have taught us that the treatment of the chronic psychiatric patient in the community involves the presenting of material support (food, shelter, clothing, medical care, etc.), the opportunity for skill development (vocational or interpersonal), an optimal social environment (an environment that neither stresses nor underchallenges the patient), an "effective" medication regimen, and a support system that adequately implements and integrates these elements of care. How this implementation and integration occur and the problems and methods involved in this task are the subject of three chapters in this section.

The three chapters differ in that each discusses a different site at which integration is to occur. What will be learned, as you read and consider each paper, is that the environment within which the care is to occur—rural, urban or community—dramatically alters the nature of the integration. This would naturally lead to a diversity of systems of care. However, since the reassignment of patients from institutional to noninstitutional settings is motivated by both human *and* political considerations, the creation of these alternative patterns of care are not always easy or sure. Huessy, for example, decries the fact that efforts in establishing integrated care appropriate for a rural setting must combat regulations often created for urban environments. He is particularly concerned about how the premature professionalization of personnel and the standardization of facilities and procedures limit the creative solution of problems required for the development of an integrated care program. Contrast, he would say, the evolution of the structured but nonformalized care provided the chronic psychiatric patient in Gheel, Belgium, with the task facing today's providers. In the extreme, providers in response to increasingly stringent regulations must create, in a steplike, all-or-nothing manner, elaborate programs of care, set in communities that have limited involvement and commitment to such programs. Rural communities, with their low population density and adequate housing, would seem to be able to avoid many of these adverse consequences, yet their potential is limited by the regulations established to ensure the quality of such programs. To Huessy, this paradox results in the loss of the essential ingredient required for integrated care, a caring relationship between the provider and patient.

Also discussed by Huessy are the advantages and disadvantages of caring for the chronic psychiatric patient in rural settings, where available resources are unavoidably dispersed. The danger of dealing with a decentralized care system is that it increases the chances that a patient will not be provided all opportunities to receive care, while the chief advantage is that it increases the chance that a person will be exposed to an optimum social environment.

Lamb's paper addresses another issue—whether or not the chronic patient can be provided integrated care in cities. He reviews what is known, but the reader cannot help but be struck by the complexity of the task of urban care and the minimal amount of supporting data (see Chapter 22). It is possible that the issue here is not to determine whether the inner city is an adequate care site, since it inevitably will be, but rather how best to provide this care. This he discusses in some detail. A primary issue discussed by Lamb is the problem of how best to allocate limited resources. He argues that the successful management of the severely disabled in the community requires a maximum commitment of resources, if integrated care is to occur.

The paper by Stein and Test describes a specific method for providing community care. Their program is designed to deal with what they consider to be the major barrier to a patient's ultimate ability to function in the community. This barrier is created when the patient is removed from the community and placed in a hospital—which consequently becomes the setting in which the patient ostensibly is prepared for independent living in the community. The authors believe that this strategy has failed. In contrast, Stein and Test believe that the effort must be directed toward sustaining the patient in the community, in contrast to preparing the patient for community living (as occurs in a hospital).

The system that Stein and Test describe includes a number of separate psychosocial therapies. For example, crisis intervention techniques are used in the initial phase of treatment to avoid having to institutionalize the patient. The patient's drug therapy is also carefully assessed and adjusted at an early stage in the treatment. Vocational assessment and training and various psychotherapies are then combined to sustain the patient in the community. Continuity of care, and integrated care, are principle objectives of this program, and are achieved by a balance between judicious application of specific treatments and innovative administrative procedures.

CHAPTER 15

SERVING LONG-TERM PATIENTS IN THE CITIES

H. RICHARD LAMB, M.D.

A high proportion of the severely mentally disabled who used to reside in hospitals are now living in the cities; many have been placed there because of the availability of large old hotels and board and care homes; others have drifted there on their own. Still another contributing factor to the concentration of these patients in the cities may be the essentially urban nature of the deinstitutionalization model (Bachrach 1977); the architects of the deinstitutionalization movement have been, for the most part, urban in their residence and orientation. In any event, the result has been the clustering of thousands of expatients in the lower socioeconomic sections of our large urban areas.

In what kind of environments do these persons now find themselves? Much has been found wanting in our cities by urban planners and other students of contemporary American society (Schneider 1979). They have described such characteristics of our cities as a deepening social alienation which calcifies human behavior, promoted by the fractured nature of urban life. It is said that the biting lesson of human alienation in urban society is that the worthiness of individual existence is ultimately identical with the worthiness of interpersonal life, the very thing which has been neglected. The covering over of land by buildings and paving in our cities is seen as removing one from vital contacts with nature, a removal often unnoticed but rarely unfelt. In our desire to use time most productively, there is concern on the part of many that both time and speed can annihilate experience, that is, rob experience of reflection, inner organization, reformulation of thought and behavior, and, ultimately, human meaning.

While these are among the crucial problems of our time, paradoxically some of them work to the advantage of many of the severely disabled in their adjustment to the community. For instance, many long-term patients have great difficulty with interpersonal relationships and closeness and are able to "get lost" and escape interpersonal demands in the faceless society of our large cities. Further, in the cities, especially in neighborhoods which are not primarily residential, bizzare behavior and appearance are generally tolerated and often go unnoticed by passers-by. And for those who need a supportive network, Cohen and Sokolovsky (1978) have demonstrated that expatients can have meaningful and supportive social networks even in a large, single-room occupancy hotel in New York City. Their data suggest that these social networks, especially when they comprise involvement with other persons in the hotel, can act to reduce hospital readmissions.

There are other, perhaps more important, advantages of an urban environment for effecting the integration of exhospital patients into community life. Public transportation is better in urban areas, and confidentiality of patient treatment is much easier to maintain in the anonymity of the city (the clinic receptionist is less likely to be your next-door neighbor). Because there is a greater population to serve and draw from in the cities, there tends to be more, and a wider variety of, treatment and rehabilitation facilities, which makes for greater flexibility in formulating treatment plans; there also tends to be a greater availability of trained staff. The broad spectrum of different kinds of housing in the cities, both existing and potential, makes it easier to set up programs to meet the needs for varying kinds of living situations for the long-term mentally ill.

On the other hand, there are a number of negative factors that come into play when serving the long-term patient in an urban environment as compared to a more rural one. Urban areas tend to be high-crime areas which are more frightening to long-term patients, as well as to the rest of the citizenry. As a result, there is a heightened fear of going outside after dark, and it becomes more important for programs to schedule activities during daylight hours. There is increased exposure to street drugs, which becomes a major problem in trying to serve this population; it can be difficult to sort out the effects of drugs from the illness itself, and one now has an additional problem with which to deal. The long-term psychiatric patient is also vulnerable to hustlers and predators of all descriptions who abound in the cities (Reich 1972).

In a small town there may be fewer facilities, but what few facilities there are may be in the same place and/or better coordinated because "everybody knows each other." This is in contrast to the fragmentation of services in the cities, which will be discussed later. Likewise, in a small town there is a potential natural supportive social network made possible by the smaller population and the fact that the residents of the town are more closely involved with each other. An example that highlights this phenomenon is the Missouri Foster Community Program in which the citizens of two small towns have taken ex-state-hospital patients into their midsts; each town has made a community project of becoming involved with these patients, providing support to them and integrating them into the life of the town (Keskiner et al. 1972). It must be noted, however, that the supportive social network of rural areas has disadvantages as well as advantages. For instance, in a rural area or small town where one tends more to mind his neighbor's business and where anonymity is hard to come by, persons have more difficulty escaping interpersonal demands when they need to. For the same reasons they are more easily labeled and stigmatized, and escape from such an identity as a mentally ill person becomes more difficult.

One frequently thinks of an urban environment as characterized by high pressure as compared to the slower pace of rural areas. Whether or not this generalization is true, we will see that there can be facilities in the heart of the largest cities which provide a low-pressure setting.

POLITICAL AND ADMINISTRATIVE CONSIDERATIONS

Implementation of new programs and upgrading of old ones have been made much more difficult by the crisis of the cities and the resulting imposition of severe fiscal constraints. Mental health services have to compete with all other public services for a shrinking total amount of dollars. Frequently in cities, the nonmental-health competition is highly vocal and organized as compared with even the most effective mental health consumer and advocacy groups. In this regard, strong community boards can be invaluable (Kellam and Schiff 1968; Polak et al. 1979). The involvement of citizens is also crucial in helping mental health administrators recognize what the priorities of the community are with regard to mental health services. Further, citizens are much more likely to work hard for services they think are vital and of high priority. At the same time, it must be recognized that finding community boards in urban areas which are not only effective, but truly representative of segments of large, diffuse metropolitan communities is much more often talked about than actually accomplished. A board composed of persons of different races and ethnic groups, of professionals and tradesmen and housewives may look representative; but often, in fact, these persons represent only themselves and a small circle of friends and associates.

While urban areas offer many advantages for the treatment and rehabilitation of the severely disabled, the whole process may get bogged down in the inefficiency and incompetence of the large, cumbersome, impersonal bureaucracies of the cities. Even in cities with highly developed services, individual agencies, both in and out of government, tend to operate in isolation. As a result, most cities have gaps in services, duplication of effort and waste of scarce monies. This fragmentation of services greatly complicates the lives of long-term patients, who must wander from agency to agency seeking the kinds of services they need. Nowhere is the role of the case manager more important than in the cities in helping to formulate the treatment plan that includes these services, and then helping to coordinate and facilitate the long-term patients' access to, and use of, these services.

The special needs of the long-term mentally ill are an issue for society generally, and receive much attention and most of their funding from federal and state governments. However, the actual implementation of these services needs to be kept at the local level, especially in the cities, if they are to be effective (Elpers 1978). And this is where major problems arise. The larger the city, the larger (and usually more inefficient) the bureaucracy. In these large bureaucratic structures, there is a tendency to overemphasize the technical administrative tasks, and the bureacracy loses sight of the importance of program policy setting and planning which are needed for the *clinical* program management. "Small is beautiful" (Schumacher 1972) should be a watchword for every level of government.

Elpers (1978) emphasizes that decentralization of programs, preferably on a geographic basis, can keep both the volume and the scope of the managers' responsibility within human dimensions. This concept of geographically based services has been advocated for many years (Stubblebine 1971; Mesnikoff 1978). But too often only lip-service has been paid to this concept, and authority has not truly been delegated to the regional administrators. The geographic definition of a service population facilitates the coordination of mental health services with other human service agencies such as welfare, social security, housing authorities and the state departments of employment and rehabilitation. When this concept is working well and the catchment area is rationally defined, there can be continuity of care and free movement of patients, records and staff among various service elements.

It must not be imagined, however, that drawing catchment area boundaries in urban areas is without problems (Whittington 1971). Frequently, such boundaries in a large metropolitan area are arbitrary, especially in dealing with the long-term mentally ill who are extremely mobile, and who move about the city with great frequency—from family, to board and care home, to family again, to another board and care home, and so on. If we are to have continuity of care for these persons, there must be flexibility so that the patient need not change his entire mental health support system every time he moves.

Getting community support often means reconciling oneself to political realities (DeSole, Singer and Swietnicki 1968). Mental health professionals may wish to dissociate themselves from certain politicians whom they do not respect or from some religious and community groups whom they regard as inflexible and too self-serving. Many mental health programs have been much less effective or even failed in their objectives because of failure to include, or deal with, these persons and groups.

PRIORITIES

Because of the crisis of the cities and the increasing scarcity of funding for human services, including limitations on money available for mental health services, priorities must be established. I feel that the highest priority should be given to the severely disabled mentally ill, and that, at the very least, what would have been spent on them had they remained in state hospitals should be made available for services to them in the community. Conversely, the lowest priority for services in the public sector should go to primary prevention, the value of which is, in most instances, uncertain and unproven (Lamb and Zusman 1979). Long-term psychotherapy with neurotics and those suffering from character disorders, the healthy but unhappy, should have an equally low priority. Not that this modality is not effective and invaluable for many persons, but the time and resources involved in serving a relatively small number of persons can make the difference between adequate and inadequate services for great numbers of long-term patients. A community mental health center then would concern itself primarily with services for the severely disabled mentally ill as well as short-term crisis intervention for more healthy persons.

Establishing these priorities would improve the image of community mental health among persons both in and out of the mental health professions; initial enthusiasm for community mental health has given way to a barrage of criticism from all quarters, much of it deserved (Zusman and Lamb 1977). Originated to deal with abysmal conditions in state hospitals and provide community treatment for exstate-hospital patients, community mental health focused instead on primary prevention, political activism and the mildly mentally ill. And nowhere has the plight of the seriously mentally ill been more apparent than in the cities, where they are congregated in great numbers and highly visible. A return to the original fundamentals, stressing that the highest priority be given to the community treatment and rehabilitation of the severely mentally ill, would go a long way toward countering the valid criticisms that these persons have been neglected by community mental health.

In a similar vein Hansell (1978) points out that in the 1960s there was an unwarranted emphasis on crisis intervention and on those who require a single episode of treatment, and lack of interest in patients such as the seriously disabled who need ongoing services in order to decrease repeated hospitalizations, monitor psychoactive medication and provide effective treatment and rehabilitation services.

USE OF NONPROFESSIONALS

Indigenous nonprofessionals have an important role in both urban and rural settings (Ruiz and Saiger 1972). Brought up among the people they are to serve and still residents of the area, they have invaluable contacts within the community as well as an understanding of the local culture or subculture. These factors, however, are not sufficient in and of themselves, and adequate training is essential. It has also been observed that the effectiveness of the worker and his closeness to the patient are more often a function of the worker's personality than of his ethnicity, residence in the community or professional role (Lowenkoff and Zwerling 1971).

The rural sense of community and small town closeness can be an important asset for mental health professionals seeking grassroots cooperation in providing care. Recruitment of volunteers—indigenous mental health care extenders—can flourish where there is a strong sense of community. However, something very similar to this can be found in the largest urban areas. For instance, the congregation of an active church, and especially one whose leadership is concerned with mental health issues, can provide a group with the same sense of community. From such a church group, one can enlist the assistance of the church as a whole in running social rehabilitation projects (Cutler 1979), or one can recruit individual volunteers for various other mental health activities. Still another important source of volunteers are the universities and colleges to be found in any urban area. Students, if carefully screened, can provide high-quality services. They frequently bring a high degree of enthusiasm and motivation and can be rewarded with college credits, letters of recommendation to graduate schools and experience that will be invaluable to them in their future careers.

CRISIS INTERVENTION

Urban areas are apt to have a wide range of resources such as walk-in clinics, day treatment centers, private practitioners, hospitals and alternatives to hospitalization. But sometimes these resources are less effective than they might be. For example, the importance of a psychiatric outpatient clinic's capability to be available immediately to severely disabled patients at times of crisis cannot be overemphasized; despite this, some clinics resist implementing the walk-in clinic concept because of their desire to have all appointments scheduled and/or their wanting to devote themselves to long-term psychotherapy.

For acute crises, alternatives to hospitalization are desirable for many persons who would otherwise be hospitalized (Lamb 1979b); these alternatives have taken a variety of forms, some especially well suited to urban settings. For a large proportion of acutely ill psychiatric patients, psychiatric hospitalization as we have known it in the past is not necessary, and these persons can be treated as effectively as—or more so than—would have been the case had they been in conventional hospitals. Patients who are not hospitalized are less likely to be labeled and stigmatized. Generally speaking, persons treated in alternatives to hospitalization tend to be less separated from the community and are less likely to lose their links with their support systems. Further, continued reliance on the hospital relieves the pressure on community programs to develop services for this population. The ability to export these patients and their problems allows professionals in the community to forget the need for community services for the acutely and chronically severely disabled. The following two examples of alternatives to hospitalization, both from urban settings, illustrate what can be accomplished.

At Lincoln Hospital in New York, the Community Mental Health Services wanted to help psychiatric patients avoid hospitalization, but had to work with limited resources in an urban catchment area characterized by poverty, crime, joblessness, school failure, high rates of physical disease and the host of other social ills that beset a slum and its inhabitants (Ruiz 1979). Their solution was a partial-hospitalization service consisting of two parts sharing the same premises, staff and facilities: a twenty-five-patient day hospital and a five-bed overnight unit. These five beds were all that stood between their psychotic patients and the state hospital located outside of the catchment area, but the service proved to be an effective alternative to hospitalization.

This program illustrates some other important issues when working in an urban setting. A major problem was that of security. The building was burglarized several times with much loss of equipment and furniture, and staff automobiles were broken into. In addition to loss of property, these events caused considerable staff insecurity. The funds that were then allocated for a security guard and other security measures could otherwise have been spent on direct services, but, generally speaking, programs operating in urban areas have no choice but to provide expensive security. Training of staff presented other important issues. As a result of the ethnic composition of this program's Hispanic clientele, much attention had to be paid to language and cultural matters, particularly in regard to the professional staff, who for the most part were not Hispanics. For instance, there were instances of emergency patients being transferred to the state hospital only because a non-Hispanic psychiatrist could not communicate successfully with them. This program, therefore, set up (1) a large-scale in-service training program primarily directed to decreasing cultural conflicts that had a direct effect on the quality of the care rendered; and (2) Spanish classes to reduce communication problems. These measures were quite effective, but the rapid professional-staff turnover forced them to maintain them on an ongoing basis, at considerable cost and diversion of resources, which again could otherwise have been used for direct service.

The second example of an alternative to hospitalization well suited to an urban setting is the Therapeutic Residential Center (TRC) model developed in Orange County California (Elpers 1979). This model treats in skilled-nursing facilities (convalescent hospitals) persons who would otherwise need acute inpatient hospital care, with the treatment staff provided by the county mental health services. These TRC's have been designated as facilities that can accept involuntary patients. Most initial evaluations are done at the medical center, which has fully staffed emergency services and serves the entire county. Patients who require locked inpatient care, or who have special needs, are admitted to that facility of forty locked adult beds. The remaining patients who require hospitalization are admitted to TRC's, which provide the equivalent of inpatient services, but at half the cost. The clinical program in the TRC is milieu oriented and includes a full range of therapeutic modalities. Psychotropic medications play an important role, as do community meetings, group and individual psychotherapy, occupational and recreational therapies, work with the patients' families, and comprehensive planning for continuing care. Each patient has an assigned primary therapist who is responsible for his or her case management. The primary therapist may be a member of any discipline, but most are mental health workers, for the most part persons with psychiatric-technician or vocational-nurse licenses and usually psychiatric hospital experience. The TRC's gross cost per patient per day of about half that of a psychiatric ward in a general hospital results in a crucial saving of scarce mental health dollars. In addition, the TRC taps all available sources of revenue, in particular Medicaid, which reduces the net cost of the mental health services further by a very substantial amount. Thus, a considerable proportion of the costs for acute care is shifted out of the state-county mental health funding system, and funds are made available for developing other mental health treatment and rehabilitation services.

LIVING ARRANGEMENTS

Long-term patients have differing housing needs and requirements depending on factors such as age, level of functioning, rehabilitation potential and degree of disability. Therefore, there should be a range of living arrangements in the community which includes transitional programs and facilities oriented towards all levels of rehabilitation as well as facilities that provide primarily long-term care (Easton 1974). As noted earlier, the wide variety of living accommodations in the cities lends itself to setting up this range of facilities. They may be highly structured in terms of program and supervision, or they may allow for a maximum degree of independence. They may be government operated or operated by private, nonprofit or private proprietary organizations. What is important is that the facilities be run by persons who know how to relate to long-term psychiatric patients, who are able to maximize their rehabilitation potential, if any, and who can provide as much nurturing and structure as the patient needs, but no more than he needs.

In my opinion there is no optimum size for facilities for long-term patients. Some do best in a small, familylike setting where there is considerable interaction with the other persons living there and with the operator of the facility. Others seem to do poorly with too much closeness and too much contact with nurturing persons and do better in a large facility where they can "get lost" when they need to and avoid interpersonal contact at times when they cannot deal with it.

Still another factor in determining choice of a facility is the extent to which a person tends to be a victim. The harsh realities and the survival-of-the-fittest environment of the cities and of some urban facilities, such as loosely supervised single-room occupancy hotels or large board and care homes, make special consideration important for the masochistic patient, who tends to put himself in positions where he can easily be taken advantage of and become a victim. Often a selected foster home or even a well supervised larger facility can make all the difference in stabilizing such a person in the community and obviating his need to flee back to the hospital.

Let us look more closely at these sheltered living arrangements. Persons in many of them have come to what one might call adaptation by decompression (Lamb 1979a). They have found a place of asylum from life's pressures, but at the same time a place where there is support, structure and some treatment, especially in the form of psychotropic medications. For a large population of long-term psychiatric patients, facilities such as board and care (boarding) homes have not only replaced, but have taken over, the functions of the state hospital. These facilities provide structure in a variety of ways. Medication management and supervision are one way; psychiatrists come to the facility and prescribe psychotropic drugs for the great majority of the residents, and the staff dispense these medications at regular times. The better staff are reasonably aware of residents who are becoming symptomatic or more floridly symptomatic, and convey this to the visiting psychiatrist, who then may adjust medications accordingly. In addition, the staff often see problems that are causing the resident to be symptomatic and may intervene by manipulating the patient's environment to ease the pressures on him. There is additional structure in the supervision of the resident's money and the disbursement of it according to the staff's estimate of the resident's ability to handle his money. Thus, facilities such as board and care homes may provide a low-pressure setting in the midst of an urban area that is usually thought of as a high-pressure environment.

In talking with residents and staff about their experiences in board and care homes, another side of this picture emerges (Lamb 1979a); some operators are seen as regarding their board and care homes almost solely as a business, squeezing excessive profits out of them at the expense of the residents. Whether or not this is true is far from clear, but having this situation overseen by a strong licensing and monitoring agency as well as by patient advocate groups would do much to reassure staff, residents and outside professionals. This applies to the physical structure, food and staff (both numbers and quality), and to the provision of, or arrangement for, treatment and rehabilitation services. Segal and Aviram (1978) suggest that certification of facilities with respect to the quality of the social environment be done by the professionals who place residents in them, together with residents' groups. Most patients see themselves as dependent on board and care home operators and feel powerless to bring about a higher quality of care. Still another factor is the unwillingness of many residents to organize because of their reluctance to be identified with other mental patients. A balance must be struck so that the board and care home operators will make a fair return on their investment and at the same time will provide adequate services to the residents. There also needs to be more careful initial screening of the operators so that only the ethical and competent are allowed in.

A high concentration of mental patients in the same geographical location should be avoided. This has happened in many urban areas of this country (Moltzen 1975; Easton 1974). In these instances the patients become highly visible and identifiable, sometimes provoking public protest that hampers or prevents their assimilation into the general community.

For those persons who are not ready for completely independent living, no other therapeutic housing program comes closer to helping long-term patients live normal lives in an urban community setting than satellite housing programs. Satellite housing may be apartments, duplexes or small single-family dwellings. The housing is leased by the residents or the sponsoring agency or coleased by both. Here patients live in small groups of two to five, without live-in staff, but with some professional supervision. And it is this supervision and support that enables these persons to achieve the closest thing possible to independent living, instead of an institutional setting such as a board and care home. Staff members assigned to satellite housing programs are available as needed for guidance and counseling, both individual and group, and are also available on a twenty-four-hour, on-call basis for crisis intervention. The existence of a large number of community apartments increases the possibility that roommates can be matched in terms of age, personality, interest and level of functioning. Shopping, cooking and housework are shared, and residents have a responsibility for paying the rent, either to the landlord directly or to the agency.

If one were given unlimited resources, one undoubtedly would not use an old, midcity, single-room occupancy hotel for seriously disabled patients. However, given the existence of these facilities and the large numbers of patients in them, it has been shown that it is possible to upgrade the level of services and quality of life by bringing treatment staff to these facilities and providing consultation to staff and welfare personnel already there (Levitt et al. 1968; Cohen, Sichel and Berger 1977). The consultation can be case consultation for the welfare workers, and consultation to help set up social rehabilitation group activities in the facility, including a resident's council. The council, a group of residents selected by their peers, can serve as liaison between the resident staff and the hotel management and/or welfare staff and can take considerable responsibility for the activity programs. The professionals who come to these hotels also do some crisis intervention and try to facilitate the use of mental health services by the residents, by meeting residents and workers arriving in mental health clinics, day treatment centers and hospitals, by guiding clients through the admission procedures and by providing historical background for hospital and clinic staff.

VOCATIONAL

The wider range of vocational facilities in urban areas makes appropriate referral easier. Thus, there is generally a choice of vocationally oriented day treatment centers, prevocational activity centers, workshops with varying degrees of expectations, extensive vocational rehabilitation counseling and testing resources, and a variety of work-experience and job-training opportunities. This is important, for a major factor in the vocational rehabilitation of long-term patients is being able to individualize their vocational plans and match each person with a program that will maximize his potential, but not exceed his capabilities. To do otherwise is to invite a failure experience and the reluctance or unwillingness to pursue vocational goals again. Frequently the absence of prevocational programs is the missing key ingredient for long-term patients.

On the other hand, a problem in the cities is that it is more difficult to make vocational placements in rehabilitation facilities and private businesses on the basis of personal and social relationships than it is in a small town. These contacts leading to work and work experience placements need to be developed by hard work on the part of vocational rehabilitation counselors and/or job placement specialists.

SOCIAL REHABILITATION

We have already described the potentially rich resources for volunteers in urban areas in churches, colleges and universities. To this should be added the various service clubs in each community, as well as persons recruited through mental health associations and volunteer bureaus. Still another important resource is the large urban school districts, in particular the adult high schools, which usually have established programs in basic education and are often willing to add courses geared to the needs of long-term psychiatric patients who need to learn the basic skills of everyday living.

When the many thousands of long-term psychiatric patients began streaming out of the state hospitals into the community, it quickly became clear that they were woefully deficient in the basic skills of everyday living. More recent experience in community mental health programs with young, chronic schizophrenics has revealed similar problems even though these patients have not spent long years in state hospitals. Their deficits in ego functioning include being unable to achieve mastery over their environment. Much of their difficulty in adjusting to the community has to do with not knowing such things as the essentials of managing their money and budgeting; how to use banking services; how to utilize the resources available to them in the community; how to use their leisure time; the fundamentals of nutrition; meal planning and shopping; how to use public transportation; the essentials of grooming; personal hygiene and sex education; and the very basic social amenities that make the difference between a life of isolation and having friends. For many patients, knowledge and skills in these areas not only make a great difference in the quality of their lives, but make the difference between being able to live independently in the community and living in a hospital or at a very low level of existence in a board and care home (Ludwig 1971).

It has been shown that entire social rehabilitation programs are operative and, at the very least, more effective outside of mental health settings. For instance, to teach the basic skills of everyday living to long-term patients in one metropolitan area, a program was set up not only on an educational model, but actually in the educational system (Lamb 1976). The class is a regular part of the adult high school, is taught by a teacher and is in a regular classroom—not in a mental health center, and the participants are called students and not patients. Mental health professionals are used only for consultation. Long-term patients begin to see that they can be like other people in the community, doing things that other people do, such as going to school. They begin to acquire an identity of student rather than patient. When they meet people and are asked what they are doing, many of the students say, "I am going to school," or "I am taking a class in personal growth education."

CONCLUSION

We have seen that in large cities, despite their seemingly faster pace and more highly pressured life styles, we can find, or construct, supportive environments that meet the varying needs of long-term patients. These may be settings with expectations for significant improvement in functioning, or settings that are essentially places of asylum from the pressures of the world for those who need them.

But if we give the severely disabled high enough priority, we can use the rich resources of our cities to provide a wide range of treatment and rehabilitation. For those who are able and willing, we can help them raise their level of functioning in all areas; for others, we can, at the very least, enhance the quality of their lives.

REFERENCES

Bachrach, L. Deinstitutionalization of mental health services in rural areas. *Hospital & Community Psychiatry* 28: 669-672 (1977).

Cohen, C., Sichel, W., and Berger, D. The use of a mid-Manhattan hotel as a support system. *Community Mental Health Journal,* 13: 76-83 (1977).

Cohen, C. I., and Sokolovsky, J. Schizophrenia and social networks: Ex-Patients in the Inner City. *Schizophrenia Bulletin* 4: 546-560 (1978).

Cutler, D. L. Volunteer support networks for chronic patients, in L.I. Stein, ed. *New Directions for Mental Health Services: Community Support Systems for the Long Term Patient* 1(2): 67-74 (1979).

DeSole, D., Singer, P., and Swietnicki, E. A project that failed, in *Mental Health and Urban Social Policy,* L. J. Duhl and R. L. Leopold, eds. San Francisco: Jossey-Bass, 1968, pp. 163-183.

Easton, K. Boerum Hill: A private long-term residential program for former mental patients. *Hospital & Community Psychiatry* 25: 513-517 (1974).

Elpers, J. R. Management and programmatic constraints on community mental health services. *Hospital & Community Psychiatry* 29: 369-373 (1978).

Elpers, J. R. The therapeutic residential center in a community mental health system. *New Directions of Mental Health Services: Alternatives to Acute Hospitalization* (1): 39-48 (1979).

Hansell, N. Services for schizophrenics: A lifelong approach to treatment. *Hospital & Community Psychiatry* 29: 105-108 (1978).

Kellam, S. G., and Schiff, S. K. An urban community mental health center, in *Mental Health and Urban Social Policy,* L. J. Duhl and R. L. Leopold, eds. San Francisco: Jossey-Bass, 1968, pp. 113-138.

Keskiner, A., and Zalcman, M. Returning to community life: The foster community model. *Diseases of the Nervous System* 35: 419-426 (1974).

Lamb, H. R. Acquiring social competence, in *Community Survival for Long-Term Patients,* H. R. Lamb, ed. San Francisco: Jossey-Bass, 1976, pp. 115-129.

Lamb, H. R. The new asylums in the community. *Arch Gen Psychiatry* 36: 129-134 (1979a).

Lamb, H. R. Changing concepts in acute twenty-four hour care. *New Directions for Mental Health Services: Alternatives to Acute Hospitalization* 1: 85-87 (1979b).

Lamb, H. R., and Zusman, J. Primary prevention in perspective. *American Journal of Psychiatry* 136: 12-17 (1979).

Levitt, L. I., Brownlee, W. H., and Lewars, M. H. A model project in community mental health: Consultation to an urban welfare center serving a single-room occupancy hotel. *Community Mental Health Journal* 4: 492-498 (1968).

Lowenkopf, E. L., and Zwerling, I. Psychiatric services in a neighborhood health center. *American Journal of Psychiatry* 127: 916-920 (1971).
Ludwig, A. N. *Treating the Treatment Failures.* New York: Grune & Stratton, 1971.
Mesnikoff, A. M. Barriers to the delivery of mental health services: The New York City experience. *Hospital & Community Psychiatry* 29: 373-378 (1978).
Moltzen, S. Showing the way in San Jose. *exChange* 3: 3-8 (1975).
Reich, R. The chronically mentally ill: their fate in New York City. Bulletin of the New York State District Branch of the American Psychiatric Association, p. 6 (Nov. 1972).
Polak, P. R., Kirby, M. W., and Deitchman, W. S. Treating acutely psychotic patients in private homes. *New Directions for Mental Health Services: Alternatives to Acute Hospitalization* 1: 49-64 (1979).
Ruiz, P. Avoiding hospitalization for the urban poor: Problems and prospects. *New Directions for Mental Health Services: Alternatives to Acute Hospitalization* 1: 65-72 (1979).
Ruiz, P., and Saiger, G. Partial hospitalization within an urban slum. *American Journal of Psychiatry* 129: 89-91 (1972).
Schneider, K. R. *On the Nature of Cities.* San Francisco: Jossey-Bass, 1979.
Schumacher, E. F. *Small is Beautiful.* New York: Harper & Row, 1978.
Segal, S. P. and Aviram, U. *The Mentally Ill in Community-Based Sheltered Care.* New York: John Wiley & Sons, Inc., 1978.
Stubblebine, J. M., and Decker, J. B. Are urban mental health centers worth it? *American Journal of Psychiatry* 127: 908-912 (1971).
Whittington, H. G. Area-wide planning, in *Development of An Urban Mental Health Center.* H. G. Whittington, ed. Springfield, Illinois: Charles C. Thomas, 1971, pp. 186-193.
Zusman, J., and Lamb, H. R. In defense of community mental health. *American Journal of Psychiatry* 134: 887-890 (1977).

CHAPTER 16

RURAL CARE: PROVIDING CARE FOR THE CHRONIC PATIENT UNDER CONDITIONS OF DISPERSED RESOURCES

HANS R. HUESSY, M.D.*

The word "rural" in the chapter heading raises many different images. For some, it evokes a bucolic scene of an Iowa farm; for others, a scene of poverty in the Mississippi Delta. For others still, it would be the ranch country of Montana. Rural settings vary as much as urban settings. There are rural as well as urban slums and areas of rural wealth similar to wealthy suburbs. Therefore, in assessing the mental health problems and needs of an area, whether urban or rural, the important factors are income level, the quality of social organization and cultural stability.

In the face of these aspects which rural and urban life have in common, we must ask ourselves, "Through the years past, have the patterns of care of the chronic psychiatric patient in rural areas differed from those in urban areas?". The answer is, probably not—at least not since our large mental hospitals were established, because they took care of chronic patients from all areas. There is some evidence that the patient's distance from a mental hospital influenced his chances for being admitted there (Person 1962). The rural patient who did not have a state hospital nearby was less likely to end up in one. The further away he lived, the greater the difficulties in getting him admitted. The problem had to be more severe before it warranted the trouble.

*With the editorial assistance of Frances Bracken.

Parenthetically, it should not be forgotten that the large mental hospital not only took care of the chronic patient in so-called back wards, but also set the patient to work maintaining the grounds and running the hospital farm, laundry and kitchen. These hospitals in fact provided a protective community, as well as a sheltered workshop. This made it very easy for the patient, no longer in an acute psychotic state, to shift from being the recipient of intensive ward care, to being a chronically disabled resident functioning within this characteristic in-hospital community.

Although this was reasonably effective practice among the hospitals before the days of antipsychotic drugs, community psychiatry originally dreamed that community care would *prevent* chronicity in patients. However, this has not been borne out by experience. Viewed retrospectively, the sheltered work in a large hospital was not such a bad mechanism for caring for the chronic patient. There are professionals who feel that instead of abolishing these hospitals, we should have upgraded their services. With improvements, the large hospitals might have worked very well indeed, and deinstitutionalization would have been needed for fewer patients. Although the patients worked for no pay and led rather limited lives, many at least felt useful. The addition of payment for work and social enrichment could have provided good quality care for many patients.

From 1960 to 1977, the Vermont state hospital population decreased from 1,450 to 350. Deinstitutionalization took place during this period. Admission to the state hospital was actively discouraged. Currently, there are close to 2,500 individuals—exclusive of children—with mental illness or mental retardation in community care homes. A comparison of the numbers of the chronically mentally ill in the treatment system shows that we have not reduced the number of patients, but we have changed the locus of their care.

I am certain that some of our success in deinstitutionalization is related to the prevailing rural character of our state. The state community care program places many chronic patients in former farm homes. These homes have extra bedrooms with the outdoors available for seasonal activities and comparative privacy.

CARE IN THE RURAL SETTING

Our community care programs have the advantages inherent in rural living. Rural life means a low density of population and usually less extreme socioeconomic segregation. The rich and the poor are likely to meet in the same school and church. Rural houses tend to be larger, thus making unnecessary the costly building of suitable facilities for small group homes for chronic patients.

The outdoors is more readily available, and the opportunity for becoming involved in activities such as gardening, wood cutting and splitting, and animal care is much greater. Whereas neighbors sometimes don't like to accept community homes, there are nevertheless fewer concerns about dangerous neighborhoods in a rural setting. Social activities like church suppers are frequent and easily accessible. Continuous care for the patient is relatively easy in a rural area because a mental health specialist can work with a number of agencies, and can therefore be responsible for a patient as he moves through a variety of services. Thus, the patient's progress is easily followed. True continuity of care is possible. Where this is not so easily possible, the different view each consulting psychiatrist has of the patient produces shifts in expectations and programming, which are often very confusing to the patient. Unfortunately, these changes are not always explained, and the patient begins to feel even more helpless with little or no notion of what is happening to him.

Transportation is one of the most difficult problems patients and professionals alike must face. Many rural areas have no public transportation. Consequently, specialized programs such as day hospitals and sheltered workshops, which require frequent patient attendance, may suffer—as does the patient who cannot make the trip from home. Professionals run into difficulty when they are expected to make calls on patients. Not only must the professional make patient calls, but visits to the small villages all over the area are necessary too. Duplicating the urban model, which requires many specialists, leads to too many professionals spending too much time on the highway. We can overcome this by acknowledging the need for fewer specialists. Rural programs require more generalists. For instance, the area public health nurse is already traveling the distant rural roads on a regular basis and could stop at the homes of some of our chronic psychiatric patients. Thus, a mental health professional would not have to travel the same road to make these visits. In travel to distant clinics, a generalist backed up by consultants available by telephone is more efficient. Instead of an adult psychiatrist, a child psychiatrist and a psychiatrist specializing in alcohol problems traveling to a small community, one generalist can do the job.

Dr. H. B. M. Murphy (1967) of McGill has shown that various culturally homogeneous communities in Canada have different tolerances for different kinds of deviance. One community extrudes hostile outbursts immediately, another cannot tolerate paranoid ideation. This type of knowledge enhances the staff's ability to place chronic patients appropriately. It is not the chronicity or severity of the illness the patient suffers but the *specific symptoms* of the illness which may determine the patient's acceptability in a specific community.

In a different light, Murphy showed that certain members of these homogeneous communities themselves underwent excessive stress, due to cultural differences, and that the excessively stressed members of this social group had higher rates of psychiatric disorder. For instance, career-oriented women experienced great pressure when living in Old-World-type French communities. Such knowledge is important when placing patients in small communities.

The success of rural group homes varies in part in relation to two factors: one—the home's proximity to a population center, and two—the area community mental health centers' relationship to each home. The first factor decides the ease with which patients can socialize outside the home. The second factor has a pervasive influence. Our community care program works well in only about half of the state because of differences in how the local community mental health centers relate to the community homes. In the successful programs, the home operators are part of the center's team; they participate in decision making. When medication changes are contemplated, the home operator is included in the discussion. Furthermore, the home operator understands that he or she is providing something precious, something no one else can provide. In the less successful programs, operators are made to feel like third-class citizens. The mental health center may require patients to appear there at certain times so that Medicaid can be billed, even if this rides roughshod over the home operator's more pressing needs. The patients also must sign agreements not to discuss in their own homes what goes on in the sheltered workshop during the day.

There are also disadvantages in a rural setting. Group therapy, currently very popular, is much more difficult in a rural setting, since it is quite likely that some private, social connections already exist between the various group members who are likely to be neighbors.

STAFFING ISSUES

Until recently, because mental health professionals tended to cluster in urban areas, rural programs were difficult to staff (Huessy

1972). Due to changing styles of residential choice, rural living is becoming more popular, but we find that new staff members can be more easily recruited in an area in which a college and/or medical center exists.

Furthermore, staff unaccustomed to rural life have difficulty in adjusting to their high visibility (Huessy 1972). Personal life becomes part of professional activity. For some this is difficult to accept. There also may be a tendency for more idealistic or perhaps even "odd" or eccentric people to come to rural areas. This is unfortunate, since rural areas have very little tolerance for "odd" professionals.

An active program of in-service education for rural staff is necessary to prevent feelings of isolation and professional stagnation. Our experience has been that it is far better to bring this education to the area. Staff members sent away for an intensive educational experience learned much about dealing with problems applicable only to the site of the session. Nothing was done to help them apply their new knowledge to their own ongoing programs.

For the energetic and innovative individual, the rural setting offers special opportunities. It is easy to develop, in any number of different ways, programs coordinating social agencies—to the mutual benefit of the agencies involved. Fewer people exist in the bureaucratic processes, so the professional not only knows, but also can easily contact the appropriate agency representative—without going through a formal chain of command. This advantage is not usually available to urban-based professionals. The rural setting also offers unusual opportunities for research, both in epidemiology and for studying the effectiveness of different patterns of care. One can try a variation in a care pattern without risking or asking for millions of dollars; and since rural populations are not nearly as mobile as urban populations, followup is much easier. An informal news network keeps one informed about much that is happening to one's patients.

Because there is little in the way of a mental health "establishment" in a rural area, great opportunities exist for trying new ways of doing things. One is continually challenged with problems which must be faced without the usual urban resources, and so one tries new approaches. In the light of this attractive opportunity, it is a wonder anyone would want to work in an urban setting!

COSTS AND OTHER ADMINISTRATIVE DILEMMAS OF PROVIDING CARE IN THE RURAL SETTING

Rural programs don't have to be expensive. Studies already made on the social cost of space (Kraenzel 1966) will help in the development of estimates of the extra cost (such as the cost for transportation) that rural life imposes on the programs. Wisconsin has pioneered in the analysis of costs of different rural programs (Test 1976). In Vermont, we have been able to achieve community care at a very low cost because we have been able to find many homes that would take from 2 to 8 patients on the model of the extended family. Most of these small-group homes are run by one family. The home operators occupy their own home and do not work a 40-hour week. They have very few employees, and this keeps personnel costs at a minimum. In contrast, as soon as such a small group home caring for 6 to 8 chronic patients is staffed by 40-hour-a-week personnel, the costs become very high, even exceeding those of a hospital. The substitute family gives way to a mini-institution in which frequent staff turnover keeps nearly everyone from making a long-term commitment to the patient, consequently losing one of the major advantages of community care.

The home operators take care of patients for a monthly fee of $405.50, a very low sum that covers the cost of food, shelter and supervision. These homes are, however, supplemented by an extensive program sponsored by the area community mental health center, which provides supervision, regular medication checks and enrichment programs involving recreational, social and occupational activities.

Often money is spent on certain services because they are reimbursable, not because they are needed. Governmental programs and third-party payers support specific services, and treatment is too often determined by the chance for a reimbursement dollar, not by the patient's needs. The patient does need room and board, and he needs medical, vocational and social therapy, which embodies enrichment and socialization experiences. Many chronic patients receive either individual or group therapy, even though they may not benefit from this. This treatment is paid for, but no one makes financial provision for caring. Most chronic patient care is financed now through third-party payers who reimburse only for room, board and treatment, not for caring. Caring is that special quality in human relationships that is not limited by work schedules and that goes beyond assigned tasks. It is what a mother provides for her children, and is something that cannot be bought from professionals. Our chronic patients no longer receive this caring from their own families. Caring for chronic patients is draining and exhausting, but it is essential. Remember the rural home operator who provides family-type care for the $405.50 per month. What he provides, beyond the necessities of life, simply isn't financed adequately. He provides caring. Particularly when state leaders insist on hold-the-line expenditures, not allowing for inflation, budget cuts will hit these homes hardest, possibly forcing their closure. The home operators, as a group, are virtually helpless because they lack any kind of political clout. No lobbyist can be afforded to represent them in the state capital. It would take a body of people large enough and with enough resources, such as the nursing home operators, for instance, to obtain the lobbying force they need.

The danger in this runs even further. By refusing to finance caring, third-party payers continually push us toward greater professionalization. Professionals are needed to diagnose, to supply professional therapies as indicated and to assess needs. But many of these needs can and must be met by nonprofessionals. Not only can professionals not supply caring, they are further handicapped because patients tend to relate to them as substitute parents. Many chronic psychiatric patients have their most severe relationship problems with their parents. Such a patient can more easily look upon nonprofessionals as peers and may be able to form more successful, less regressive relationships with them. The indigenous worker was originally introduced to supply such caring. However, for economic reasons, and because he was faced with an alleged need for quality control, he became a professionalized paraprofessional, complete with a diploma. And now third-party payers will foot the bill for almost any therapies, even if unproven, as long as they are provided by professionals carrying certification of one kind or another. Consequently, we add more therapy to make up for the lack of caring, even though therapy can never substitute for caring.

During the heyday of community mental health, more was felt to be better. We need to study how much is best. Phil May's (1968) studies lend little support to many of our favorite therapies. How many of these therapies do you suppose are used simply because they are reimbursable? And while third-party payers practically guarantee payment for inpatient care, payment is inadequate for time-consuming outpatient care. Insurance will pay $10,000 a month per patient to a private psychiatric hospital, but not the necessary $1,800 a month for a patient in a therapeutic community.

Most of us have a general notion of what a community is. But in many ways, federal regulations for community mental health programs violate the concept of community (Hodges 1967). Recently, Vermont was being forced to join three truly separate independent communities into one administrative unit. Why? Because federal regulations on population of a catchment area insist. This adds an extra layer of administrative costs with no benefit to patient care. Federal rules do not care whether an administrative setup is successful. Rules are rules, and those designed for urban settings are inappropriately enforced in rural settings. Thus, major administrative changes have been mandated at considerable cost without benefit to the patient. These federal regulations, whose benefits may have been established in an urban setting, can't begin to suit rural areas. For the sake of the patient, we cannot afford to be as nearsighted as the people writing the rules in Washington. We must respect the genuine community and work with it despite federal regulation. It is only in the genuine community that one can achieve integration of all human services.

As I said before, having specialists in rural areas is not financially reasonable. Our need for generalists though, runs head-on against federal regulations. A social worker may work each day of a week under a different federal program for a group of projects. The worker has to fill out different worksheets for each grant, and no two ask for the same information. We can safely say that the mental health of these agencies is so poor that they cannot even agree on a standard form! Their rules, designed for urban settings, are destructive to rural programs. One program has five annual site visits! That's a poor way to save money.

Third-party payers insist on maintaining standards set only in ways which are easily measurable, mainly physical standards of buildings. Standards easily lead to standardization; we have the need for a great variety of different community care facilities that are not yet ready to be standardized (Huessy 1969). The worry is that as the regulations become more stringent and exacting, the small group homes will be gradually eliminated because they cannot meet the physical standards of an institution. Regular close personal monitoring will ensure good quality control, including caring. Present standards ignore caring and emphasize physical standards and diplomas.

Professionalization limits the intensity of interaction with the patient. The psychotherapist is not truly the patient's friend. He does not invite him home for the weekend. But who will provide the caring for these chronic patients whose family ties have been broken? I do not believe that anyone can do it on an indefinite basis. It requires a continual succession of people willing to give of themselves for a limited time. They must also give of themselves in a way which interferes with their own desires and their own pleasures. Unless we build this into our programs for long-term care and find ways to finance it, we can soon expect the mini-institution in the community to become a replica of the chronic ward in the state hospital.

The VA Hospital in Albany, New York, demonstrated deinstitutionalization 30 years ago. When the enthusiastic director moved on, it did not take long before the program succumbed to inadequate supervision by her less enthusiastic successor. The community care programs are subject to budget cuts, mandated federally at the insistence of third-party payers or state and local government. The enrichment and social support services will be the first to be cut because they are hard to justify quantitatively. That would leave us with many chronic mini-wards scattered throughout the community. Let us hope more rational financing can protect us from that day. Now the care of chronic patients is divided between social welfare and mental health. Within each of these departments there are multiple sources of finances—federal, state and local. Uncoordinated policy changes could alter these financial resources and destroy the delicate balance of the programs.

Innovation is one of the watchwords of today; and yet what we are concerned about in providing caring for our chronic patients is nothing new. The need for caring relationships for our patients is as old as humanity. Innovation often seduces us into thinking that we can, through some professional technique, supply human caring in a way which will not give us or any of our colleagues any pain.

The financial picture is unnecessarily bleak not only for community aftercare programs, but also for their beneficiaries, the patients. We must not forget that many chronic patients can still work—in state hospitals as well as in a rural setting or elsewhere. However, the patient is at a financial disadvantage on several fronts. The chronic patient who can sustain a job is often penalized by losing his pension benefits as soon as he or she is employed. This may guarantee decompensation. From the money he or she is able to earn, the patient cannot pay for the social support system he needs to maintain his level of functioning. Further, under the current situation, the chronic patient who obtains employment loses his Medicaid and cannot pay for his drugs. We would like to propose a special

Medicaid program to pay for antipsychotic medication and necessary social support systems for chronic patients. The patient could thus achieve employment and sustain it.

Now some chronic patients can again work within the state hospital. Many years ago, we did not pay them. Now we do. These people work when they can, are paid for their work and convert to patient status easily should the need arise. Often they resume their paying work while still patients. In years gone by, chronic patients were the major work force of our state hospitals, but were, unfortunately, exploited. Now the state hospital is becoming a sheltered workshop.

THE DELIVERY OF CLINICAL CARE

Let us examine some clinical lessons about chronic patients in general. One of our experiences is that chronic patients do better if they do not go home until after a lengthy stay in a transitional facility. Relatives seldom consider the patient capable of independence when he returns from the hospital. They change their expectations only after they have seen him functioning in a nonhospital setting for some time.

Careful review of every chronic patient's entire record is extremely important when taking over the care of a patient. There are many manic-depressives, for instance, being treated as chronic schizophrenics; and the necessary clues may be found farther back in the patient's history. We have also found that chronic patients with a childhood history of minimal brain dysfunction may be greatly helped, and consequently they can adjust more easily to a transitional facility if their MBD is treated also. Adult MBD's are helped by the same medications that helped them in childhood.

What else can be done for chronic patients who would benefit from community care? Over the years, we in Vermont have frequently employed the principle of complementary programming. In this, the needs of one group of people are met not by the hiring of a professional but by matching these needs with those of another group. The use of college students as volunteer big brothers and big sisters and the use of foster grandparents with high-grade retardates are two examples of this type of programming. As a result, the needs of both the providers and recipients are met in the common activity. Some of the social activities of aftercare can be provided in a nursing home, for instance. Nursing homes need enrichment, and the chronic psychiatric patient can often find satisfaction in what he can do for the chronically physically disabled. The English have demonstrated successfully how high-grade mental defectives can care for autistic children, and how in nursing homes the elderly disabled patient can gain satisfaction from relating to a mentally retarded child. In turn, the mentally retarded child can do simple tasks for the elderly disabled. There must be many more opportunities for complementary programming.

There are other workable plans enabling some patients to become productive. In Canada, some industries allow two mothers to take one job. They assume responsibility for the job between them and thus can be flexible with their hours, accommodating to illness or special events at home. Some of our chronic patients could fill shared jobs. In England, all employers must hire a specific percentage of the disabled. If we really mean to make our chronic patients into full members of our society, then we must pass similar legislation.

I believe one of the major disabilities of the chronic schizophrenic is an inability to switch among social roles. Our aftercare programs should be designed to minimize multiple social role requirements. Simple societies appear to be able to set up unitary social roles for their schizophrenics. Perhaps this accounts for the apparent infrequency of chronic schizophrenia in simple societies. Our society, on the other hand, requires us to fulfill multiple social roles and to switch easily among these roles. Our insistence on forcing chronic patients into multiple social roles may contribute to their difficulty in coping with our society. Consequently, there is a limit to the enrichment programs that should be built into aftercare programs. Our enrichment programs aim to push the chronic patient into living life as we think it ought to be lived, but not perhaps as the schizophrenic can live it. As I read the data (Vargish 1966), some very simple economical aftercare programs achieve results comparable to those of very expensive ones. More is not necessarily better, and we should strive not for complexity but for simplicity.

If positive expectations are essential for successful treatment, how can you help a chronic patient? Forget the long-term prognosis and set up instead a flexible list of goals to be reached one step at a time. You cannot predict how many steps any patient will be able to make, but you can have positive expectations for one step at a time.

Our aftercare work is divided among three major groups. First, there are the chronic patients who have been in the hospital for many years. They require the largest percentage of our efforts. The second group consists of patients who have recently become chronic, despite our best efforts. And third, we have patients to whom we supply intermediate facilities because these people seem to have the potential for achieving independent living. They all need caring. Sometimes, other patients can supply some of this. Chronic patients can be handled in a variety of ways—with the goal of lifetime care, rapid rehabilitation or any number of alternate objectives; therefore, we must be careful to determine which patient is best suited for which program. Many years ago we (Huessy 1969) described the many types of community care feasible. We must learn how to design community care homes for these various purposes, and also how to decide which kind of care a patient needs. We have tended to think of all community care homes as interchangeable. We need transitional facilities to help ease the patients from the hospital back into the community. We need long-term boarding homes which will supply a social support system to a patient who can earn a living but who cannot maintain his own social support system. We need group homes for patients who may have the potential for rehabilitation over a long period of time. In short, we must learn to assess the needs of the patient and then match him to the appropriate home. A patient with rehabilitation potential should not go to chronic care. We need homes which may accommodate decompensated patients briefly to eliminate their admission to an inpatient service. Some homes work to maintain the status quo; others put pressure on their guests. Different homes for different patients: there is a great deal of research potential here.

Missouri (Keskiner 1972), in an attempt to improve community acceptance of chronic patients, has attempted to involve community representatives in planning improvements in care. This would be especially valuable in communities at some distance from mental health resources. The project was called the Foster Community Project and in some ways attempted to copy Gheel, Belgium, the original foster community for psychiatric patients.

Vermont has a long history of concerning itself with the chronic psychiatric patient in the community. *The Vermont Story*, a book describing some of this early work, appeared in 1961. At that time, Vermont had three psychiatric halfway houses, one halfway house for the retarded, and Spring Lake Ranch, a therapeutic community built around work. Over the years, we have reported on the effectiveness of minimal aftercare programs (Vargish 1966) and on the many different types of halfway houses (Huessy 1969) for which we see a real future.

Dr. Milton Mazer's book, *People and Predicaments* (1976), is an excellent description of the mental health problems of a rural community. In this book, he describes his experiences as the only psychiatrist on Martha's Vineyard, an island off the coast of Massachusetts. He was more than just a psychiatrist; he was the director of mental health for the island. In a book of ours called *Mental Health with Limited Resources*, which appeared in 1966, we described many intriguing projects that had been carried out in rural mental health before that time. For a historical review of rural mental health starting in 1922, see Huessy, in Barten and Bellak, *Progress in Community Mental Health*, 1972. Rural health has now become a federal priority (DHEW 1978), and I believe there will be growing opportunities for adequately funded and professionally satisfying work in rural areas.

We talk of research, demonstration and evaluation. I would invite you to consider stable rural areas like Vermont as possible laboratories. I believe the rural settings will produce better models for urban care. A new pattern of care can be tried in a limited area for comparatively little money. If it cannot be made to work there, it is unlikely to work in an urban setting. Urban problems of slums, social and racial segregation, urban renewal and many extraneous events make urban care demonstrations almost impossible. An unforeseen urban-renewal project, for instance, could destroy a research demonstration project. We can follow our patients with ease. Vermont is covered by community services. Questions can be researched for much less money. The arguments raised in this chapter beg for proof. If NIMH wants the maximum demonstration or evaluation for its dollar, Vermont or a similar rural area is the place.

BIBLIOGRAPHY

Chittick, R. A., Brooks, G. W., Irons, F. S., et al. *The Vermont Story: Rehabilitation of Chronic Schizophrenic Patients.* Burlington, Vermont: Queen City Printers, Inc. 1961.

DHEW. *The Mental Health of Rural America* U.S. Govt. Printing Office, 1973.

Director, National Institute of Mental Health. *A New Day in Rural Mental Health Services.* DHEW, 1978.

Hodges, A., Fritz, K., and Fasso, T. The realities of geographic space in rural mental health programming. Public Health Reports No. 5 (May 1967) p. 386-388.

Huessy, H. The general practitioner's contribution to after-care, in H. Huessy, *Mental Health with Limited Resources,* New York: Grune & Stratton, 1966.

Huessy, Hans R. *Mental Health with Limited Resources.* New York: Grune & Stratton, 1966.

Huessy, Hans R. Beyond the half-way house. *The International Journal of Social Psychiatry* 15(3): 235-39 (1969).
Huessy, H., in *Progress in Community Mental Health*, Vol. II, H. H. Barten, and L. Bellak, eds. New York: Grune & Stratton, 1972, pp. 199-220.
Huessy, H. Tactics and targets in the rural setting, in *Handbook of Community Psychology and Mental Health*, Golann and Eisdorfer. New York: Appleton-Century-Crofts, 1972.
Keskiner, A., Zalcman, M. Y., Rupert, E. H., and Vlett, G. A. The foster community: A partnership in psychiatric rehabilitation. *A. J. Psych.* 129: 3 (September 1972).
Kraenzel, F., and MacDonald, F. *The Social Cost of Space as a Criteria in the Distribution of Federal Grants*, Bozeman, Montana, Montana State University (1966).
May, P. *Treatment of Schizophrenia*. New York: Science House, 1968.
Mazer, M. *People and Predicaments*. Cambridge and London: Harvard University Press, 1976.
Murphy, H. B. M., with Marcel Lemieux. "Quelques considérations sur le taux Elevé de schizophrenie dans un type de communauté Canadienne-Française. *Can. Psych. Assoc. Jrnl.* 12 (numero spécial): S72-S81 (1967).
Person, P. H. Geographic variation in first admission rates to a state mental hospital. Public Health Reports 77: 719-731 (1962).
Test, M. A., and Stein, L. I. Practical guidelines for the community treatment of markedly impaired patients. *Community Mental Health Journal* 12(1): 72-82 (1976).
Test, M. A., and Stein, L. I. Use of Special Living Arrangements: A Model for Decision-Making, presented at NIMH-sponsored working conference, *Community Living Arrangements for the Mentally Ill and Disabled: Issues and Options for Public Policy*, held at Rosslyn, Virginia, September 22-24, 1976.
Vargish, F. A community after-care project, in *Mental Health with Limited Resources*, H. Huessy. New York: Grune & Stratton, 1966.

CHAPTER 17

THE COMMUNITY AS THE TREATMENT ARENA IN CARING FOR THE CHRONIC PSYCHIATRIC PATIENT

LEONARD I. STEIN, M.D.
MARY ANN TEST, Ph.D.

"No man is an island, entire of itself." The fact that man must have others in order to survive has been recognized for some time and has been stated in many ways. Current phrasing used by social scientists to describe how this interdependence is manifested are "social networks" and "community support systems." Indeed, in order to survive we must be skillful in developing our support systems.

Long-term psychiatric patients are no different from the rest of us in needing a support network to maintain themselves in their environment. Unfortunately, however, their emotional disabilities are so serious and persistent that, without special help, they are unable to develop and maintain such a network. Long-term psychiatric patients generally do poorly when living in the community; they live isolated lives, experience frequent crises and have numerous readmissions to hospitals. This "revolving-door" pattern is, in large part, a consequence of their inability to create and sustain a support system. It is our belief that remedying this problem requires a major shift in strategy for treating the chronic psychiatric patient.

In the past, whether our treatment took place in the hospital or in the community, our efforts were directed toward *preparing* patients for community life. In general, the research has shown that

Some material for this chapter was published in *Alternatives to Mental Hospital Treatment*, Stein and Test (eds.), Plenum Publishing Corp., New York, 1978; *Archives of General Psychiatry*, vol. 37, April 1980; *New Directions for Mental Health Services*, Jossey-Bass, no. 2, 1979.

both inpatient treatment and community treatments which attempt to help the patient prepare himself for independent living in the community have not succeeded. Specifically, although intensifying inpatient treatment leads to improved inpatient behavior and more rapid discharge from the hospital, it has an insignificant effect on posthospital adjustment (Anthony 1972). And likewise, *time-limited* community-based programs are useful to patients only as long as the patient is involved in treatment (Test & Stein 1978). The research of others, as well as our own research and clinical experience, has convinced us that we must change our treatment strategy from *preparing* patients for community life to *sustaining* patients in community living. To shift from a preparatory to a sustenance strategy also requires that the treatment arena shift from some specialized site where the patient gets "treated" to the community as a whole where the patient is living. Therapy is not delivered out of the context in which the patient is living with the hopes that what is learned will generalize to the patient's life outside of the therapy setting. But instead, therapy is delivered where the patient is living; in his home, in his neighborhood, at his supermarket, at his place of work, etc. The aim is to teach the patient what he needs to know, where he will be using it. In addition, this approach recognizes that those people who come into contact with the patient, such as his family, his landlord, his employer, his friends, etc., play an important role in influencing the patient's functioning. Thus, the treatment includes these persons as important actors in the patient's life, and therefore sees working with these persons as just as important as working with the patient himself.

This chapter presents a conceptual model, based on patients' needs, for developing programs directed towards sustaining patients in community life. It then describes a treatment program entitled Training in Community Living (TCL) that was based on this model and developed as an alternative to mental hospital treatment. The TCL program won the American Psychiatric Association's Gold Achievement Award in 1974. The remainder of the chapter reports the first year's results of a controlled experiment which compared TCL with our present system of treatment, namely, short-term hospitalization plus traditional kinds of aftercare programming.

CONCEPTUAL MODEL

It is our contention that the inadequacies of current models of community treatment are caused by the fact that they do not effectively address certain factors required by patients to achieve a satisfactory life in the community. Absence of one or more of these factors leads to a tenuous community adjustment that keeps patients on the brink of rehospitalization. These requirements were derived from our clinical experience, and similar ones were also clearly delineated in a paper by Mechanic (1978); they are as follows:

1. *Material resources—food, shelter, clothing, medical care, recreations, etc.* Community treatment programs must assume responsibility for helping the patient acquire these resources.
2. *Coping skills to meet the demands of community life.* These are the kinds of skills we all take for granted, such as using public transportation, preparing simple but nutritious meals, budgeting money, etc. We are convinced that the learning of these skills must take place *in vivo* where the patient will be needing and using them.
3. *Motivation to persevere and remain involved with life.* Our patients experience a good deal of stress, and their motivation to remain in the community becomes easily eroded. A ready available system of supports to encourage the patient, to help him solve real life problems and to help him feel he is not alone and that others are concerned about his welfare is crucial in keeping his motivation intact.
4. *Freedom from pathological dependent relationships.* We define a pathological dependent relationship as one which inhibits personal growth, reinforces maladaptive behavior and generates feelings of panic in its members when its loss is threatened. Many of our patients have been pathologically dependent on families or institutions all their lives. Unfortunately, hospitalization deepens pathological dependency, and upon discharge the patient is often returned to a highly conflictual family situation where the ingredients for another crisis and hospitalization are omnipresent. This cycling has been termed the revolving-door syndrome. In order to break that cycle, community programs must help the patient become free of pathological dependent relationships, and in so doing must provide sufficient support to keep the patient involved in community life and encourage growth toward greater autonomy.
5. *Support and education of community members who are involved with patients.* An important factor influencing patient behaviors, and thus community tenure, is the ways in which community members (family, law-enforcement personnel, agency people, landlords, etc.) relate to patients. Community programs must

provide support and education to these community members to help them learn to relate to patients in a manner which is both beneficial for the patient and acceptable to the community.

6. *A supportive system which* assertively *helps the patient with the above five requirements.* Chronically disabled patients are frequently passive, interpersonally anxious and prone to develop severe psychiatric symptomatology. Such characteristics often lead these patients to fail to keep appointments and to "drop out" of treatment, particularly when they are becoming more symptomatic. Hence, a program designed for their care must be assertive in involving patients in their treatment program and must be prepared to "go to" the patient to prevent drop-out. Additionally, it must actively insure continuity of care among treatment agencies, rather than assume that a patient will successfully negotiate the often difficult pathways from one agency to another on his own.

TREATMENT PROGRAM

TCL is a clinical research program that radically departs from the present system of short-term hospitalization plus aftercare. It is unique among "alternative to the hospital" programs in that, unlike the others which accepted only patients whose families were willing to take them back home (Langsley and Kaplan 1968; Pasamanick et al. 1967; Rittenhouse 1970), TCL accepts an *unselected* sample of adult mentally ill patients coming to the state hospital for admission. As will be described in more detail in the evaluation section, the patients are people who by and large have a long history of poor community adjustment with multiple admissions to the hospital.

The treatment program was designed to attend to the very requirements discussed in the last section. Its base of operation is the community, and its goal is to help patients develop and maintain a satisfactory community adjustment. Use of the hospital is virtually eliminated. The program will be described in terms of work with patients, work with families, work with the community and a description of the staff and how it functions. Finally, a case study is presented to illustrate the operation of the program.

Work With Patients

Patients coming to the hospital for admission are immediately interviewed by a member of the community staff, and are then taken from the admissions office to the community to begin their treatment program. Every effort is made to avoid hospitalization, with use of hospital reserved for patients who are imminently suicidal or homicidal, or who require doses of medication high enough to necessitate the hospital's structured environment. In the rare instances when hospitalization is used, it is of short duration so that "community treatment" can begin with minimal delay.

The community treatment approach focuses directly on an in vivo teaching of coping skills as well as treatment of the acute problem that precipitated the patient's coming to the hospital. The patient's "treatment" consists of participation in a full schedule of daily living activities in the community with pharmacotherapy utilized where appropriate. The therapeutic input from staff consists of motivating, supporting and often being "by patients' sides" day and evening. More specifically, staff members "on-the-spot" in patients' homes and neighborhoods teach and assist them in daily living activities such as laundry upkeep, shopping, cooking, restaurant utilization, grooming, budgeting and use of transportation. Additionally, patients are given sustained and intensive assistance in finding a job or sheltered workshop placement, and staff then continue daily contact with patients and their supervisors or employers to help with on-the-job problem solving. Furthermore, patients are aided in the constructive use of leisure time and the development of effective social skills by staff "prodding" and by staff support of their involvement in relevant community recreation and social activities. This frequently includes staff members accompanying patients to such functions until the patients are comfortable enough to attend by themselves. In all these activities, a "can do" philosophy is transmitted from staff to patient, with the assets of patients stressed and symptomatology down-played. Daily, even hourly, contact of staff with patients is emphasized initially and is gradually diminished according to each patient's progress in the treatment program. Even after there is relatively little staff contact, staff remain aware of the patient's functioning and are *assertive* in intervening early at the first sign of regression. Thus, the treatment model is efficient. The patient gets specifically *what* he needs, *when* he needs it, and it is provided to him at the site of *where* it will do the most good.

The medical needs of our patients were carefully attended to as well. Each patient received a thorough physical examination, chest X ray, and the usual blood work and urinalysis routinely done for patients admitted to hospitals. The patient's medical status was carefully monitored while in the program, and treatment was provided when indicated.

We believe that an important therapeutic effect of the program is the tremendous amount of support patients experience through their day-to-day contacts with staff during the activities mentioned above. Over time patients learn that the staff members indeed care about them and are concerned with them as individuals.

Work With Families

Work with families is primarily directed towards breaking pathological dependency ties. With married patients structured meetings with patient and spouse are held to facilitate increased symmetry in the relationship. Most of the patients, however, are unmarried. In these cases families (parents, parent surrogates, siblings) are evaluated to determine whether the patient's problems are significantly contributed to by a pathological family relationship. When this is found to be the case, a highly specialized treatment approach termed "constructive separation" is utilized (Marx, Test and Stein 1973). Operationally, it consists of meeting with family and identified patient, describing the community treatment program to family members and then explaining to them in a firm, though supportive manner that the patient's living with or receiving any support whatsoever from his relatives would be antithetical to the program's goals. Specific guidelines are set up to regulate interactions such as visits, phone contact and letter writing. Frequently, complete curtailment of these activities for an indefinite period of time is requested. Both parents and patient are given enormous support in maintaining the "separation," with staff being constantly available to families to provide guidance and reassurance. Finally, structured visits between patient and family are initiated when the patient has gained sufficient independence to relate to his family in a more adult-to-adult fashion.

Work With Community

A program of this nature could not survive without the community being carefully prepared for its implementation. Prior to beginning clinical work with patients, conferences were held with every relevant community agency to establish the closest of working relationships. We described our program in detail and helped them understand what we wanted to achieve. We clearly outlined the role we expected them to play, which briefly stated, encompassed the following:

1. We did *not* expect them to be mental health workers.
2. We did expect them to operate solely in their own area of expertise; i.e., we wanted police to do police work, landlords to be landlords, etc.
3. We advised them to respond to our patients as they would to any other citizen.
4. Finally we gave them our phone number and encouraged them to call us at any time, 24 hours a day, if they felt they needed our help. We assured them that we would be constantly available.

Our major effort was to influence them to respond to patients in a manner that would promote responsible behavior rather than reinforce maladaptive modes of coping with stress. For example, if a patient's behavior was disruptive to other tenants in his apartment building, we would encourage the landlord to talk to the patient directly about his behavior and to tell him he would be evicted if it continued. This is in contrast to the community's usual response, which is to see to it that the patient's disruptive behavior leads to rehospitalization. That action implicitly gives the patient the message that he is not responsible for his behavior, teaches the patient a maladaptive mode of coping with stress and leads to a hardening of the chronic patient role.

We received excellent cooperation from the community. We believe the most important factors positively influencing community cooperation were living up to our commitment by responding promptly whenever called and not asking community members to change their social or professional roles.

The Staff

To carry out the program, we retrained a typical mental hospital ward, i.e., psychiatrist, psychologist, social worker, occupational therapist, nurses and aides. As outlined above, this staff spend their time dispersed throughout the community working with patients in their homes, places of work, supermarkets, recreational facilities, etc., helping them learn the requisite skills necessary to sustain a satisfactory community adjustment. The staff gather twice a day at the community headquarters, a rented house in downtown Madison, to share information, revise treatment programs as necessary and plan the next shift's work schedule. There are two shifts so that the program is well staffed from 7:00 A.M. until 11:00 P.M., seven days a week. A member of the professional staff remains on call at night to provide 24-hour coverage for patients as well as community agencies.

Utilization of mental hospital personnel in this kind of extrohospital program has advantages as well as disadvantages (Stein and Test 1976). The advantages include experience in, and commitment to, working with severely ill patients and an orientation towards working with patient *behaviors* as well as feelings and cognitions. Additionally, they have experience in a team approach and have a willingness to rotate shifts so that the program can be operational at all times. The major disadvantage lies in making the transition from working in a highly structured hospital setting, where there is relatively little in the way of individual decision making, to working in the inevitably unstructured setting of the community, where a great deal of initiative and willingness to make decisions on the spot becomes vital. Fortunately, with training and support this transition could be made, and staff have increasingly welcomed the taking on of increased responsibility. Moreover, working in a program where the fruits of their labors are demonstrable has proven most gratifying to them.

Case Example

The following case illustrates how the program was operationalized:

John, a 30-year-old, single male, was brought to the hospital by his parents for voluntary admission. They brought with them admission papers signed by a physician, stating that the patient was in need of hospital treatment. This hospitalization would have represented the sixth hospital admission for John, with an accumulation of 11 prior months in a psychiatric hospital. John had been living at home and had been unemployed for the past year. Prior to that he had a poor work history, having had many jobs, none lasting more than 6 months. Although he had lived away from home several times for very brief periods, he virtually lived as a "child" in his parental home, contributing nothing financially to the support of the family. Since his last discharge, the patient had been maintained on phenothiazine medication and was seen at a mental health clinic as an outpatient for periodic medication checks. Over the past two months he had become increasingly irritable and irrational, and had precipitated frequent arguments with his parents. During this time he began missing mental health center appointments, and it was questionable whether he was taking his medication faithfully. This whole pattern was one that the family had become very familiar with, and in the past it had invariably led to the patient being hospitalized.

When John came to the admissions office, the hospital registrar picked up an envelope which *randomly assigned* the patient either to the extrohospital, Training in Community Living program or to the acute treatment ward in the hospital. In this case, the envelope indicated "Training in Community Living," and the registrar called our community-based program headquarters to inform us that our patient was in the admissions office.

Almost immediately a psychiatrist and nurse came out to meet John and the family. It was soon evident that John was in the midst of a schizophrenic episode. Although he was somewhat withdrawn, he was cooperative during the interview and spoke of hearing voices that told him that the F.B.I. was keeping him under constant surveillance and that they were able to monitor all his thoughts. He was, however, not imminently suicidal, homicidal or in need of such high dosages of phenothiazines as to necessitate the structure and nursing care of the hospital. Therefore, hospitalization was ruled out. Our program was then described to John and his family; they agreed to accept a nonhospitalization treatment approach, and they were taken down to the community headquarters where plans were initiated for John's treatment program.

The immediate plan included increasing John's medication, arranging for him to stay at the YMCA at night until a more permanent community living arrangement could be worked out and giving the family instructions that we would essentially "take over" with John—requesting, at least for the time being, that they curtail all contact with him in order to prevent the continuation of the pathological relationship between John and his family. For support, the family was encouraged to get in touch with us whenever they wished and were given a 24-hour-per-day contact phone number. The rest of the afternoon and evening John spent time with the staff, going to supper with a staff member, going to the YMCA to rent his room and going to an evening activity with another staff member, as well as receiving a thorough physical examination.

The next morning he was picked up by a staff member and taken to breakfast at a nearby coffee shop. Later than morning he met with the vocational rehabilitation counselor, who felt John could benefit from a workshop experience. That afternoon he was taken over to one of the community's sheltered workshops and allowed to look the place over. Plans were then made with him to work the next day.

Within a week John was clinically much improved, and he indicated that he wanted to move into a rooming house where he could have kitchen privileges. Staff spent time with him, looking through the classified ads and visiting prospective housing sites. After choosing a place to live, staff time was allocated to help John learn how to keep his place livable, plan simple menus, shop for food and budget his money.

Staff time was also allocated to help John discover leisure time activities and to make use of those in which he manifested an interest. At the onset staff frequently accompanied him to these social-recreational activities.

During his first month in the treatment program, John's performance in the sheltered workshop continued to improve, and he was becoming more autonomous in his living situation. His family did require repeated reassurance that John was able to manage without continuous supervision, and they were strongly supported for not seeing John and reinforcing his dependency in other ways.

However, not unexpectedly, difficulties arose. The day after John received a very positive evaluation at the workshop indicating that he was close to being ready for competitive employment, he got into an argument with the floor supervisor at the workshop and walked off the line. Since he was on a contingency program where he got paid only if he worked, he did not get that day's pay. John then stormed into the program's headquarters and demanded money for supper. A staff member spent the next hour with John going over the events at work, attempting to delineate resolvable problem areas, but emphasizing to him that he would not receive money he did not earn. The next morning he did not show up at the sheltered workshop. A staff member immediately went to his place of living and urged John to get out of bed and to get back to work. Although he complied at that time, within the next two weeks several more disruptive episodes occurred—one at work; the other at the rooming house, eventuating in his eviction. Finally, John appeared at his parent's home asking to move back in with them. All these episodes were handled firmly and consistently. He again was held to the contingency program at work; he learned most directly that certain behaviors would lead to eviction from his residence; his family was given extra support to help them resist John's becoming dependent on them again; and most important, *John found that this gamut of disruptive behaviors would not get him back into the hospital!* Our consistent message to him was that while we were always available to help him learn to adapt to the community, we could not be coerced into treating him as an "irresponsible child."

Twelve months after his entering the program, work with John continued. He was in a competitive job, but still required some support from us, implemented by our getting together with him several times a week to talk about how things were going at work. He also still needed some help in learning to effectively budget his money. Overall, John was managing his autonomous living arrangement quite well, and he did his own shopping and meal preparation. At that point in time, we spent approximately two hours per week with him. He was no longer struggling against us, and his family had come to see him as a person with more potential than they believed possible. They appeared to experience satisfaction in having played their part in letting John "grow up," and they were relieved not to have him as a continuous burden. John has ties with several community agencies. His medication is being given via depot injection by the Visiting Nurse Service. He takes part in an aftercare program sponsored by the Mental Health Center and utilizes the city's Community Center for recreational activities. As each day of independent community living passed, even during the inevitable "ups and downs" he underwent, John's ties to the "sick role" lessened.

EVALUATION

The TCL model is being rigorously evaluated by comparing it with a control group receiving progressive in-hospital treatment plus community aftercare. An explication of the research design and evaluation instruments follows.

Subjects. Subjects for the study consist of all patients seeking admission to Mendota Mental Health Institute for inpatient care who meet the following criteria: (1) residence in Dane County, Wisconsin (consisting of the city of Madison and surrounding area); (2) age 18 to 62; (3) any diagnosis other than severe organic brain syndrome or primary alcoholism.

Experimental Design. Subjects meeting the above criteria are randomly assigned to either the experimental (community treatment) or control group by the admissions office staff. Control subjects are treated in the hospital for as long as deemed necessary and are then linked with appropriate community agencies. Experimental subjects do not enter the hospital (except in rare instances), but instead receive the TCL approach for 14 months, after which they receive no further input from the experimental unit staff. Assessment data on all patients are gathered at baseline (time of admission) and every 4 months for a span of 28 months through face-to-face interviews by a research staff that operates independently of both clinical teams. For experimental subjects who were hospitalized, these data are included in the results reported. Thus, *no* patients were excluded from the study on the basis of severity of symptoms or for any reason other than failure to meet the three specified admission criteria.

Description of the Control Treatment. Patients assigned to the control group are immediately screened by a member of the hospital's acute-treatment unit serving Dane County. The patients are usually (though not necessarily) admitted to the hospital, where they receive progressive treatment aimed at preparation for return to the community. The Dane County unit serves as a stringent control for the experimental program, as it has a high staff-to-patient ratio and offers a wide variety of services: inpatient partial hospitalization, and outpatient followup. It is by no means a custodial unit, its median length of stay being only 17 days. In addition, the unit makes liberal use of aftercare services available in Madison for its discharged patients.

Assessment Instruments. Assessment instruments used in the study are the following: (1) Demographic Data Form—to collect standard demographic data on life situations and economic variables; (2) Short Clinical Rating Scale (French 1970)—a measure of symptomatology; (3) Community Adjustment Form—measures the patient's living situation, time spent in institutions, employment record, leisure-time activities, social relationships, quality of environment and subjective satisfaction with life; (4) Rosenburg Self-Esteem Scale (Rosenburg 1965)—a self-report measure of self-esteem. Measures taken at the subsequent 4-month intervals are the Short Clinical Rating Form, the Community Adjustment Form and the Rosenburg Self-Esteem Scale.

RESULTS

The results reported here represent those on 65 experimental (E) and 65 control (C) subjects through their first year in the study. In tables and discussion below, N's of less than 65 are the result of

Table 1 Characteristics of the Two Treatment Groups at Time of Entry Into the Study

Characteristic		E Group (N = 65)	C Group (N = 65)	Significance
Sex				
Male		36	36	
Female		29	29	n.s.*
Marital Status				
Single		30	30	
Divorced or Separated		17	18	n.s.*
Married		18	17	
Age (years)	$\overline{X}$	31.46	30.77	n.s.**
	SD	10.49	11.29	
Prior Time in Psychiatric Institutions				
(months)	$\overline{X}$	16.65	12.52	n.s.**
	SD	30.99	28.91	

*Tested at .05 significance level (chi-square)
**Tested at .05 significance level (T-test)

missing data in cases where it was impossible to obtain the scheduled followup interview because patients were not available or did not cooperate. Through assertive data collection, however, 89% of all possible interviews were completed.

Characteristics of the Sample. Characteristics of the sample at the time of entry into the study appear in Table 1. This table indicates that the E and C groups were quite similar on basic demographic factors. About 73% of the patients in both groups were either single, separated or divorced; the mean age was fairly young (approximately 31); and patients had accumulated substantial prior time in psychiatric institutions before presenting for the current admission. Additionally, data not included in Table 1 indicated that the E and C groups did not differ significantly on any of the major measuring instruments administered at time of admission, with the exception of the Rosenburg Self-Esteem Scale, which will be discussed later.

Decision to Hospitalize. Among the most significant data bearing on feasibility are the numbers of patients in each group hospitalized at Mendota during the first year in the study and the amount of time

Table 2 Number of Subjects Hospitalized at Mendota During the First Year Post Entry Into the Study

		E Group (N = 65)	C Group (N = 65)	Significance
Not Hospitalized		53	7	p. <.001*
Hospitalized		12	58	
Mean number of days for those hospitalized	$\overline{X}$	11.17	36.60	p.<.001**
	SD	18.12	41.75	

*Chi-square
**T-test

spent there. Data on the number of subjects hospitalized appear in Table 2. In the E group, only 12 of 65 patients were hospitalized at Mendota at any time during their first year in the study, whereas in the C group, 58 of 65 were hospitalized at Mendota. The mean number of days spent at Mendota by the subjects in each group also are shown in Table 2. Not indicated in the table is the additional fact that 34 of the 58 C patients hospitalized were *readmitted* at least once, for a readmission rate of 58% in the first year. Thus, many of the patients treated in the traditional manner were becoming involved in the familiar revolving-door syndrome.

Living Situation. Data gathered on living situations of subjects indicate that throughout the first year E subjects spent very little time in psychiatric institutions as compared to C subjects. This avoidance of use of the mental hospital for the E patients did not lead to a greater use of medical or penal institutions or of supervised living situations in the community. In fact, the E group spent significantly more time than the C group in independent living situations in the community.

Also, E subjects spent increasing time in psychiatric institutions in the 12-month period as compared to the 4- and 8-month periods. Additional data indicate that 97% of the psychiatric institutional time at 12 months was due to 6 patients who left the program against our advice and then gained admission to institutions other than Mendota. Since, at the time they left the program, none of these patients were psychotic or in acute difficulty, our judgment is that had they continued in the program, hospitalization would have been avoided.

Table 3 Mean Percentage of the First Three Data Collection Periods Spent in the Various Employment Situations+

		4 months		8 months		12 months	
		E (n = 61)	C (n = 60)	E (n = 61)	C (n = 60)	E (n = 57)	C (n = 59)
Unemployed	$\overline{X}$	33.76***	61.74	22.97***	53.97	30.31	56.76
	SD	36.48	37.04	36.23	42.93	41.34	43.31
Sheltered	$\overline{X}$	26.68***	5.06	22.50***	2.00	22.39***	1.10
	SD	38.33	13.53	37.69	9.79	38.64	8.24
Competitive Employment	$\overline{X}$	39.63	33.20	54.52	44.03	47.30	42.14
	SD	42.29	36.03	46.27	43.07	45.86	42.69

+Difference between E and C groups within each of the data collection periods that are significantly different are indicated by an asterisk(s) between the two means:
***$p < .001$

Employment Status. Data concerning time spent in various employment categories by subjects in both groups are displayed in Table 3. It can be seen that E subjects spent significantly less time unemployed and significantly more time in sheltered employment than did C patients. There was no significant difference between groups in percentage of time spent in competitive employment situations. Additional data, however, indicate that the E approach did indeed have a favorable effect on competitive employment. Table 4 demonstrates that during two of the three data-collection periods, E subjects earned significantly more income through competitive employment than did C subjects. Other data indicate that this difference was probably the result of the fact that E subjects spent significantly more time in full-time competitive employment situations than did C subjects, who spent more time in *part-time* competitive employment.

Leisure-Time Activities, Social Relationships and Quality of Environment. Leisure-time activities and social relationships were not measured across the entire 4-month data-collection periods, but instead were assessed at the 4-, 8-, and 12-month followup interviews by asking subjects a series of objective questions about specific activities they had engaged in during a designated interval of time preceding the interview (such as the past three days, last week, last month). The two scales developed from these items to measure

Table 4 Mean Amount of Competitive Income (Dollars) Earned by Ss in Both Groups During the First Three Data Collection Periods+

	4 months		8 months		12 months	
	E (n = 61)	C (n = 59)	E (n = 61)	C (n = 59)	E (n = 57)	C (n = 59)
$\overline{X}$	610.00	308.80	872.30*	436.00	759.8*	418.90
SD	1053.40	622.80	1260.00	834.00	1063.5	711.60

+Significant differences between E and C groups within each of the data collection periods are indicated by an asterisk between the two means.
*p<.05

leisure-time activities revealed no significant differences between the E and C groups at any of the three data-collection points. Likewise, several of the scales measuring social relationships revealed no significant differences. One scale measuring contact with trusted friends, however, revealed that E subjects had significantly more contact ($p<.05$) than did C subjects at the 12-month period. Additionally, the mean score for E subjects on a scale measuring social groups belonged to and attended in the last month is significantly greater than the mean score for C subjects at all three of the data-collection points.

Quality of environment was measured by asking subjects about the number of meals they regularly ate, the quality of their living situation and whether they had a number of common creature comforts (such as private bath, radio, television set, easy chair). There was no significant difference between groups on these measures.

The above-cited results on leisure-time activities, social relationships and quality of environment are important since they indicate that even though E patients were spending a significantly greater percentage of their time in the community, there was no reduction in their quality of life as compared to C patients. On some measures, in fact, their social adjustment was enhanced.

Satisfaction with Life and Self-Esteem. The patient's subjective satisfaction with various aspects of his or her current life situation (such as living situation, friends, food, work and the like) was tapped through use of an eight-item self-report scale adapted from work by Fairweather and others (1969). Scores on the items were summed to produce a total satisfaction score, and the mean scores of the E and C groups revealed E subjects to be significantly more satisfied with their present life situations than C subjects at the 12-month data collection point ($p<.05$).

Table 5 Significant Differences Between E and C Group Means On Items of the Short Clinical Rating Scale+

Items	4 months	8 months	12 months
Depressed Mood	—	—	.01
Suicidal Trends	—	—	.001
Anxiety or Fear	.001	.01	.01
Expression of Anger	—	—	—
Social Withdrawal	—	—	—
Motor Agitation	.05	.01	—
Motor Retardation	—	—	—
Paranoid Behavior	—	—	.001
Hallucinations	—	—	—
Thought Disorder	—	.01	.001
Hyperactivity-Elation	.05	—	.01
Physical Complaints	—	—	—
Global Illness	.05	.001	.01

+Items on which the means of E and C groups differed significantly are indicated by the above figures which represent the level (p) of statistical significance.

In *all* cases of significant differences, C subjects were *more symptomatic* than E subjects.

Self-esteem was measured by a ten-item scale and a single total score was derived as described by Rosenburg (1965). On this measure the E group revealed significantly higher self-esteem than C subjects at baseline ($p<.05$). While the two groups may have actually represented different populations on this variable, it would seem unlikely that they did so in view of the fact that E and C groups differed significantly at baseline on no other variable. An alternative explanation is that since this measure was taken a few days after the patient's admission to the study, a lower self-esteem in the C group may be related to the fact that almost all C patients were initially hospitalized, whereas almost all E patients were kept in the community. Subsequently, both T-tests and analyses of covariance of self-esteem scores at the 4-, 8- and 12-month data-collection periods revealed no significant differences between E and C groups.

Symptomatology. Symptomatology was measured through the Short Clinical Rating Scale (French 1970), a thirteen-item scale filled out by the program evaluator after a mental-status examination of the patient. The severity of twelve different symptoms was assessed (on a nine-point scale), along with a final item assessing global illness. Scores on the individual items were analyzed separately since there was no rationale for either totaling or weighting the separate items to form a single score. Means of the E and C groups on each of the thirteen items were compared at the 4-, 8- and 12-month periods, using analysis of covariance with the baseline score serving as the covariant. Results of these analyses appear in Table 5. It can be seen from the table that at each of the three data-collection points E subjects revealed less symptomatology than C subjects—indeed revealing better functioning on seven of the thirteen scales by the 12-month period. Additional data are being analyzed to shed light on the reasons for this favorable outcome.

COMMENT

The lack of an effective model for treating the chronically disabled psychiatric patient stands out as one of the major health care problems of this decade. This chapter argues that the solution to this problem rests in shifting our strategy of treatment from one of *preparing* patients for community life to one of *sustaining* patients in community living. The results here provide support for this framework in which community programming is based on the concepts of *assertively* helping patients to: (1) acquire material resources, (2) learn necessary coping skills in vivo, (3) gain sufficient support to stay motivated and involved with treatment and (4) free themselves from pathological dependent relationships. The TCL program is an example of a program based on these principles.

The results clearly indicate that the TCL program is an effective alternative to mental hospital treatment for a large majority of the adult mentally ill patients now being admitted to our public mental hospitals. Specifically, virtually without use of the hospital it was possible to treat in the community an *unselected* group of patients presenting for admission to a state mental hospital. While most of the control subjects were admitted to the hospital, and many subsequently readmitted, almost all experimental patients experienced a sustained community tenure without suffering the disruption of life and the reinforcement of symptomatic behavior frequently incurred through hospitalization. In addition and most importantly, the data indicate that their sustained community living was not gained at the expense of their quality of life, level of adjustment, self-esteem, or personal satisfaction with life. Instead, relative to control patients, the experimental patients showed enhanced functioning in several significant areas and manifested less subjective distress and greater satisfaction with their lives.

Treating the chronically disabled psychiatric patient in the community, however, does raise questions of social and economic cost which are of crucial importance in the making of policy decisions. Much concern has been expressed over the possible burden placed on family and community members by programs emphasizing community treatment in place of hospital treatment for severely disturbed patients. In a study reported elsewhere (Test and Stein 1980), we investigated the social cost to the family and community. One subjective and six objective measures of burden placed on family members of patients in both groups were obtained. Community burden was assessed through police records of frequency of patient arrests, number of suicidal gestures requiring medical attention and frequency of emergency-room use. All measures showed that the total in-community program resulted in no more burden on family or community than the traditional approach. We believe that the large amount of support provided to patients, families and community members in the experimental approach is an important factor in explaining these results. We also carried out an economic benefit-cost analysis comparing the TCL alternative with the traditional approach of short-term hospitalization plus aftercare (Weisbrod, Test and Stein 1980). An attempt was made to identify as fully as possible all of the forms of potential benefits and costs, to monetize them whenever possible and to quantify in nonmonetary indicators those which could not be estimated in monetary terms. Results indicated that the *total* cost of treating the E group was $8,093 per patient per year as compared to $7,296 per patient per year for the C group. Importantly, 40% to 50% of the costs were in forms other than direct treatment costs. On the other hand, valued benefits (primarily earned income from competitive employment) favored the E group, $2,364 per patient per year as compared to $1,168 per patient per year for the C group. The net difference between groups was quite small, $396 per patient per year favoring the E group. Thus, considering all the forms of benefits and costs which could be converted to monetary terms, the TCL program was certainly economically feasible.

Although the TCL program was designed as an alternative to hospitalization and every effort was made to minimize hospital usage, the hospital was used, albeit for very brief periods, for 18% of the patients. Thus, it is clear that the hospital does have a role to play in the treatment of the chronically disabled psychiatric patient. We believe our study is useful in helping define what the hospital's role can optimally be. The role of the hospital, for any community, must be seen in the context of what kinds of programming are available in the community for the chronically disabled psychiatric patient. Although hospitalization has undesirable effects on patients, there may be greater patient harm and certainly greater burden to the community if use of the hospital is denied on principle without providing adequate community programming in its place. The more comprehensive the community program, the less the need to use the hospital. With a program such as TCL available, we believe the hospital need be used only for the following:

1. For protection of the individual or others when patients are imminently suicidal or homicidal. Care must be taken not to hospitalize patients who use self-destructive behavior as a means of getting help. This presents a very burdensome clinical judgment, but one that can be learned and made if the clinician is willing to do so. In our experience, if the patient is provided with the support he needs, the danger is minimal.

2. For patients whose psychosis is so severe that they require the structure and good nursing care only a hospital can provide. The goal here is to medicate the patient and interrupt the psychotic process as quickly as possible. We have used the hospital for this purpose with patients in the midst of a very manic episode or highly disruptive schizophrenic episode where we were unable to insure that the patient was being adequately medicated. Length of hospitalization in these cases was rarely over two weeks and often a matter of days.

Importantly, we found that psychosis per se was not necessarily an indication to hospitalize. We were able to successfully treat many patients presenting as acutely psychotic without use of the hospital. In short, given adequate community programming, we recommend use of psychiatric hospitalization only in the two specific instances described above.

We made strong efforts with all our patients to integrate them into the fabric of the community. Initially we had the hope that they would succeed sufficiently to disappear among the rest of us and to no longer need to see themselves or be seen by others as patients. Indeed, this did happen in a few cases. The majority, however, continue to require a wide variety of services, including psychiatric services, social welfare service, housing, financial aid, sheltered employment, recreational and the like. They continue to see themselves as patients and are so perceived by others. The crucial difference, however, is that a support system is continuously available to them to help them normalize their lives and optimize their functioning to a significantly greater degree than they have achieved in the past. Some patients, of course, experienced crises and exacerbations of their psychoses. Early intervention in these cases brought remarkably rapid resolution of these problems. One aspect of our program that cannot be overemphasized is our commitment to monitoring all our patients so that intervention can be instituted at the first sign of trouble.

Although we have come to respect the severity of our patients' disabilities, we continue, in most cases, to set expectations for improved functioning and to provide sufficient support to help the patient move toward greater autonomy. Most of our patients will require some help from us for the rest of their lives, and some will need an increasing amount of help as time passes. We have learned that "cure" is not a useful concept in thinking about most of our patients, and that growth, stability and adequate quality of life, or even prevention of deterioration, are worthwhile goals in the treatment of such individuals.

REFERENCES

Anthony, W. A., et al. Efficacy of psychiatric rehabilitation. *Psychology Bulletin* 78: 447-456 (1972).

French, M. H., Heninger, G. R. A short clinical rating scale for use by nursing personnel, I. Development and design. *Arch Gen Psychiat* 23: 233-240 (1970).

Langsley, D. G., and Kaplan, D. M. *The Treatment of Families in Crisis.* New York: Grune & Stratton, 1978.

Marx, A. J., Test, M. A., and Stein, L. I. Extrohospital management of severe mental illness. *Arch Gen Psychiatry* 29: 505-511 (1973).

Mechanic, D. Alternatives to mental hospital treatment: A sociological perspective, in *Alternatives to Mental Hospital Treatment,* L. I. Stein and M. A. Test, eds. New York: Plenum Publishing Corp., 1978.

Pasamanick, B., Scarpitt, F., and Dinitz, S. *Schizophrenics in the Community: An Experimental Study in the Prevention of Hospitalization.* New York: Appleton, Century, Crofts, 1967.

Rittenhouse, J. D. Endurance of effect: Family unit treatment compared to identified patient treatment, in *Proceedings of the Annual Convention of the American Psychological Association,* Washington, DC, American Psychological Association, 1970, Vol. 2, 535-536.

Rosenburg, M. *Society and the Adolescent Self-Image.* Princeton, NJ: Princeton University Press, 1965.

Stein, L. I., and Test, M. A. Retraining a hospital staff for work in a community program in Wisconsin. *Hosp. Community Psychiatry* 27: 266-268 (1976).

Test, M. A., and Stein, L. I. Community treatment of the chronic patient: A research overview. *Schizophrenia Bulletin* 4(3): 350-364 (1978).
Test, M. A., and Stein, L. I. An alternative to mental hospital treatment, III. Social cost. *Arch Gen Psychiatry* 37: 409-412 (1980).
Weisbrod, B. A., Test, M. A., and Stein, L. I. An alternative to mental hospital treatment, II. Economic benefit-cost analysis. *Arch of Gen Psychiatry* 37: 400-405 (1980).

PART V

ADMINISTRATIVE ISSUES IN THE APPLICATION OF TREATMENT PRINCIPLES

EDITOR'S COMMENTARY: PART V

The chronic psychiatric patient receives care in a society that has limited resources, which have to be distributed across many settings. In addition, this society has codes of behavior—legal systems that protect individuals and govern the relations between people. The complexity of both the legal and economic systems and the limitations of the patient are such as to justify that an individual be available to serve as advocate in order to ensure that the chronic patient has access to adequate care. The three chapters in this section deal with these issues as they apply to the chronic psychiatric patient in the community.

Benefit-cost analyses for assessing the care the chronic psychiatric patient receives in the community have been rarely reported, yet they need to be if such programs are to be continued in the face of competing demands on limited resources. Rubin summarizes the available literature, and in so doing highlights the important issues in this area. If mental health workers could tell economists which programs were more effective than others, then resources could be allocated to ensure maximum benefit. However, supporting programs which are most effective does not ensure an equitable distribution of resources, especially for programs which deal with specialized problems for limited numbers of individuals. Thus, *efficiency and equity* are often in conflict.

Rubin points out that defining what is equitable is a political task that requires public participation, whereas economists tend to focus on maximizing the efficient use of resources. He proposes several solutions; first, he suggests that equity be defined on the basis of what is best for society as a whole, as opposed to individuals. Alternatively, he suggests that different groups be given preferential weightings. An example would be to spend more money for the most seriously ill (see Lamb's article in this book) even though the most benefit from therapy would accrue to the least or moderately ill. In both cases, efforts at establishing equity would reduce program benefits, although total societal benefit may not be reduced.

A final point Rubin makes is that the very impetus for deinstitutionalization may have been purely economic. State governments forced by court order to improve care in state run institutions may have opted for deinstitutionalization instead of assuming the increased financial burden required to improve care. This creates the impression that deinstitutionalization effectively reduces the responsibility that the state has for the chronic psychiatric patients. Thus, ensuring the rights of this often dependent individual in the community becomes considerably more important.

As Kopolow points out, community based care, if anything, increases the vulnerability of the patient, and a host of new (noninstitutional) problems can develop that require *active* programs to ensure the quality of care the chronic psychiatric patient receives. Advocacy programs provide such active support. The advocate represents the individual in ongoing judicial settings, as a spokesperson for the patient's rights, as the person who ensures that the patient has access to mental health services and as the person who campaigns for changes in legislation or administrative procedures. The advocate helps patients during transitions (e.g., from institutions to the community, from one type of residence to another) and in practical transactions. The unique characteristic of the advocate is his commitment to the individual and concern for the protection and welfare of that individual.

While the advocate attempts to protect the rights of the patient, the judicial system both defines and protects these rights. As Evans states, a series of judicial decisions have changed our notions about the right of chronic psychiatric patients to treatment, as well as their right to refuse treatment, and their right to social access (e.g., right to work). These decisions have accelerated the deinstitutionalization process, first by making it explicit that if a person is held involuntarily in an institution, he has the right to treatment. If such treatment is not available, the individual may be released from the institution, assuming he is capable of surviving safely in the community. Next, courts have decided that a person cannot be civilly committed if the person can receive care in a less restrictive environment. This places the institution and the state in the position of having to prove that the person cannot safely receive care in the community. A patient's right to refuse treatment has also been substantially supported, although specific conditions under which the interest of the state can prevail have also been clarified.

CHAPTER 18

BENEFIT-COST ANALYSIS AND THE CARE OF THE CHRONIC PSYCHIATRIC PATIENT IN THE COMMUNITY

JEFFREY RUBIN

Increasing public concern and amounts of resources are being devoted to the problems of individuals with long-term physical and mental impairments (LaPorte and Rubin 1979). Many of the physically and mentally disabled have conditions that are not subject to cure. While the impact of the impairments on daily living may be diminished through various types of medical, social and economic interventions, it will not ever be possible to totally relieve the burdens imposed on these individuals by their conditions.

One segment of the long-term care population, the chronically mentally ill, has been the subject of growing interest at both the policy and research levels (Department of Health and Human Services 1980; Talbott 1978). The recognition that this group of people will require a wide range of services over a long period of time has forced policy makers and mental health professionals to rethink their approach to the financing and provision of mental health services. Perhaps the most critical problem brought on by the need to offer long-term care for the chronically mentally ill in the community is the required coordination of program benefits and service providers (Glenn 1978). Uncertainty about program effectiveness, confusing regulations concerning eligibility and the dysfunctional aspects of their condition complicate the choice the mentally ill must make about services. While the case-management individual approach to mental health services is the most efficacious way of treating the patient, the case manager is still faced with decisions about how to utilize a limited set of resources.

How to provide individualized and optimal care for each patient and how to do this with the limited resources available for all patients describe the economic question to be answered. The ultimate solution to the economic problem, of course, can only be accomplished after questions about the efficacy of alternative (community) therapies are also answered. It also should be stated that the fundamental economic problems arise out of the limits on resources and are only partially related to problems in financing of services.

To many clinicians and other community mental health providers, the significance of the economic question is difficult to appreciate. Perhaps the easiest way to overcome their uneasiness is to remind them that the economic question is answered every day in every decision they make. In mental health care, as with other expenditures of limited resources, numerous (but usually implicit) benefit-cost analyses must be made. In fact, implicit or intuitive decision making is by far the most efficient way to handle the great majority of allocation decisions. One purpose of this chapter is to show why some explicit benefit-cost and cost-effectiveness studies are worth doing. We will also explore some of the difficulties that arise in undertaking these types of program analyses.

Following an introduction to problems of resource allocation, we turn to some of the methodological and practical problems in conducting a benefit-cost analysis. Finally, a few important studies will be reviewed, not so much for their results, as for their technique.

PRINCIPLES OF RESOURCE ALLOCATION

The resources available for the production of goods and services consist of manpower, natural resources and physical or capital goods. Because these resources are limited, it is impossible to produce all the things we want. Thus, choices have to be made regarding which outputs will be produced. In making these choices, we incur a cost in the sense that the inputs are not available for other uses. In principle, benefit-cost analysis provides a criterion by which decisions about resource allocation can be made (Sugden and Williams 1978). A thorough accounting of all benefits and costs associated with all possible projects would enable us to select those uses of resources that are optimal. The allocation would be optimal in the sense that, for a given outlay, correct project selection would insure that net benefits would be maximized. There would be no other allocation that would produce more benefits.

The allocation of resources resulting from adherence to the principle of maximum net gain does not take into account the distribution of resources. There is no assurance that an efficient allocation of resources will also lead to an equitable distribution of those resources (Okun 1975). In fact, in many cases the dual objectives of efficiency and equity are in conflict. Among economists, there is a strong preference for dealing with the efficiency problem while leaving the resolution of equity problems to the political sector. The grounds cited for this preference are that efficiency is a more neutral, value-free principle to which general acceptance is accorded, whereas equity or fairness in the distribution of resources is a value-laden concept on which agreement is difficult to achieve. We will return to these issues when the uses of benefit-cost analysis are discussed.

Until now benefit-cost analysis has been discussed in the context of total social resource allocation. The problem facing the clinician searching for the best use of a limited budget is conceptually the same, but with a much more restricted set of choices. Consider the situation where some unit of government is given a budget and required to serve a group of the chronically mentally ill. Disregarding the equity and measurement problems for the time being, the economic issue is one of choosing people to serve and a way to serve them so that net benefits are maximized. Satisfying this objective requires knowledge about the efficacy of different treatments, the benefits and costs of the treatments, and the benefits and costs for people with different personal characteristics and mental conditions. With sufficient information, it would then be possible to select clients and treatments that maximize net benefits.

The same basic model could be applied in a variety of contexts. For example, a series of benefit-cost analyses could be done for each possible treatment for an individual. Alternatively, benefit-cost analyses, by putting widely divergent projects on a similar footing through monetary quantification of benefits and costs, could be used to decide whether to increase the mental health budget or some other activity. For purposes of this chapter, we will restrict the discussion to the application of benefit-cost analysis to decisions about alternative kinds of community care. Note that in making this restriction, we are side-stepping the institution-community dichotomy. We accept as a given the decision to deliver care in the community for some proportion of the chronically mentally ill.

MEASUREMENT OF BENEFITS AND COSTS

The measurement of benefits and costs involves two separate considerations: the theoretical determination of what to treat as a benefit and cost and the quantification of the benefits and costs. Furthermore, the answers to both questions depend on the perspective of the decision maker. For any individual or agency affected by a project, there is a unique set of costs and benefits incurred by that entity. For example, consider the use of a psychiatrist's services financed completely from a program such as Medicaid. For the individual receiving the service, there is no cost, but there is a benefit in the form of mental health care. For the government there is the cost of reimbursing the psychiatrist whereas a possible benefit might be a future reduction in services and transfer payments if the individual is helped.

The broadest perspective is to consider the costs and benefits in the context of total social resources. In this case, the emphasis is on the creation and use of resources. When resources are used up in the delivery of psychiatric services, society incurs a cost in the sense that these resources are not now available for any alternative use. Generally, the simplest method to value these foregone opportunities (i.e., the cost) is to take the dollar charge for the service as a measure of the cost of using the resource. Although this may not always be the most accurate measure of real cost, it is likely the most easily adduced. Another problem arises when the resource is used but when no charge is involved. While on the surface the resource may appear to be free, this is not so. The point is that as long as the resource had some alternative use, there is a cost in using it, regardless of whether or not a charge is levied. One example of such a resource is the time of the client. From both the client and social perspective, the time spent in therapy is a cost because some alternative use of that time must be foregone. The clearest case is when hours of work are reduced, but there is a cost, albeit perhaps not as great, even if the alternative is a period of leisure time.

Similar kinds of vexing problems arise in the consideration of benefits. Again, what constitutes a benefit depends upon the perspective from which the study is being conducted. The standard approach to measuring social benefits is to consider the value of what is produced as a result of the project. Generally, value is determined by what people would willingly pay for the output. In the case of community mental health care, one possibility is to determine what consumers would pay if the service were billed directly to the client.

Often clients are not asked to pay, and furthermore, a lack of income would require them to seek a loan to pay for services. The failure of capital markets to develop in such cases would further complicate an assessment of benefits.

Even with these problems, it may be possible to devise reasonable proxies for benefits by attempting to measure the gain to an individual from the project. The implication is that the individual would be willing to pay an amount up to the net benefits he *expects* to receive from the project. For programs designed to return an individual to work, the wages he will receive over and above wages received had there been no project are a first approximation to benefits. In health programs, there is an added element to benefits: the improvement in health status. Without charging for the service, there is no direct way to measure this component of benefits. One option is to look at what similar people are paying for similar services (when no wage increase is expected, as for someone working full-time or someone who does not seek employment) and to use that payment as a proxy for the pure health benefit.

Another important point to consider is the difference between a preprogram estimate of benefits and actual benefits. Although benefit-cost analysis has been most often used in mental health policy and analysis as a postproject evaluation tool, ultimately the correct use of these studies is as a guide in making expenditures to different programs. To be able to choose among alternative programs, we must have information on the expected benefits and costs for each of the programs. To the extent that previously evaluated projects are being proposed, we can develop reasonably good estimates based on historical evidence. For programs not yet operational, a large part of the allocation decision involves guess work. Since the program is new, and because the lack of a control group will confound attempts to measure benefits precisely, it is wise to view the allocation process as an iterative procedure during which adjustments in program design and resources are made to improve performance.

Even when decisions are based on previously evaluated programs, some important problems remain. For example, since personnel in an operating program will differ from that in an experimental program, the evaluated program is never perfectly replicated when it is copied elsewhere. There is a strong possibility that even though client differences can be accounted for through control groups, the professional staff in the experimental program may be uniquely suited to the operation of the program. In all likelihood, it is these professionals who developed and designed the experiment to fit their own skills.

Another complicating factor is imposed on the benefit-cost analyst because of the chronic nature of the client's condition. The program may involve a series of services delivered periodically over the client's lifetime. As of yet, there are no long-term controlled studies involving continuing service provision. Furthermore, even if the program is short-term or a one-time service, the chronicity of the client requires us to consider the program's effects on clients and the behavior of any control group over a number of years. Again, no such long-term followup and evaluation, in the context of benefit-cost analysis, has yet been done.

The problems associated with benefit measurement in mental health programs have led several researchers to suggest the use of cost-effectiveness analysis (Johnson 1977). With cost-effectiveness analysis, it is not necessary to put a monetary figure on benefits. In place of the dollar value of benefits, some other unit of output is estimated. Generally, the output measure is in terms of physical units produced (e.g., the number of rehabilitated people). For mental health care, the use of a physical output measure is not feasible. Even a traditionally used measure in health care evaluation such as the number of lives saved does not appear satisfactory for programs for the chronically mentally ill. (Programs specifically directed toward suicide prevention are an exception.)

An alternative to the number of lives saved might be the increase in the number of days free of the disabling aspect of the mental illness or the improvement in functioning as measured by various tests of mental health. Obviously, the objectives of the program manager have a lot to say in the choice of an appropriate output measure. Whatever measure is chosen can then be used in the evaluation of different programs. By examining output per unit cost, we can decide what distribution of resources across the different programs will maximize output for a given outlay. But cost-effectiveness analysis does not help us determine the most efficient size of a project. Because we are not considering the dollar value of benefits, there is no direct way to determine if the benefits of an additional unit of service outweigh the extra costs needed to produce the service. In place of such considerations, the judgment must be made as to whether or not a particular increase in a mental health test score is worth the cost. When this decision is not made by the customer (who may also not be bearing the cost), there is no guide as to what constitutes the efficient level of service.

One other problem that often arises in cost-effectiveness analysis is the use of inputs as a proxy for output. For example, the number of hours of counseling or therapy is an input in the production of better mental health and not an output. To use such a measure in a cost-effectiveness study is to make an unwarranted assumption about the link between inputs and outputs when in fact that is exactly what we wish to test.

The method of analysis selected hinges a great deal on how well defined and measurable the benefits of the program are. Moreover, the correct measurement of cost is also essential in making the study results valid. Often costs are recorded for accounting purposes. As a result, the data are not available to measure the true cost of a program. Specially designed evaluations can overcome this problem by planning ahead to collect the required data.

The benefits and costs and the perspectives of the analysis are all important to understanding the difference between actual and ideal policy decisions. Although a mechanical value-free economic analysis, assuming the data were available, would inform us as to the socially ideal use of resources, this is no guarantee that such a policy will be enacted. In many cases, it is the benefits and costs as perceived by the decision-making unit that determine the actual allocation of resources. As we have seen earlier, these benefits and costs can be very different from the social benefits and costs. Furthermore, we should keep in mind that client willingness to participate in any program is an important factor. And while social benefits may greatly outweigh social costs, this is no guarantee that individual benefits are above individual costs. These are the kinds of considerations that have given rise to the so-called "disincentive problem" in rehabilitation programs. Available evidence suggests that for some clients a successful return to work is not the most rational choice because the loss of disability, welfare and medical benefits makes the return so costly to the individual (Berkowitz 1980). This disincentive problem is one of the reasons Congress has had to mandate participation in a rehabilitation program for Disability Insurance and Supplemental Security Income recipients, rather than rely solely on individual motivation to make use of such services.

Even if the disincentives to individual participation in community psychiatric care are not a serious problem, the question of individual, versus program, benefits and costs may be important for decisions. For example, if the alternative programs require different forms and amounts of individual participation, we might expect that the efficient assignment of individuals to programs will be complicated by the possibility that individual preferences may not coincide with the assignment decisions. One option would be to alter the programs to change individual benefits and costs so that there is greater agreement between individual preferences and the efficient use of resources. An example of one such adjustment is recent legislation allowing rehabilitated individuals to maintain eligibility for health care benefits for a period after rehabilitation (U.S. Congress 1980). This bill would lower the cost to the individual of returning to work, thereby encouraging participation in the rehabilitation program. Of course, the use of this kind of restructuring to compensate for individual costs is limited by the amount of net resources available for compensation.

In summation, the recognition of differences in benefits and costs depending on perspective is critical to understanding recommended policy actions and individual and agency reactions. Identifying the socially most efficient method to provide psychiatric services in the community is not enough. Steps must be taken to ensure individual participation and agency cooperation. Without such actions, postprogram evaluations may fail to live up to preprogram expectations.

APPLICATIONS OF BENEFIT-COST ANALYSIS

Despite the methodological and measurement difficulties apparent in the application of benefit-cost analysis to evaluation of mental health programs for the chronically mentally ill, there is an increasing effort to assess the economic value of alternative therapies. The emphasis in recent studies has been on the choice between institutional care and community care (Murphy and Datel 1976). The economic differences between alternative community therapies are still unresolved. To the extent that court orders and professional opinion continue to support community care, the economic studies of institutional versus community care are of limited importance. It may soon be that mental health providers really will have no choice as to where care is delivered. As rules for commitments are tightened and institutional length of stay declines, the important choice will be from among the great variety of community programs (Robinault and Weisinger 1978). What is not yet determined is the comparative assessment of these alternative community programs. In the short review of these studies that follow, the emphasis will be on questions of method and the possible uses of the findings in resolving the debate on which types of community programs are economically efficient.

The Wisconsin Study

The most recent and complete economic analysis of a community mental health program involved 130 clients. The benefits and costs of an experimental community care program were compared with the benefits and costs of institutional care (Weisbrod, Test and Stein 1980). Half of the clients were randomly assigned to a control group, and half were assigned to the experimental group. For purposes of selecting from among alternative community therapies, the missing element is additional clients assigned to a variety of community therapy programs.

For our purposes, we need not go into all the details of the experimental and control program. A fuller description of the programs and their results is reported elsewhere (Stein and Test 1980). The conceptual basis for the project grew out of the project directors' belief that only when a complete, wide-ranging set of services are offered are clients likely to remain in the community. Furthermore, an active and assertive support team was necessary to keep the patient in the program and ultimately in the community.

The experiment consisted of comparing outcomes for clients going through 14 months of the community program to the outcomes for a control group receiving traditional hospital and aftercare services. Rather than entering the hospital, the clients in the experimental group were assigned to the community program. The program consisted of training in activities of daily living, employment assistance and support services for family members. Although a wide range of outcome measures are reported, we will concentrate on the benefit-cost analysis that was conducted.

Issues in Cost Measurement

The calculation of costs and benefits is quite explicitly detailed (Weisbrod 1979; Weisbrod, Test and Stein 1980). Costs are broken into nine categories including some items for which no monetary estimate could be made. The nine categories are direct treatment, indirect treatment, law enforcement, maintenance, family burden, other family burden, burdens on other people, illegal activity and

Table 1 Benefits and Costs Per Patient in an Experimental Community Mental Health Program*

	Control Group	Experimental Group
Costs		
Direct Treatment	$3,138	$4,798
Indirect Treatment	2,142	1,838
Law Enforcement	409	350
Maintenance	1,487	1,035
Family Burden	120	72
Benefits		
Earnings	1,168	2,364
Net Benefits	-$6,128	-$5,729

*This table is a summary of Table 1 in Weisbrod, Test and Stein, p. 401.

patient mortality. Benefits are comprised of earnings, labor market behavior, improved consumer decision-making and patient mental health. A summary of the results is presented in Table 1.

Direct treatment costs include inpatient, outpatient and experimental program expenditures. The hospital costs reflect operating costs, costs of capital and an implicit charge for use of the building and land.

One problem that has proven difficult to resolve, in efforts to estimate mental health costs (National Institute of Mental Health 1977; Weisbrod 1980), is the measurement of the extra (marginal) costs associated with serving one client. In the Wisconsin study, average cost rather than the more theoretically appropriate marginal cost is used. Marginal cost is preferable because it is the cost that will be saved or expended if the individual leaves or enters a program. When a client is released or added to the program, average cost may differ from the actual marginal cost saved or added. The distinction is not critical if the choice is between total programs such as all institutional care or all community care. The distinction is important when individual clients are being released to a community program. For example, one less client in a large institution may lead to a savings of less than average cost, while the addition of a client to a small community program may require new treatment personnel with an additional cost greater than average cost. Weisbrod suggests that for the programs he was studying marginal and average costs may be nearly equal.

A related issue affecting costs is the matter of scale. Costs of a program vary as the size of the project changes. As a program grows, average costs can be expected to decline. Hence, measurement of costs should be done in light of these scale effects on costs. In the Wisconsin study, the cost estimate was based on the middle year of the project because the author felt that was when the most efficient production occurred.

The indirect costs consisted of the other social and medical-service costs of the clients. The largest differences occurred in the use of other hospitals. The control group relied much more heavily than the experimental group on hospital care. This would suggest that the experimental program services acted as a substitute for hospitalization.

Other indirect costs included law enforcement costs and maintenance costs. The inclusion of cash payments such as SSI and AFDC is somewhat unusual in a social benefit-cost study and deserves some close scrutiny. As noted earlier, a social benefit-cost analysis is concerned with resources created or used up. Maintenance or transfer payments involve taking dollars from taxpayers and making payments to recipients. No real social benefits or costs are involved. In general, therefore, changes in transfer payments are ignored in social benefit-cost analyses.

In the Wisconsin study, it was decided to include such costs. This is an important point because the experimental program required $564 per person less in transfers. Since net benefits favor the experimental program by $399 per person, the resolution of the methodological problem of transfer costs has significant implications for the determination of the relative efficiency of the treatment alternatives.

The argument in favor of including transfer payments as costs relies on recognizing that the payments will be used for food, clothing and shelter. If a differential in living costs is attributable to the program, then it may be necessary to use a part of maintenance payments to account for the differences. Estimating the correct differential is complicated when maintenance payments are not independent of family status. For example, a father returning home to live with his wife and children would be eligible for dependent benefits under Supplemental Security Income. Thus, clearly a portion of transfer payments are unrelated to maintenance costs for the individual. In addition, disability insurance benefits are not affected by institutional status, and hence their payment cannot be considered a program cost.

Another problem is that part of hospital costs are for maintenance expenditures. Theoretically, these expenditures are not a cost of mental illness and should be deducted from hospital costs. What we should determine is the differential cost of maintaining oneself due to the different treatment programs. It does not appear that including total transfer payments satisfactorily answers that question.

Issues in Benefit Measurement

Benefit calculations in community mental health programs are made difficult by the inability to put improvements in mental health in monetary terms. In the Wisconsin study, monetary benefits are included in terms of wages from earnings. Other benefits were measured differently. For example, clinical symptomatology and patient satisfaction with life are valuable outputs of mental health programs. The results can be implicitly valued by asking how much of a monetary difference in benefits and costs could be compensated for by a particular improvement in these mental health measures. While this cannot be done by the analyst-observer, it is one of the kinds of factors entering an individual's decision to seek care through a community program or in an institution.

Uses of Benefit-Cost Studies

In using and interpreting the results from a study like the one in Wisconsin, several limitations must be recognized (and were recognized by those who conducted the study). The results are of value in comparing the two programs tested. Other untested alternatives may be better. Furthermore, the limited duration of the project means the full effects of the programs over a lifetime are not measured. Another difficulty is the generalizability of the findings to other settings and with other providers. It is likely that the providers of care in an experimental program were highly motivated to work for the program's success. It was probably their belief in the program that first made them consider the experiment. The results might be different if the program were widely implemented with different staff.

The relative success of the control and experimental programs differed greatly by diagnosis. Finer breakdowns by age, sex and other characteristics, (e.g., prior institutionalization) help pinpoint who is the best target for which program. Efficient client selection for a wide range of community and institutional programs is not going to be easily accomplished, but this study clearly documents the need to distinguish benefits and costs for specific groups of clients.

Clearly, we have a long way to go in conducting an ideal set of benefit-cost studies to compare community mental health programs. Although the Wisconsin study is a valuable contribution to the small literature on mental health program evaluation, it alone cannot be the basis for selecting between the wide variety of available programs. As indicated earlier, benefit-cost analysis aids the policy maker in choosing among the tested options. But the efficiency of the numerous untested options remains uncertain. Therefore, if we wish to select the most efficient way to serve different clients in the community, many such options need to be evaluated. For example, residential arrangements and staff involvement could be altered to determine if net benefits can be increased.

Virginia Study

As with the Wisconsin program, the purpose of the Virginia project, called Service Integration for Deinstitutionalization (SID), was to shift the care of the chronically mentally ill from institutions to the community. The basic feature of the program was the coordination of resources of twelve state agencies through use of prerelease client assessments and community-based advocates (Datel and Murphy 1976).

The SID project differed in some significant ways from the Wisconsin project. In Virginia, clients were not randomly assigned to a control and experimental group, but instead the assessment team evaluated clients and made recommendations as to release or retention. Without a control group, it is not possible to be certain what would have happened without the program. Also, the clients consisted of persons currently institutionalized, and not clients just entering the mental health system as in Wisconsin. Although the projects are not comparable, some important methodological and measurement issues were raised in the Virginia study that make it a project worthy of review.

The terminology used in the Virginia project confuses the traditional distinction between governmental and social perspective (Murphy and Datel 1975). Although it was claimed that a social benefit-cost analysis was done, in fact the study includes all governmental benefits and costs. It falls between a purely social benefit-cost study and a calculation of just benefits and costs to government. Another problem arises from the decision to delete the information on failures (that is, those clients who returned, or were likely to return, to the institution). This approach implies that the program could be run elsewhere without any failures. When the inevitable percentage of failures turns up, we will find the program producing less net benefits than suggested by the study.

One problem that was not resolved in the Wisconsin study, but was examined in Virginia, was how to include benefits and costs due to the project but occurring after the project terminated. Since projects may have different patterns of costs and benefits over a client's lifetime, limiting the time period of the study may not give a true reading of the efficiency of alternative projects (U.S. Dept. HEW, 1975). For example, if an initial period of institutionalization led to less long-term, but greater short-term, use of hospitals than an initial assignment to a community program, then the benefit-cost results would favor a different program depending on the time period studied. The difficulty in calculating total lifetime benefits and costs is that most program evaluations are not able to track clients and collect data very long beyond the completion of the service components of the program. Yet, given the nature of the chronic patient, it is obvious that costs will continue long into the future.

In the Virginia study, the authors used estimates by counselors to project costs and benefits for 10 years. This method is limited by counselor capacity to correctly judge what will happen in the future. It would be wise to compare those counselor projections with the actual costs and benefits. It is especially critical in the long-term assessment of benefits and costs to have a control group. Without such a control, we cannot be certain what costs and benefits should be attributed to the program.

Recognizing that benefits and costs would differ greatly by client situation, the authors stratified the clients by housing status (as a proxy for disability), employability and primary source of funds. If the results confirmed the expectation of differences in benefits and costs, then client selection would become important in maximizing net benefits.

The authors compared the costs and benefits of the community program with the institutional alternative. Six cost and four benefit categories were identified. The costs included community support services, client maintenance, service integration, deinstitutionalization costs, lost economic productivity of family members and community-related costs. No dollar value was assigned to this last category because it covered such intangibles as "fear, confusion and misunderstanding about placement of SID clients in the community" (Murphy and Datel 1976, p. 167). The benefit categories included the institutional costs saved, increased economic productivity and client and community psychological improvements. Again, this last category of benefits was not measured in dollar terms.

These benefits and costs were estimated for 52 successfully deinstitutionalized clients, of which 38% were mentally retarded. As with the Wisconsin study, the authors found that the net benefits of deinstitutionalization were positive, with the average net benefit per client for the 10-year period being $20,800.

Although both studies provide economic support for community rather than institutional care, caution should be exercised in making claims for vast savings from closing all public mental institutions. At this stage in the application of benefit-cost methodology to mental health programs, a great many questions remain unanswered. Both studies show how important certain program features are in attaining a positive net benefit. In particular, better success in getting the chronically mentally ill into labor markets, including sheltered workshops, will improve the economic return to community care programs. By breaking down total benefits and costs into their different components, we can identify those areas most suitable for cost control and benefit gains.

SOME CONCLUDING COMMENTS

Problems of comparability in method plague any attempt to reach a general conclusion about benefits and costs of alternative community therapies. What is needed now is a benefit-cost study of a large sample of clients released or diverted from institutions. Clients should be randomly assigned to a number of competing types of community programs. In a sense, psychiatrists and others responsible for referral to community programs probably use benefits and costs implicitly as a guide in making their recommendation. But there is no doubt that what is considered a benefit and cost does not accord with the real costs and gains for society. The first step in improving on this haphazard allocation is more knowledge of the effectiveness of the available therapies (Glasscote 1978). There is probably a close correlation between economic benefits and the success of different therapies. Information on costs could then be used to make determinations of the most efficient programs for different clients. At this point, it would be necessary to design public and private financing programs so that patients flow into the efficient program. In principle, if done correctly, we would then find mental health dollars producing the greatest possible net benefit.

Even if we assumed away the methodological, measurement and financing problems, there would be an important equity question to resolve. Both studies reviewed in this chapter found a wide variation in benefits and costs by client characteristics. If benefit-cost analysis is applied as a tool to gain an efficient allocation of resources, then some potential clients will not be served. An emphasis on efficiency requires that clients be selected to maximize net benefits. Since services for different clients produce different outcomes, net benefits will vary across clients. Efficiency, therefore, implies preference be given to some clients at the expense of others. For example, as research progresses, it is conceivable that the results will favor people with particular diagnoses, backgrounds and family situations. The aged, those with little work experience and people with personality disorders are some of the clients who might be rejected because net benefits could be expected to be negative.

There are a number of possible solutions to the equity dilemma. (This kind of equity problem is not inherent to mental health but arises in all public expenditure decisions.) One solution would be to ignore benefit-cost patterns for individuals and to seek instead efficiency at a program level, where all clients are (not necessarily equally) represented. Another solution is to weight benefits to certain groups more highly than others (Musgrave and Musgrave 1980). This method indicates a social preference for one group over another. For example, the weights could be correlated with severity of illness.

The problem with each of these options is that they guarantee less total measurable net benefits than is possible. To the extent that society is "willing to pay" for equity with fewer net benefits the problem is lessened. Unfortunately, there is no way to measure society's preference for equity. One other solution to the equity problem also requires a difficult accounting technique. Recall that benefits and costs include only those effects quantifiable in dollars. The community programs have many other consequences, most notably, improved patient mental health. If this outcome is valued, then selection of clients could be adjusted for the health variable. Although net dollar benefits are diminished, in an overall sense the program will be efficient because "true" net benefits will be maximized.

With any of these adjustments, there will probably still be persons who will not "succeed" regardless of expenditures. Even though efficient allocation of community mental health resources requires that no services be provided for that person, society may wish to provide aid for this person from any number of other sources. Also, as the technology of mental health care changes, so too do the benefits and costs of serving different clients. In fact, one could argue that the deemphasis on institutions in the past twenty-five years came about as governments, professionals and individuals reacted to changing benefit-cost patterns due to available drug therapies and changes in financial payments for mental health care. Even the litigation of the past decade began with the notion that states could be expected to respond to financial incentives (Rubin 1978). Some proponents of the legal approach argued that as courts mandated more expensive care, states would react by making less use of institutions (Ennis 1975).

As evidenced by the review in this chapter, solving the allocation problem is immensely difficult. Benefit-cost analysis simply cannot eliminate the human element from the decision of who to serve and how. What this form of economic analysis can contribute is more information. Used correctly, a good benefit-cost study can result in people receiving the services that do the most (economic) good. But it would be foolish to rely on this technique alone. Community mental health care is not like building a dam or a bridge. At this stage in the application of benefit-cost analysis to community mental health services, there are too many unresolved problems to justify its use as the sole instrument for making allocation decisions. What benefit-cost analysis can do is to add to the clinician's medical decisions the necessary economic considerations. Furthermore, documentation of the economic value of mental health care will give advocates an effective weapon in the political arena. When done well, benefit-cost analysis can mean that more and better mental health services will be available to more people. It is this promise of improvements in efficiency that justifies further efforts to measure the benefits and costs of community mental health services for the chronically mentally ill.

REFERENCES

Berkowitz, Monroe. *Work Disincentives.* Institute for Information Studies, 200 Little Falls Street, Suite 104, Falls Church, VA 22046 (1980).

Datel, William, and Murphy, Jane. A service-integrating model for deinstitutionalization. *Administration in Mental Health*: 35–45 (Spring 1975).

Ennis, Bruce. The impact of litigation on the future of state hospitals, in *The Future Role of the State Hospital,* J. Zusman and E. Bertsch, eds. Lexington, Mass.: D. C. Heath and Company, 1975, pp. 83–89.

Glasscote, Raymond. What programs work and what programs do not work to meet the needs of chronic mental patients?, in *The Chronic Mental Patient* John Talbott, ed. Washington, DC: The American Psychiatric Association, 1978, pp. 75-85.

Glenn, Trevor. Exploring responsibility for chronic mental patients in the community, in *The Chronic Mental Patient,* John Talbott, ed. Washington, DC: The American Psychiatric Association, 1978, pp. 173-193.

Johnson, William G. *A Model for the Economic Evaluation of Mental Health Care.* Paper presented at American Psychological Association Convention, San Francisco, 1977.

LaPorte, Valerie, and Rubin, Jeffrey, eds. *Reform and Regulation in Long-Term Care.* New York: Praeger Publishers, 1979.

Murphy, Jane, and Datel, William. A cost-benefit analysis of community versus institutional living. *Hospital and Community Psychiatry* 27: 165-170 (March 1976).

Musgrave, Richard, and Musgrave, Peggy. *Public Finance in Theory and Practice.* Third Edition. New York: McGraw-Hill Book Company, 1980.

Okun, Arthur. *Equality and Efficiency: The Big Tradeoff.* Washington, DC: The Brookings Institution, 1975.

Robinault, Isabel, and Weisinger, Marvin. *Mobilization of Community Resources: A Multi-Facet Model for Rehabilitation of Post Hospitalized Mentally Ill.* 2nd Edition. New York: ICD Rehabilitation and Research Center, 1978.

Rubin, Jeffrey. *Economics, Mental Health and the Law.* Lexington, Mass.: D. C. Heath and Company, 1978.

Stein, Leonard, and Test, Mary Ann. Alternative to mental hospital treatment: I. Conceptual model, treatment program, and clinical evaluation. *Archives of General Psychiatry* 37: 392-397 (April 1980).

Sugden, Robert, and William, Alan. *The Principles of Practical Cost-Benefit Analysis.* Oxford, England: Oxford University Press, 1978.

Talbott, John, ed. *The Chronic Mental Patient.* Washington, DC: The American Psychiatric Association, 1978.

U.S. Congress. House. *Social Security Disability Amendments of 1980.* Conference Report, Report No. 96-944, 96th Congress, 2nd Session, May 13, 1980.

U.S. Department of Health, Education and Welfare. National Institute of Mental Health. *Determining Costs of Community Residential Services for the Psychosocially Disabled.* Series B. No. 13. DHEW Publication No. (ADM) 77-504. Washington, DC, 20402, 1977.

U.S. Department of Health, Education and Welfare. Rehabilitation Services Administration. *The SID Report,* Vol. 5. Cost Benefit Analysis. Grant No. 15-P-55896/3-02, 1975.

U.S. Department of Health and Human Services. First Draft of *National Plan for the Chronically Mentally Ill.* Washington, DC, July 1980.

Weisbrod, Burton. *A Guide to Benefit-Cost Analysis, As Seen Through a Controlled Experiment in Treating the Mentally Ill.* University of Wisconsin-Madison, Institute for Research on Poverty. Discussion Paper No. 559-79, 1979.

Weisbrod, Burton, Test, Mary Ann, and Stein, Leonard. Alternative to mental hospital treatment: II. Economic benefit-cost analysis. *Archives of General Psychiatry* 37: 400-405 (April 1980).

CHAPTER 19

ADVOCACY IN THE COMMUNITY

LOUIS E. KOPOLOW, M.D.

The past decade has witnessed dramatic changes in the mental health system under the banner of the "patient rights and advocacy movement." This movement, spearheaded by members of the medical and legal professions and by expatients, has sought protection of basic human, clinical and civil rights, an end to patient abuse and the creation of a more responsive mental health system. The initial focus for rights and advocacy activities has been in public institutions where patients have been housed and all too frequently neglected. In recent years, there has been a shift in attention from hospital-based mental health care to the delivery of services in the community. Here too patients and their advocates have found it necessary to battle for the basic protections, entitlements and opportunities enjoyed by other citizens not stigmatized by the label mentally ill. Before describing mental health advocacy in detail, it would be valuable, in order to understand the strategies and priorities of each of the advocacy approaches, to review briefly some of the major events in the evolution of the nation's mental health system which led to the development of the advocacy movement.

HISTORICAL PERSPECTIVE

During colonial times, the insane poor were left to the discretion of local communities. If they were seen as harmlessly deranged, society's main fear was that they would become public charges. To prevent this from occurring, the mentally ill were subjected to whippings and banishment, and were forced to wander and beg. If they remained in a community, incarceration in the local jails or poorhouses was frequently their treatment.[1]

The last part of the eighteenth century marked the development of new approaches to the treatment of the mentally ill. Philippe Pinel pioneered a more humane treatment of the patients at Bicêtre and Salpêtrière. With moral treatment developed at York Retreat in England under Samuel Tuke, patients were treated with respect and kindness, but also with firmness, in an atmosphere allowing them quiet time before their return to open society.

Moral treatment was carried to America by a Quaker clergyman, Reverend Thomas Scattergood, and became the dominant approach used in mental hospitals during the first half of the nineteenth century. Great success, as high as 90% improvement in symptoms, was reported by early practitioners of moral treatment. This treatment was accomplished by removing the patient from his family and community at the onset of his illness and placing him in a peaceful rural retreat—the asylum—where, under the absolute control of his physician, he lived a tightly disciplined existence and engaged in useful employment.[2]

This era of humane and hopeful treatment was short-lived, as the resources of the asylum were soon overburdened by the great influx of impoverished immigrants from Europe and a growing population of chronic patients. Moral treatment began to fade and was replaced with custodialism. Overcrowding and disorder created justification for mechanical restraints and punishments which grew in usage and severity.

The failings and increasing harshness of public asylums, however, did not lead to their dismantling. Overcrowding worsened as chronic patients remained indefinitely, and loose commitment laws facilitated the extrusion of the mentally disabled who were not tolerated by an increasingly urban society. Efforts to improve conditions were sporadic and progress was slow and uneven. Despite numerous books and exposés, including Clifford Beers's *The Mind That Found Itself* (1936),[3] Deutsch's *The Shame of the States* (1948)[4] and Marcy Ward's book *Snake Pit* (1946),[5] later made into a movie, the period of custodialism continued well into the first half of the twentieth century.

By the mid 1950s, discontent with the situation in state mental hospitals was widespread. The resident population had soared to 550,000, and approximately 2 out of every 5 hospital beds were located in state and county mental hospitals. The president of the American Psychiatric Association declared in 1958: "I do not see how any reasonably objective view of our mental hospitals today can fail to conclude that they are bankrupt beyond remedy."[6]

The recognition that society was failing to provide an adequate or even humane system of services to care for its mentally ill citizens led Congress to establish the Joint Commission on Mental Illness and Health in 1955. This commission advocated the goal of community-based mental health care accessible and responsive to the needs of all citizens. Its report specifically attacked the philosophy of large state hospitals and recommended providing psychiatric services in the community to reduce the need for prolonged or repeated hospitalization. In 1963, the CMHC Act was passed, and the first federally funded CMHCs were developed.

As a result of the development of community mental health centers, the discovery of tranquilizers and growing professional acceptance of outpatient treatment, the mental hospital population has dropped markedly over the past two decades. The resident population of state and county mental hospitals in 1975 was only one third of the number in 1955. In 1955, there were 558,922 patients compared to 191,391 resident patients in 1975.[7] It should, however, be noted that although fewer patients reside in mental hospitals, many of those who are discharged return for subsequent readmissions.

The clinical factors cited above reflect only part of the story for the decreased hospital census. Social and legal economic factors have converged during the past ten years to accelerate the deinstitutionalization process. This process involves the removal of hospitalized patients from the institutional setting and their transfer to the community, the prevention of hospitalization of those persons who are considered potential candidates for less restrictive alternative treatment and the expansion of community-based services for the treatment of these persons. Despite the decrease in numbers of individuals in various public facilities, the old problem of inadequate facilities, insufficient or poorly trained staff and dehumanization continue to plague many of the nation's public hospitals. Equally disturbing is the discovery that these same problems have followed the discharged patient in the community. In its response to the General Accounting Office's report on discharged patients, the Public Health Service declared, "Although we have succeeded in drastically reducing the size of inpatient population in public mental hospitals, new patterns of exclusion, neglect, and abuse, have developed 'in the community.' "[8,23]

Aftercare programs or resources for continuing care have not always been available to assist patients leaving hospitals. Adequate coordination of services has also frequently been lacking in those facilities functioning as alternatives to hospitalization. In addition, many discharged patients do not have the physical or economic means, the motivation or the understanding to obtain needed help from an extraordinarily complex mental health and social welfare system. The result is often a social or psychiatric crisis resulting in rehospitalization. Various newspapers which in the past have exposed problems of neglect and mistreatment in public institutions are now finding this same situation in the community. A *New York Times* editorial (April 8, 1974) entitled "Civil Liberty for What?" stated:

> If there were anything that could be described as even reasonably adequate aftercare for discharged mental patients, the civil libertarians would have a case. Certainly they have the right to condemn the failure of the huge State institutions to serve a purpose which is more than custodial. But what kind of crusade is it to condemn sick and fearful people to shift for themselves in an often hostile world. . . . What are needed are open halfway communities. . . . The idea is neither novel or utopian, just costly.[9]

Those patients who do succeed in connecting up with a "board and care" facility frequently find that their problems, rather than ending, have just begun. Priscilla Allen, a member of the President's Commission on Mental Health, described from her own experience and personal observation the plight of many residents of board and care facilities. Here the most fundamental needs, such as fresh, nutritious food, safety, cleanliness, space, and adequate medical and psychiatric care, were not met. In her paper "A Consumer's View of California's Mental Health Care System," she gave examples of how some boarding home operations oppress and exploit residents by opening their mail and taking or mishandling benefit checks. The atmosphere in the home is often repressive; residents are afraid to express themselves or protest their situations because of the threat of rehospitalization for those acting-out, troublesome or uncooperative clients.[10]

Conditions such as these exist because patients living in the community are not experiencing the same protection under the law enjoyed by other citizens. While the legal advocate (whose functions will be more extensively described later) has expanded the scope of patients' rights in hospitals, such rights have frequently not been extended to the mentally ill in the community. Monitoring the quality of life and enforcing patient rights in a hospital setting may be easier than in the community. This, however, should not excuse a failure to establish effective mechanisms to protect

Table 1

1. The right to voluntary, personalized treatment by qualified staff, medical as well as mental health.
2. The right to be fully informed about treatment and services, including the nature, purpose and side effects.
3. The right to participate fully in treatment decisions that affect them, including planning for and evaluating treatment and services.
4. The right to be informed of their rights, including instruction on how to use appeal and complaint procedures.
5. The right to have advocates who will act on behalf of the clients' interests and provide continuity of services if the clients wish this.
6. The right to confidentiality of records.
7. The right to be treated with dignity and respect by service providers who take seriously the clients' opinions, views and priorities.
8. The right to be free of coercive elements in the treatment or service process.
9. The right to refuse treatment or services and be informed thereof.
10. The right to fully utilize all economic rights and benefits, earned and unearned.
11. The right to a humane psychological and physical environment, which includes nutritious food, safety, adequate shelter.
12. The right to equal protection under the law, including the services of a lawyer.
13. The protection of economic rights.
14. The clients' rights as rent-paying tenants.
15. The right to information.[11]

client rights both in and outside of mental health facilities. The bill of rights composed by Priscilla Allen addresses the unique needs and problems of patients living in the community. These rights are listed in Table 1.

In general, Allen asserts that persons living in the community utilizing mental health services as outpatients are entitled to all the rights that ordinarily accompany citizenship unless these persons are subject to specific legal limitations. Unfortunately, although one may be entitled to such rights, unless one can ask or demand them, they will not necessarily be granted.

For the large numbers of individuals discharged from public institutions, the need for advocacy support to assure rights is as great in the community as in the hospital. This population of citizens suffers from a triple hardship—first, as produced by their illness, which at times makes it difficult for them to effectively articulate their needs; second and far greater, as caused by society's prejudging of their capacities; and third, as a result of the stigma associated with their mental condition, resulting in a low priority being given to their demands. In addition to these factors, the complexity of the mental health support and treatment system and the difficulty of implementing change make the need for advocates paramount in the nation's mental health services delivery system.

The need for advocates to represent the interests of the mentally ill has been well documented. In the 1978 Report of the President's Commission on Mental Health, advocacy was identified as a major goal when the report stated:

> We are keenly aware that even the best-intentioned efforts to deliver services to mentally disabled persons have historically resulted in well-documented cases of exploitation and abuse. For this reason, an effective advocacy system must be created to protect the rights of all who receive services.[12]

While advocacy has the potential to change the rhetoric of patients' rights into reality, the term itself is unfortunately not well understood and has resulted in unnecessary disagreements and antagonism among mental health professionals, attorneys and consumers.

FORMS OF ADVOCACY

Advocacy has a number of meanings, depending on the interests and the priorities of the various groups using it. In the classic sense it means "to summon to one's assistance, defending or calling to one's aid." The present-day connotation of conflict or antagonism is not inherent in the basic concept, but rather results from the manner in which some advocates pursue their duties.[13] In this chapter, advocacy refers to efforts by an individual to secure services that the client wants or requires, to safeguard and exercise the client's rights, or otherwise to pursue or protect the client's interest. The ultimate responsibility and loyalty are to the client.

The functions of mental health advocates cover a broad range of activities and require not only the skills of attorneys, but those of mental health workers, paraprofessionals, concerned citizens and expatients. Table 2 describes some of the tasks performed by advocates.

It is clear from a listing of functions that advocacy is not a purely legal function. While it is obvious that it is the responsibility of the legal profession to advocate for legal rights of patients, this term also has other useful meanings within the mental health services

Table 2

Some of the tasks performed by advocates are:

1. Providing information concerning individual rights and how to protect them.
2. Receiving complaints of rights violations and inadequate provision of services.
3. Referring clients to social service and/or mental health agencies.
4. Representing individuals in a range of settings (meetings, hearings, etc.).
5. Promoting adoption of legislation and regulations which improve services for the mentally disabled and/or protect their rights.
6. Providing training and backup support to volunteers and mental health staff advocates.

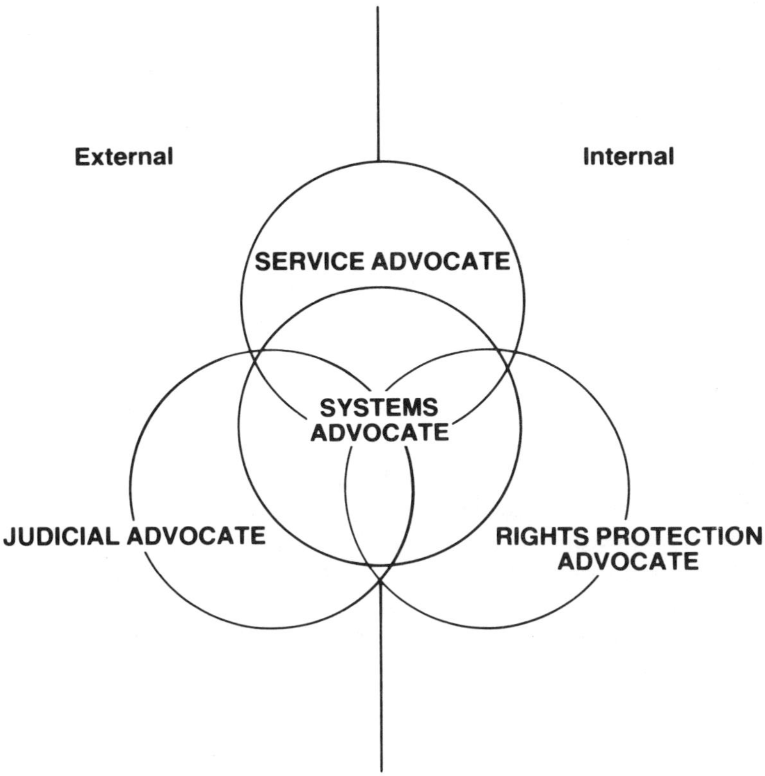

Figure 1

delivery system. After a patient's rights have been established, and attorneys have been made available to patients to ensure their protection, other issues remain which cannot and should not be resolved through the legal system. Such issues include sensitizing mental health staff to basic patients' rights issues, advocating for improvement in environmental conditions, encouraging use of alternative community services and lobbying for adequate resources to treat the nation's mentally ill citizens. These additional activities influencing the quality of the day-to-day life of mental patients can be more effectively dealt with through administrative and legislative routes than through legal intervention.[14]

To perform all the necessary tasks of mental health advocacy, no one approach is adequate. Advocacy approaches are distinguished from one another by the basic strategies they employ to assure and advance the interests of their clients. These strategies manifest themselves in judicial advocacy, rights protection advocacy, service advocacy and systems advocacy (see Fig. 1).

JUDICIAL ADVOCACY

Since the early 1960s much of the credit for spearheading action to create a more responsive mental health system goes to the civil liberties attorneys. These attorneys, sensitized to the problems of discrimination and denial of freedom by their civil liberties work, became increasingly conscious of the deprivation experienced by America's mentally ill citizens. Such citizens, while guilty of no crime, could be denied freedom and held in mental health institutions where they might be treated against their will, neglected or abused. Conditions in many public institutions encouraged these attorneys to bring various lawsuits to halt abusive practices and to assure adequate standards of care. The judicial advocate has responded to the needs of the mentally ill through one of two methods: 1) case-by-case individual representation or 2) class action litigation. It is through the latter approach that the legal advocate has had the greatest impact.

The court had historically maintained a hands-off policy regarding major mental institutions such as public hospitals. However, spurred by the activist stance of the Supreme Court, headed by Chief Justice Earl Warren, and by the activism of civil liberties attorneys, lower courts began hearing cases previously considered beyond the scope of judicial expertise. Judicial advocates, with the frequent assistance of concerned mental health professionals, have brought numerous suits on a wide range of constitutional issues, such as the right to treatment, the freedom from cruel and unusual punishment, the right to the least restrictive alternative to hospitalization, the right to refuse treatment, etc. While each of these suits has had an impact on mental health services, two of them, *Wyatt* v. *Stickney*[15] and *Dixon* v. *Weinberger*,[16] are of particular importance and deserve further examination.

The decision in *Wyatt* v. *Stickney* went substantially beyond previous decisions in the area of right to treatment. The case was brought against the mental health commissioner and the Hospital Administrator of the State of Alabama, where employees were fired from Bryce Hospital as a result of budget cuts. The issue before the court was that such cuts would threaten the quality of care and deny patients the right to treatment. The decision laid down by Judge Johnson stated that there is a constitutional right to treatment, that this right also pertains to the mentally retarded and, most importantly, that the court assumes responsibility for promulgating objectives—measurably and judicially enforceable standards by which the ultimate right to treatment can be practically implemented. The standards included minimum staff-patient ratios, nutritional requirements, the abolition of peonage, provisions to ensure humane psychological environment and treatment plans and programs.

Another case representative of the scope of class action judicial advocacy is *Dixon* v. *Weinberger.* This decision (March 1976) held that residents of St. Elizabeths Hospital in Washington, D.C., which is federally funded, have the right to receive treatment in the least restrictive, most appropriate facility. As a result of the *Dixon* decision, 43% of the patients at St. Elizabeths were ordered released to appropriate community facilities. Unfortunately, even today alternative resources are still inadequate to handle the patients who qualify for less restrictive treatment.

While the litigation approach has been essential in initiating the momentum of the patients' rights movement, it is also becoming increasingly clear that the court cannot provide the standards and the review mechanism that assure good patient care and regard for their rights. As Joel Klein, a past Mental Health Law Project attorney has noted, "Everywhere there has been litigation . . . changes in staffing, changes in facilities, changes in procedures—often at considerable cost. There is little evidence that the care of patients is improved or that their rights are any more respected."[17]

The litigation approach, while spectacular in terms of news coverage and exposure value, has had mixed results in improving the nation's mental health system. Litigation has created a sense of urgency and a reordering of outdated priorities in the nation's mental health system, which the other large and complex bureaucracies tend to be slow to change. Emphasis on custodial care and neglect of patients' rights are increasingly being replaced with requirements for active treatment programs and protection of the legal, clinical and human rights of all patients. The judiciary has succeeded where well-meaning governors, mental health commissioners and citizen committees have failed in focusing legislation to appropriate needed resources for improving the mental health delivery system. In addition, the litigation approach has produced such positive results as increased sensitization of the public to the plight of the mentally ill, and has led to the release from hospital of many individuals who were confined without treatment or who should more appropriately have been cared for in less restrictive alternative facilities. On the negative side, litigation and judicial intervention into the mental health system have led to mass discharges without adequate aftercare planning, have retarded the development of alternative care programs by redirection of funds into improving existing institutions and facilities, and have caused the departure of many mental health professionals who did not wish to have their names immortalized in a lawsuit or to work under the pressures of judicial review and policy making. In summary, the basic problem with the litigation approach has been its inability to carry through a comprehensive implementation plan to solve the problems existing within the mental health system, its difficulty in dealing with day-to-day administrative complaints, and its tendency to discourage rather than encourage an atmosphere of collaboration and cooperation among the providers whom judicial decisions most directly affect.[18]

Major suits such as those described above may result when a judicial advocate seeking to represent his or her client's wishes realizes that this goal might be more successfully accomplished through class action rather than individual case litigation. The judicial advocate's ultimate loyalty and responsibility, however, is to the client. The advocate must attempt to determine what the client wants, try to persuade the client to adopt the course of action that seems indicated to the counsel and then either attempt in good faith to attain the wishes of his client or withdraw from the case.

The judicial advocate will perform a wide range of functions, including representing the client in commitment proceedings, lodging complaints about specific violations of patients' rights in order to obtain redress and, in general, providing the client with the legal expertise necessary for handling multitudinous problems of the property transfers, wills, etc., which may concern an institutionalized individual.

In commitment proceedings, the judicial advocate must take an adversary stance that follows the expressed wishes of the client, even if this precipitates the release of a person who needs treatment. Reflecting this approach, the *Yale Law Journal*, in a scholarly article on the role of the attorney in commitment process, stated:

> If hearings are to bring meaningful procedures designed to arrive at fair deposition based on a full representation of the facts, the lawyer must act as an adversary. Otherwise, the idea that due process is being accorded the mentally ill individual will stand as little more than pretense.[19]

While the primary function of a judicial advocacy program lies within the realm of judicial procedures and legal rights, the scope of action may at times branch into areas of primary concern to rights protection advocates (grievance resolution) and service advocates. In carrying out expanded activities, as well as in pursuing its day-to-day tasks, a judicial advocacy office needs a multidisciplinary staff that includes attorneys, psychologists, nurses and consulting psychiatrists. This need for the skills of other professionals in assuring patients' legal rights has been recognized by Michael Perlin, J.D., Director of the New Jersey Division of Mental Health Advocacy. He has stated, "Although the role of the lawyer in the mental health arena is both a proper and necessary one, and is one which must and should expand, it is impossible for only lawyers to do the job."

In order to be able to represent the client's needs effectively, the judicial advocacy program must be independent of providers of mental health treatment and external to the service delivery system. Such independence might be achieved through the creation of legal advocacy programs in various mental health facilities funded by organizations such as the American Bar Association Commission on the Mentally Disabled, or by the Legal Services Corporation. Another more effective approach would be the creation of a program such as New Jersey's Division of Mental Health Advocacy. This program is located in the cabinet-level Office of the Public Advocate and has the dual function of individual case representation and the bringing of classification suits when appropriate. In less than five years of operation, New Jersey's Division of Mental Health Advocacy has served

12,000 individuals with success in 3 out of every 4 cases (success is defined as attaining the client's objective). In addition, the program has been responsible for cases resulting in court decisions defining and expanding patients' rights in areas of right to treatment, right to refuse treatment, right to periodic review and due process for institutionalized patients, right to vote, patients' right to access to their records, and others.[20] Another approach to protecting the legal rights of patients nationally has recently been explored by the Department of Health Education and Welfare. During 1979 a number of demonstration projects in mental health advocacy began to be funded and evaluated to provide the Secretary of HEW with information upon which to base future legislation.

Judicial advocacy has had such an impact on the mental health system, that to many mental health professionals the concept of advocacy is synonymous with litigation and other activities of attorneys. While this perspective may have had some accuracy at the beginning of the advocacy movement during the early '60s, it is not the case today with the growth of rights protection services and systems advocacy programs across the country.

RIGHTS PROTECTION ADVOCACY (RPA)

The second major advocacy strategy which has developed in recent years is rights protection advocacy. This approach requires the establishment within the mental health service delivery system of an effective operating mechanism to protect and advance the full range of patients rights and to correct abuses when they occur.

The rights of patients in treatment facilities may be established in several ways. These include:

1) The incorporation of formal bills of patients' rights into state mental health codes.
2) The adoption, administratively by departments, of such codes.
3) The establishment by court decisions of various rights which must be respected.
4) The evolution within mental health divisions or facilities of various codes refined through experience.

After patients' rights are established through any of the above procedures, it is the job of the RPA to assure that these rights are translated from a set of abstract principles into concrete guidelines and procedures. How this is done varies from state to state, but there are a number of common characteristics worth noting. In general, the RPA will carry out his/her duties by establishing procedures for grievances and appeals, and by facilitating access to an external legal system when necessary. Specifically, the RPA will:

1. Investigate complaints from patients, friends, relatives and staff members;
2. Initiate grievance procedures based on his/her own observation;
3. Attempt to resolve complaints or remedy grievances through direct negotiation with hospital staff;
4. Bring the issues directly to the attention of an institution director or mental health division director if the issues cannot be resolved to the patient's satisfaction;
5. Assure and facilitate the patient's access to external legal assistance if the issue cannot be resolved within the mental health service system.

The individual responsible for carrying out the activities of RPA is frequently an attorney, mental health professional or other concerned citizen employed by the mental health service system. The advocate is usually not involved in direct treatment activities and, in the better state programs, is not under the authority of the director of the facility in which he or she is working. While being "in" but not "part of" the mental health facility gives the RPA a number of benefits, these may come at the cost of the complete confidence of his or her client. On the positive side, by being an employee of the mental health department, although not of the facility, the RPA will have easier access to patients and their records than would an outsider. He or she will be able to participate in program policy development and will have a collegial relationship with the administrator, which engenders trust and cooperation rather than defensiveness, and which fosters the ability to identify problems without outside pressures or publicity. Because the RPA will have an office located in the facility and will be readily accessible to patients, speedy and responsive action to complaints will be possible. The informal nature of RPAs and their solutions to grievances, the familiarity with treatment facility routine and ongoing contact with facility staff all help to assure the patient an effective advocate on his/her behalf.

Along with these benefits of being with the system, come a number of problems for the RPA. Based within a facility, the RPA will be subject to certain pressures common to workers in any institution, which may limit his or her scope of action. The advocate will always be in a potential conflict-of-interest position, since advocating for a client may mean advocating against one's employer.

At times, pressures from coworkers can be difficult to resist, and pressures from higher-status colleagues can be unbearable. Furthermore, working in an institution, an advocate's responses to similar complaints may become institutionalized, and his or her view of the picture may become myopic. Thus, despite the effectiveness of a rights protection advocacy program in solving complaints about daily living and in promoting improved care, it is essential that there be adequate linkage with an independent, external legal advocacy system, such as the one described previously. Such a linkage would assure that any complaint not resolved to a patient's satisfaction could be appealed to the courts (a right enjoyed by all citizens).

In the development and monitoring of grievance procedures, the RPA must organize programs to educate and sensitize facility staff regarding the nature of patients' rights and the best way to assure them. As Joel Klein has so eloquently noted, "All the litigation has been unable to assure patients of what they need most—respect and kindness." The RPA's training program, however, will at least alert staff to aspects of the patient's perspectives toward treatment.

One state which has a comprehensive rights protection program is Michigan. The Michigan Office of Recipient Rights (ORR) was established to guarantee rights delineated by the State Mental Health Code, statutes and administrative rule. The ORR reports to the director of the Department of Mental Health. Its staff of rights advisors across the state investigates apparent violations of rights and acts to resolve disputes. Although the program's initial thrust was in the hospital setting, the ORR has expanded to community programs and presently has 40 offices of recipient rights in the community.[21]

SERVICE ADVOCACY

Another advocacy approach, and the one which is having the greatest impact on present and former patients living away from institutions and in the community, is service advocacy. Service advocacy is the process by which one person or group of persons assists or represents present or former patients in securing public benefits and services as well as protecting their human and civil rights. These benefits, services and rights are essential if newly discharged patients are to function independently in the community.

Unfortunately, few people seeking public benefits have either the rudimentary understanding of the programs or the skills required to use them effectively. The problem is magnified for discharged mental patients who are less able to advocate for themselves as a result of their illness or the dependency produced by institutionalization. Many of these patients share common characteristics, including the need for continual contact with the mental health system, impaired capacity to seek and perform regular employment, reliance on psychotropic drugs, lack of self-confidence, impaired ability to seek and use sources of support, possible continuance of psychiatric symptoms, such as delusions, hallucinations and episodes of acting-out behavior, and limited abilities to act on their own behalf. As a result of these factors, reintegration into the community is very difficult for many formerly hospitalized psychiatric patients.

Within institutions, patients have their basic needs for food, shelter, recreation, medical services and rehabilitation organized for them in one setting. In the community, however, they must rely on a complex system of public benefits and social services in order to survive. The responsibility for the care and support of discharged mentally disabled persons is, according to a report by the General Accounting Office, "diffused among several local state and federal levels of Government which have established separate agencies to provide most of the resources to fill their needs."[22] Programs implemented by these agencies include Social Service programs, Supplemental Security Income, Social Security, General Assistance, Veterans Benefits, Medicaid, Medicare, Public Housing and housing subsidy programs.

Although these programs exist in order to provide benefits to individuals meeting certain conditions of need or disability, certain factors make obtaining entitlements a difficult and complicated process. Such factors include "a lack of commitment of 'mainstream' human service agencies to providing needed resources and services for mentally disabled persons," confusing and forbidding application procedures, rejection or termination of benefits because of poor agency administration rather than provision of the law, and lack of access to legal or paralegal assistance in appealing denial of rights and benefits. To overcome these obstacles, patients living in the community need the assistance of the service advocate.

While primarily concerned with assuring the client of his/her just entitlements, the service advocate's activities may at times overlap the functions of the judicial advocate or rights protection advocate. In a like respect, the legal or rights protection advocate may under certain circumstances take on some of the roles of the service advocate; e.g., when a client's claim for services is denied, a judicial advocate may bring suit against the agency administrating the program, or the rights protection advocate may explore various benefit programs to assure an individual the right to the least restrictive alternative to hospitalization.

With the increasing numbers of people with disabling mental health problems returning to life in the community, the particular skills of the service advocate become especially important. The activities of the service advocate fall into five categories of operations:

1. Identification and location of benefits to which a client may be entitled;
2. Assistance to client in preparation and submission of application for benefits;
3. Coordinating the various social, rehabilitative, medical and other programs with which the client is involved, with the goal of enabling the individual to function as normally as possible in the community;
4. Negotiating problems arising between clients and various agencies administrating benefits and service programs;
5. Identifying legal and social problems and making proper legal and social referrals.

In performance of these tasks, the service advocate must have skills and experience in dealing with the complex social, legal and economic problems faced by discharged mental patients. Daily activities may fall on a continuum ranging from calling an agency for information, to representing the client in informal negotiations or at formal administrative proceedings, to developing and reviewing legislative proposals, to improving benefits for the client. The service advocate can be an attorney, mental health professional, paraprofessional, consumer or anyone else who helps an individual or group exercise rights and obtain legitimate benefits. The breadth of activities of the service advocate is so great that he or she can function independently of the service provider as in the case of the advocate in the Community Support Program, or as part of the system as in the situation of the court-screening patient advocate in community mental health centers. A brief description of these two developing national programs provides good examples of the scope of service advocacy.

Through the Division of Mental Health Service Programs, the National Institute of Mental Health has established a new pilot program—the Community Support Program (CSP)—to improve services for adults with chronically disabling mental health problems. A Community Support System is defined in NIMH guidelines as a "network of responsible people and coordinated resources committed to the goal of assisting a vulnerable population to meet their needs and to function as normally as possible in the community."[23]

The Community Support Program, which presently is funded through contracts to 39 states and the District of Columbia, identifies advocacy as an essential mechanism in the coordination and utilization of resources for the "benefit of the client." The "Definition and Guiding Principles for the Community Support Program" notes that advocates will be able to meet the following client needs:

1. A dependable resource person to whom to turn when assistance is needed or a crisis arises, who will protect the client from exploitation, represent the client as necessary, and espouse the client's cause in necessary contacts with service agencies.
2. Assistance in obtaining and making appropriate use of entitlements as citizens or residents of their respective communities.
3. A clearly defined and accessible grievance procedure.[24]

When the advocacy capacity of the CSP is fully implemented, it can serve as a model of service advocacy for the country.

Another example of a national program which has many aspects of service advocacy incorporated in it is the court-screening and advocacy operations of community mental health centers. Public Law 94-63, enacted in January 1976, required centers to establish court-screening procedures and to assure potential patients of the least restrictive alternatives to hospitalization. This requirement has been implemented by a number of centers in a fashion consistent with the philosophy and activities of the service advocate.

The individual (the patient advocate) in a CMHC who is assigned the task of coordinating court-screening programs and assuring that the least drastic and most clinically appropriate community services are found, must work closely with a number of community agencies and a variety of different professionals. To accomplish this task, the advocate must be aware of the existing community resources and understand legal rights of patients relative to hospitalization. In addition, the CMHC in which the advocate works will have to develop procedures and screening standards for guidance in diverting potential inpatients to less restrictive alternatives. Effective utilization of community alternatives requires close cooperation between the patient advocate and elements of the community interested in providing alternative services. The advocate will work closely with existing community agencies and community support programs where they exist to assure that all possible resources have been explored. Thus, in addition to identifying appropriate clinical resources in the community, the patient advocate may also serve to help the patient, with court approval, overcome bureaucratic obstacles to obtaining such services.

SYSTEMS ADVOCACY

The fourth advocacy approach, and the one which could have the greatest impact on the future direction of the delivery of mental health services, is systems advocacy. This approach encourages change in the mental health services system. While each advocacy group discussed above—judicial advocacy, rights protection advocacy and service advocacy—has a change component, systems advocacy focuses more directly on system-wide reorganization.

The other three advocacy approaches focus on implementing rights already guaranteed by the Constitution, state laws, government regulations and administrative directives. Systems advocacy works toward changing mental health care delivery. Systems advocacy can come from within a facility (hospital, CMHC, etc.) or from the outside. People working inside the facility, such as administrators, ombudsmen and mental health care workers, can advocate for change in the system by negotiating through administrative channels. People working outside the institution, such as attorneys, expatient groups and public interest groups, can also effect change in the internal administration of a delivery system through the impact of pressure, legislation and litigation. In the broader delivery system, advocates can encourage expanded services and/or changes in service direction for the mentally disabled population. The systems advocacy approach also offers a forum for new and sometimes radical ideas. Attorneys, public interest groups, the news media and coalitions of interested parties can work to change existing laws, or write new legislation to expand or reallocate mental health budgets and to develop alternate solutions to the problems of mental health care delivery.

In addition, systems advocates can educate the public to eliminate the stigma of mental illness for present and former patients. Rosalynn Carter, Honorary Chairperson of the President's Commission on Mental Health, concluded in 1978 that "There is no challenge more important than addressing the problem of stigma." The stigma often lasts far longer than the mental disability and may compromise the expatient's rights in the areas of housing and employment, as well as his/her general social adjustment and well-being. This, then, is one issue of great importance for advocates of change in mental health systems to address.[25]

In order for change agents to deal effectively with legislators and administrators, they need skills in lobbying and negotiating, the ability to generate publicity, and innovative planning to improve programs, legislation and funding.

One example of a systems advocacy program is the Sharing Life in the Community (SLIC) Program. In the spring of 1975, advocates from the Three-County East-Metro Area of Minnesota came together in coalition to advocate for the development of community-based services that would lead to independent community living for previously hospitalized patients. The coalition included individual advocates from the Department of Public Welfare, service providers, clients and relatives of clients. As they began to work, they involved as many people as possible from different agencies, groups and associations. As a result of this systems advocacy effort, the state legislature provided SLIC with $350,000 in funding to establish their program and provide one year of service. Participants in this successful program stress the importance of organization, the cooperative efforts of many representative groups, the focus on a single issue and perseverance.[26]

SUMMARY

The four advocacy approaches—judicial advocacy, rights, protection advocacy, service advocacy, and systems advocacy—must be coordinated. Their common effort will assure a logical continuum of advocacy services for the patient. Working in cooperation, they can help ease the transition of patients from institutions to community settings not only by advocating for their discharge when appropriate, but also by advocating for the provision of necessary services and aftercare planning to follow the patient. They can help maintain expatients on a level of optimal functioning in the community by assuring entitlements to the full range of federally mandated services which are the rights of all citizens, and by reducing stigmatization through public education. They can help prevent unnecessary readmission to the hospital by protecting clients' rights and by helping them meet their needs in the community.

Advocates work to assure that mental health systems do what they are supposed to do for patients: respect their constitutional and statutory rights (judicial advocacy); protect their personal rights and privileges and correct abuses (rights protection advocacy); help them to secure all appropriate entitlements (service advocacy); and serve them by changing system-wide policies when these no longer adequately respond to patient needs (systems advocacy). The four advocacy components play different roles in each patient setting; however, they will be most effective when they join efforts and create partnerships which encourage easy referral from one advocacy group to another.

The major challenge of all advocates in the community is to obtain for their clients or patients the rights or services to which they are entitled. While their approaches may differ, all advocates will share a common loyalty and commitment to their clients. The advocate role will require courage in the face of opposition, persistence in dealing with obfuscation and tolerance in working with often suspicious clients and hostile staff. The advocate will at times feel isolated and frustrated, but will be sustained in this important work by the recognition that without his/her efforts, many of the clients' concerns, fears and wishes would not be heard, attended to or resolved. The advocate's immediate goal is assuring patients' rights, but the larger mission is to be a change agent in creating a more responsive mental health system that is sensitive to the human wants, clinical needs and legal rights of patients. The rhetoric of patients' rights can then be made a reality.

NOTES

1. Deutsch, A. *The Mentally Ill in America.* New York: Columbia University Press, 1949.
2. Rothman, D. J. *Discovery of the Asylum.* Boston: Little, Brown, 1971.
3. Beers, C. *The Mind That Found Itself.* Garden City, N.Y.: Doubleday, 1936.
4. Deutsch, A. *The Shame of the States.* New York: Harcourt, Brace, 1948.
5. Ward, M. *Snake Pit.* New York: Random House, 1946.
6. Solomon, H. C. Presidential address. *Amer. J. Psychiat.* 115: 1-17, (1958).

7. National Institute of Mental Health, Memorandum #6. Resident Patient Rate in State Mental Hospitals. June 27, 1977.
8. Public Health Services Comments on the Draft of General Accounting Office Report. *Improvements Needed in Efforts to Help Mentally Disabled Return to and Remain in the Communities.* Oct. 15, 1976.
9. Civil liberty for what? Editorial in *New York Times,* April 8, 1974.
10. Allen, Priscilla. A consumer's view of California's mental health care system. *The Psychiatric Quarterly* 48(1) (1974).
11. Allen, Priscilla. A bill of rights for citizens using outpatient mental health services, in *Community Survival for Long-term Patients,* Richard H. Lamb, ed. San Francisco: Joseph-Boss, Inc.
12. Report of the President's Commission on Mental Health. Washington, D.C.: GPO, 1978.
13. Kopolow, Louis, and Bloom, Helene, eds. *Mental Health Advocacy: An Emerging Force in Consumers' Rights.* Washington, D.C.: GPO, 1977.
14. MacLean, Colleen. General Counsel, Department of Mental Health of Tennessee. Personal Comments. Nov 1978.
15. *Wyatt* v. *Stickney.* 325 F. Supp. 781 (M.D. Ala. 1971).
16. *Dixon* v. *Weinberger.* No. 74285 (C.D.D.C. Feb. 14, 1974).
17. Klein, Joel. *Mental Health and the Law: Too Much Courting and Not Enough Caring.* Presented at Meeting of Southern Regional Educational Board. Atlanta, Ga., 1976.
18. Kopolow, Louis. Op. cit. 13.
19. The role of Counsel in the Civil Commitment Process: A Theoretical Framework. *Yale Law Journal,* 84: 1540 (1975).
20. Perlin, Michael, and Van Ness, Stanley. *Mental Health Advocacy—The New Jersey Experience in Mental Health Advocacy: An Emerging Force in Consumers' Rights.* Washington, D.C., GPO, 1977.
21. Coye, Janet. Michigan's system for protecting rights. *Hospital and Community Psychiatry.* 25(5) (May 1977).
22. *Returning the Mentally Disabled to the Community: Government Needs to Do More.* Report to the Congress by the Comptroller General of the United States. GAO, HRD-76-152. Washington, D.C. 1976.
23. Public Health Services Comments. Op. cit. no. 8.
24. Turner, Judith. *Comprehensive Community Support Systems for Adults with Chronically Disabling Mental Health Problems: Definition Components and Guiding Principles.* A Working Paper based on NIMH Conference. NIMH, Jan 10, 1977.
25. Kopolow, Louis. *Shall We Wait to be Sued: The Malpractice Madness.* Paper delivered at Annual Meeting of American Psychiatric Association. Atlanta, Ga., May 9, 1978.
26. Schmidt, Don. *The Minnesota Experience in Mental Health Advocacy: An Emerging Force in Consumers' Rights.* Washington, D.C., GPO, 1977.

CHAPTER 20

JUDICIAL DECISIONS AND THE CHRONIC PSYCHIATRIC PATIENT

MARIEN E. EVANS

This chapter deals with the various confrontations of the chronic psychiatric patient with the legal system and the effect of recent judicial decisions upon those confrontations. While the most compelling of the recent decisions include the right to treatment, the right to treatment in the least restrictive setting and the right to refuse treatment, less provocative but equally important decisions have affected living arrangements, employment opportunities, contractual relationships, marriage and voting rights and conservatorship and guardianship proceedings.

I. THE AMERICAN JUDICIAL SYSTEM

Since not all decisions have equal meaning, an adequate evaluation of the impact of recent judicial decisions, such as those apparently establishing the right to refuse treatment, requires knowledge of the American judicial system. That system, in reality, consists of two separate systems, the state and federal. There are 50 separate and distinct state jurisdictions, each of which consists of, with some variations, three levels. The first level is the trial court, usually the county court, in which a legal proceeding is begun. The proceeding may be criminal or civil in nature. Most often these proceedings involve civil or criminal violations of state laws or of rights guaranteed by state and federal laws. It is at this level, the trial court level, that an individual, group,[1] * or governmental body seeks redress for wrongs sustained by private persons or by society as a whole. That redress may consist of money damages, the enforcement of the right by injunctive relief or punishment for a wrong against society. After receiving the evidence, a decision or verdict is rendered by the jury in accordance with the instructions of the presiding judge, or, in jury-waived trials, by the judge, who acts both as fact finder and interpreter of the law. Decisions of trial courts are not published in any recognized compilation and are not truly binding in future cases.

The second level of courts which is common to most states is the appellate level. Judges of appellate courts (known as courts of appeal or appeals courts) review the decisions of the trial courts for errors in interpretations of law upon the request or appeal of the party who is dissatisfied with the decision of the trial court. Only where the decisions appear to be completely contrary to the evidence presented at the trial will the appellate court make a judgment regarding the facts presented. The appellate court may affirm the decision of the trial court, it may reverse the decision or it may remand the case to the trial court for further proceedings in accordance with the decision. The decisions of the appellate courts, unless overturned by a higher appellate court upon further appeal, are binding in future similar cases.

The decision of the appellate court may be reviewed by a higher appellate court, the state supreme court, if certain criteria are met. Those criteria vary from state to state, but commonly depend upon the importance of and/or the novel character of the issues raised. Decisions of state supreme courts establish the law of that state, but they have no extraterritorial effect. That is to say, for example, a decision of the California Supreme Court effects directly only future actions in the state of California. When, however, there is no case precedent in a state, the court may—but is not required to—adopt the ruling of another state supreme court. A very recent example of the

**Class action suits are brought by named individuals on behalf of a group or class of persons too numerous to name individually, when there are questions of law or fact common to the class, when the claims of the named individuals are representative of the claims of all the members and when the named persons will adequately protect all the membership of the class.*

latter principle was the *Saikewicz**[2] decision in which the Massachusetts Supreme Judicial Court considered and rejected the approach taken by the New Jersey Supreme Court in the *Quinlan*[3] case. Frequently, however, where no precedent exists in state law or federal law, a court examines the principles of the case before it and the principles involved in analogous situations and applies the law of the analogous cases.

The federal system is identical to that described above. The federal trial court is the District Court. The appellate courts, of which there are eleven, are the Circuit Courts of Appeal, and the final decision is rendered by the United States Supreme Court. Federal district courts are vested with jurisdiction or authority over federal crimes, admiralty and bankruptcy—as well as a variety of other civil actions where jurisdiction rests upon a specific grant of federal jurisdiction by Congressional act, upon the fact that a general federal question is involved or upon the fact that litigants are residents of different states. Where federal laws are involved or where the parties reside in different states, federal and state trial courts have the authority to render decisions. In certain cases involving civil rights, Congress has determined that three federal judges must decide the case, even though the action must be initiated in the District Court where a single judge presides.

As in the state system, the Federal Circuit Court of Appeals reviews the decision of the trial court for errors of law. Additionally, the federal intermediate courts are vested with the authority to review administrative actions. Such jurisdiction is usually granted by the statute which establishes the particular administrative agency.[4] Since the various circuits are not bound by interpretations of law other than those of the Supreme Court, or, where applying state law, the interpretations of the law of the state by the state supreme court, a discrepancy may exist in the applications of law in different parts of the United States. Final resolution of these discrepancies is made by the United States Supreme Court.

The United States Supreme Court is authorized by the Constitution of United States[5] to decide cases arising under the Constitution, the laws of the United States and treaties arising thereunder. The Supreme

**Both Saikewicz and Quinlan involved the rights of terminally ill, incompetent patients to reject heroic measures initiated to save their lives.*

Court is also empowered to review the final judgments and decrees rendered by the highest court of a state,[6] either through appeal or by *certiorari. Certiorari* as a means to obtaining review by the Supreme Court differs from an appeal in that an appeal invokes obligatory jurisdiction, whereas *certiorari* is granted only if four justices agree that there are special and important reasons for review of the case and no statutory right to review exists.

Decisions of the Federal Courts of Appeal may also be reviewed by the United States Supreme Court. Whether the appeal or request for review is from a state court decision or a federal court decision, the pronouncement of the U.S. Supreme Court is final and binding on all future similar cases, unless and until the Supreme Court reverses or modifies its decision. The binding effect of such decisions is referred to as *stare decisis.*

"Law" arises usually in one of two ways; by legislative enactment of a statute or by judicial decision (common law). The common law comprises the body of those principles and rules of action which derive their authority from usage and custom or from the judgments and decrees of courts recognizing and affirming and enforcing such usages and customs. In rare instances, law may originate from an "advisory opinion." An advisory opinion is issued by a court upon the request of the legislative or executive branch of government on matters which have not yet resulted in litigation. Although a few state supreme courts[7] are empowered to issue such opinions, the United States Supreme Court is denied that power. An example of an advisory opinion resulting in the formation of law is the familiar M'Naughton Rule test of criminal responsibility. In the M'Naughton case the British House of Lords submitted certain questions about unsoundness of mind to fifteen English judges. The Rules consist of the replies to the questions propounded to the judges.[8]

Limits on the generalizability of legal findings as suggested in the preceding paragraphs should be kept in mind in the following discussions.

II. DECISIONS REQUIRING DEINSTITUTIONALIZATION

A. Right to Treatment Cases

In the 1966 landmark case *Rouse* v. *Cameron,*[9] the Washington, D.C. Court of Appeals held that persons involuntarily committed under the 1964 Hospitalization of the Mentally Ill Act have a right to a *bona fide* attempt at treatment and noted that the denial of that right might have constitutional implications. While *Rouse* has been cited as having created a constitutional right to treatment, in reality the decision confirmed the right to treatment mandated by the District of Columbia ordinance, not the Constitution of the United States. Similarly, in the 1968 case of *Nason* v. *Superintendent of Bridgewater State Hospital*,[10] Justice Cutter, writing the majority opinion for the Massachusetts Supreme Judicial Court, questioned the confinement of mentally ill persons who had not been adjudged guilty of crimes without affording them reasonable treatment. Again, while the court did not specifically find a constitutional right to treatment on the part of such persons, it did hold that "a program for Nason's appropriate treatment [shall] be determined by competent doctors in their best judgment within the limits of permissible medical practice and is to be followed diligently."[11] The court further determined that if adequate treatment were not provided within a reasonable period of time, the legality of Nason's future confinement might be presented to the county court.

Subsequently, four federal district courts held that there exists a constitutional right to treatment on the part of persons involuntarily civilly committed to state mental hospitals.[12] In the widely cited case of *Wyatt* v. *Stickney (Wyatt* v. *Anderholt)*, guardians of patients confined at Alabama Bryce Hospital and employees of that hospital alleged that involuntarily committed handicapped patients were not receiving treatment for their illnesses. Chief Judge Johnson held that the involuntarily committed patients "unquestionably have a constitutional right to receive such individual treatment as will give each of them a realistic opportunity to be cured or to improve his or her mental condition."[13] In a subsequent order in the same case, Judge Johnson held that the mentally retarded patients have a constitutional right to "such individual habilitation as will give them a more useful and meaningful life and to return to society."[14]

The Fifth Circuit Court of Appeals sustained Judge Johnson's finding of a constitutionally guaranteed right to treatment on the part of involuntarily civilly committed patients. In its opinion the Court of Appeals relied upon its holding in *Donaldson* v. *O'Connor*,[15] which it had decided a few months earlier and which was subsequently reversed by the United States Supreme Court[16] on the question of a constitutional right to treatment. In the *Donaldson* case the Fifth Circuit Court held that

> [W]here a nondangerous patient is involuntarily committed to a state mental hospital, the only constitutionally permissible purpose of a confinement is to provide treatment and such a patient has a constitutional right to such treatment as will help him be cured or to improve his mental condition.[17]

In reviewing the *Donaldson* decision, the United States Supreme Court concluded that the "difficult issues of constitutional law dealt with by the Court of Appeals are not presented by this case in its present posture."[18] Instead the court stated that a finding of mental illness alone cannot justify custodial confinement and that a state cannot "constitutionally confine without doing more, a nondangerous individual who is capable of surviving safely in freedom by himself or with the help of willing and responsible family members or friends."[19]

Thus, the Supreme Court refused to find a constitutional right to treatment on the part of nondangerous, involuntarily committed mentally ill; rather, the court found that the act of confining civilly committed nondangerous persons in the absence of efforts to provide treatment for the mental illness is a violation of the patient's right to freedom and liberty. A literal reading of the *Donaldson* case would require the release of nondangerous, mentally ill persons into the community on *two conditions*: 1) *where there is no treatment available within the institution*, and 2) *where the persons are capable of surviving safely within the community.*

B. *The Right to the Least Restrictive Treatment*

> Perhaps the most basic and fundamental right is the right to be free from unwanted restraint. It seems clear then, that persons suffering from the conditions of being mentally ill, but who are not alleged to have committed any crime, can not be totally deprived of their liberty if there are less drastic means for achieving the same goal. . . . We believe that the person recommending full-time, involuntary hospitalization must bear the burden of proving (1) what alternatives are available; (2) what alternatives were investigated; and (3) why the alternatives investigated were not deemed suitable. These alternatives include voluntary or court-ordered outpatient treatment, day treatment in a hospital, night treatment in a hospital, placement in the custody of a friend or relative, placement in a nursing home, referral to a community mental health center, and home health aide services.[20]

Thus, Judge Sprecker, speaking for the three-judge Federal District Court in *Lessard* v. *Schmidt*,[21] set out the requirement that less drastic means of treatment than commitment be investigated. The same requirements were enunciated in the earlier cases of *Lake* v. *Cameron*,[22] *Lynch* v. *Baxley*[23] *Wyatt* v. *Stickney*,[24] and in numerous subsequent cases which challenged the constitutionality of state commitment statutes. In 1975, in the case of *Dixon* v. *Weinberger*,[25] Judge Robinson liberally interpreted the District of Columbia's 1964 Hospitalization of the Mentally Ill Act as guaranteeing the right to the least restrictive treatment to patients at St. Elizabeth's Hospital. Judge Robinson held that the least restrictive treatment doctrine included alternative sites for treatment such as "nursing homes, personal care homes, foster homes and half-way houses."[26]

These decisions, together with the philosophy of the Community Mental Health Act of 1970,[27] following upon the heels of the development of potent, effective psychoactive medication, have motivated state mental health agencies to sponsor community-based programs for the treatment of the nondangerous mentally ill and infirm. Consent decrees entered in several recent cases involving the institutionalized mentally retarded and mentally retarded of state institutions[28] have given rise to regulations and standards for the establishment of community residences and for the provision of community aftercare for those former residents of state institutions.

However, as the subsequent discussion will reveal, the developing law of the right to refuse treatment may seriously jeopardize the efforts of mental health planners to continue the movement of the chronically ill psychiatric patient from the institution to the community for care.

C. *Right to Refuse Treatment*

Premised upon the doctrine of informed consent is the emerging doctrine of the right to refuse treatment. The doctrine of informed consent is based upon the fundamental concept that "[e]very human being of adult years and sound mind has a right to determine what shall be done with his own body. . . ."[29] Although suits charging failure by a physician to adequately disclose the risks and alternatives of proposed treatment date back a half-century, the doctrine was refined during the past decade in such cases as *Canterbury* v. *Spence*[30] and *Cobbs* v. *Grant*.[31] In the first of these cases, the *Canterbury* court set forth the standard for disclosure as the divulgence of all risks which potentially affect the patient's decision.[32] The court in *Cobbs* distinguished between common-law battery and negligence in informed consent cases.[33] Where the physician obtains consent for one type of therapy and consequently administers a substantially different treatment for which consent was not obtained, the physician may be found to have committed battery. However, when an undisclosed potential complication results from therapy or the occurrence of a known but undisclosed risk of the treatment, the physician has not exercised due care to disclose pertinent information and has thereby acted negligently.

Applications of the principle of informed consent are found in the leading right-to-refuse-treatment cases such as *Kaimowitz* v. *Department of Mental Health*,[34] *In Re Quinlan*,[35] and *Saikewicz* v. *Superintendent of Belchertown State School.*[36] *Kaimowitz* established the principle that mentally ill patients are not competent to consent to the extreme treatment of psychosurgery because of the irreversibility of the procedure, because of the experimental nature of the procedure and ". . . because of the inherent inequality in their positions [as patients]."[37] As the result of the *Kaimowitz* case, several states have enacted legislation aimed at protecting the rights of patients for whom psychosurgery is proposed.[38]

Subsequent decisions have noted that psychoactive drugs may have effects as long lasting and possibly as irreversible as psychosurgery.[39]

A less startling but equally important case affirming the right to refuse treatment is that of *Winters* v. *Miller*,[40] which held that a mentally ill patient has the right to refuse medication if ingesting the medication would violate the patient's religious precepts. In its decision, the court stated that where First Amendment religious beliefs are involved and where there is no strong showing of a state interest* (in this case there was no indication that the patient was dangerous to herself or to others), and in the absence of an adjudication of incompetency, treatment could not be forced upon the patient. In a recent affirmation of the First Amendment right to refuse treatment, the Court of Appeals for the District of Columbia held that a Christian Scientist had the right to refuse medication even

*In enforcing First Amendment rights, courts invariably balance the individual's rights with the interest of the state in preserving life or protecting the rights of other citizens.

though incompetent and hospitalized for an emergency. The court held that the decision whether to force acceptance of medication must be made in accordance with the doctrine of substituted judgment. That doctrine requires the court to substitute itself for the incompetent and act on the same motives and considerations.[41] In this case the court found that the patient was opposed to the administration of medication, and since the medication would not save the patient's life, the state's interest in preserving life was not sufficiently strong to warrant an invasion of the patient's right to religious freedom.

Very recently, two federal district courts, on the basis of the constitutional right to privacy,[42] have upheld the rights of the institutionalized mentally ill to refuse treatment in the form of psychotropic medication. In the first case, *Rennie* v. *Klein*,[43] Judge Brotman of the United States District Court for the District of New Jersey actually issued three separate opinions. This case involved a 38-year-old, highly intelligent man who was involuntarily committed to the Ancora Psychiatric Hospital in New Jersey. This was his twelfth admission, and his admitting diagnosis was manic-depressive illness, circular type.

At the time of this case, New Jersey law seemed to say that involuntarily committed mental patients did not have a right to refuse medication.[44] *Rennie* challenged the constitutional validity of New Jersey law by seeking an injunction pursuant to 42 USC s 1983.[45] Rennie had attempted to refuse medication because of the side effects of akathesis and wormlike movements of the tongue. In November 1978, Judge Brotman preliminarily ordered that Rennie not be forcibly medicated except in emergencies.[46]

In examining the right to privacy, as in the right to religious freedom, the court must look to whether that individual right is overridden by strong state interests. The court here examined the state interests which could negate the patient's right to refuse treatment in nonemergencies and found two state interests which could conceivably override the individual's interest in privacy. First, the police power of a state allows it to protect its citizens from harm. Thus, if Rennie were a danger to others or out of control, forcible treatment might be justified to protect other patients from harm. Second, the doctrine of *parens patriae* not only allows, but requires, a state to protect those of its citizens who are unable to protect themselves. Since the *parens patriae* doctrine may be invoked only when a patient is unable to care for himself, and since mental illness is not necessarily equal to incompetence, the state cannot excuse forced medication on the basis of *parens patriae* unless a determination of incompetency is made. In making such a determination, the fact finder must establish the degree to which the underlying mental illness contributes to the incompetency. On this occasion, Judge Brotman issued no permanent injunction, but retained jurisdiction of the case, allowing continued administration of a maintenance dosage of medication.

On December 12, 1978, Judge Brotman in a supplementary opinion noted that Rennie's condition had deteriorated significantly since his November 1978 ruling. At this time, the court found that Rennie's competency was substantially lessened, and that his refusal to take antipsychotic medication should be overruled. The court further noted that the only less-restrictive alternative to the medication (Thorazine) was constant restraints.[47]

In his third opinion, issued September 15, 1979, Judge Brotman affirmed the plaintiffs' (at this time members of a class action including Rennie) constitutional right to refuse medication. That right could be denied, but only after due process had been provided to the patient. The due process requirement would be met by the holding of a hearing presided over by an independent psychiatrist rather than a judge or an administrative hearing officer.[48] Thus, the *Rennie* case established procedural safeguards intended to insure the need for the medication.

The second recent decision holding that involuntarily committed mental patients have a constitutional right to refuse treatment is *Rogers* v. *Okun.*[49] In *Rogers*, Judge Tauro of the United States District Court for the District of Massachusetts recognized a constitutional right to refuse treatment for mental illness in the absence of an emergency. In this case the plaintiffs representing a class of mental patients sued physicians and officers of a state hospital for allegedly subjecting them to unauthorized treatments. The plaintiffs complained that the defendant physicians' policy of administering medications and secluding the patients in nonemergency situations violated their rights to privacy as well as the standards of accepted medical care. The crux of the plaintiffs' claim was that in all but emergency situations, the mentally ill are competent to decide whether to refuse treatment.[50]

In arriving at his decision, Judge Tauro considered three preliminary questions: (1) whether mentally ill are competent to refuse treatment; (2) whether it is proper for a guardian to refuse treatment for the patient; and (3) whether there exists a right to refuse treatment in an emergency.

On the issue of competency, Judge Tauro stated:

> the weight of evidence persuades this court that although committed mental patients do suffer at least some impairment of their relationship to reality, most are able to appreciate the benefits, risks, and discomfort that may reasonably be expected from receiving psychotropic medication . . . [i]ndeed, a fundamental concept for treating the mentally ill is the establishment of a therapeutic alliance between psychiatrist and patient. Implicit in such an alliance is an understanding and acceptance by the patient of a prescribed treatment program.[51]

On the issue of a guardian's refusing treatment on behalf of the patient, Judge Tauro did not find compelling the defendants' argument that the right to refuse treatment is a personal right which cannot be relinquished by a guardian. Rather, the court stated that such reasoning would force the incompetent patient to make the sort of decisions he had been adjudged unable to make.

Viewing the question of refusal of treatment in an emergency, the court first defined emergency. Judge Tauro rejected the defendants' proposal of the psychiatric definition of emergency, which includes evidence of suicidal behavior, assaultiveness, destruction of property, intense anxiety, panic, bizzare behavior, acute or chronic emotional imbalance having the potential for interference in the patient's daily functioning, and conditions needing treatment to prevent or decrease the possibility of additional suffering or rapid worsening of the clinical status. Rather, the court adopted the position that "a committed mental patient may be forcibly medicated in an emergency situation in which failure to do so would result in a substantial likelihood of physical harm to that patient, to other patients or to staff members of the institutions."[52]

Contrary to the holding of Judge Brotman, Judge Tauro did not establish a requirement for a due process hearing to determine whether an emergency actually existed, but seemed to leave that determination to the physicians having the care of the patients. Thus, these decisions again illustrate the need to examine local decisions on any issue before determining the rights and responsibilities of an individual in a particular situation.

Fearful that the Rogers decision will result in patients having been committed for the purpose of treatment refusing treatment yet remaining in the institution—a situation which would violate the *Donaldson* holding,[53] and which would seriously impede the movement toward deinstitutionalization—the Massachusetts Attorney

General has appealed the decision. Deinstitutionalization is predicated upon community-based care, including outpatient care and acute psychiatric care in general hospitals. The *Rogers* decision may negatively impact upon that movement, forcing hospitals to provide separate accommodations for those committed patients who refuse treatment and who thus do not meet the *Donaldson* criteria of capability of surviving in the community alone or with the help of friends or relatives. Alternatively, such patients may invoke the *Donaldson* doctrine and demand to be discharged from the hospital.

III. DISCRIMINATION AGAINST THE CHRONIC PSYCHIATRIC PATIENT

A. *Housing*

Even before discharge from an institution, the chronic patient faces one of the first legal issues of deinstitutionalization. In attempting to provide care for the deinstitutionalized patients, state and community mental health agencies have established or funded halfway houses, foster homes and boarding houses. The use of group residences including halfway houses during the care, treatment and rehabilitation of mentally handicapped persons is a product of the 1960s decade of deinstitutionalization. These facilities, together with community mental health services, may avoid the harmful effects of institutionalization and provide a needed transitional housing after institutional care.

Halfway houses, group homes and other community residences are operated by nonprofit organizations, governmental agencies and private persons. Vital to the success of foster and group facilities is their homelike atmosphere and normative environment. Social groups and community contacts, as well as access to therapeutic facilities, assist in the transition to independent community living.[54] However, local or municipal ordinances establishing single-family and other residential areas have been interpreted to exclude foster or community residences because the intended residents would fail to meet the definition of "family" that frequently specifies a blood, marital or adoptive relationship. For example, in the case of *Newark* v. *Johnson*,[55] a New Jersey court upheld a single-family ordinance restricting occupancy to persons related by blood, marriage or adoption against a family desirous of caring for foster children. In

Browndale International Ltd. v. *Board of Adjustment*,[56] a Wisconsin zoning ordinance defining family as "any number of individuals related by blood or marriage or not to exceed five . . . persons not so related living together on the premises as a single housekeeping unit, including domestic servants . . ." was invoked to bar the establishment of several homes for the care and treatment of emotionally disturbed children. These homes were intended to be operated by house parents and other professional staff. The trial court (the court having primary or original jurisdiction over actions to enforce laws, regulations and ordinances or to restrain such enforcement) ruled that the homes would be single-family residences if each housed no more than five children. However, the Wisconsin Supreme Court reversed that ruling on the grounds that the proprietor was in business and hence the homes would not be used exclusively for residential purposes. That court specifically ruled that "therapeutic home arrangements" are nonresidential usage.[57] The United States Supreme Court refused to review that decision, in effect agreeing with the Wisconsin Supreme Court.

By refusing to review the *Browndale* decision, the Supreme Court appears to have extended its ruling in the *Village of Belle Terre* v. *Boraas*.[58] In *Belle Terre*, six unrelated college students had sought to rent a house in an area zoned for single-family residences. The village ordinance defined a "family" as including any number of related persons living together but including only two unrelated persons living together. The Supreme Court, in reviewing the lower-court decision, held that the ordinance was a rational means of achieving legitimate objectives of preserving a "quiet place where yards are wide, people few, and motor vehicles restricted."[59]

On the other side of the coin, New York State courts have been far more receptive to the establishment of community group care residences, perhaps because New York was in the forefront of deinstitutionalization. In *East House Corporation* v. *Riker*,[60] the court reversed a board of adjustment's dismissal of the corporations' request for a special exception from the zoning ordinances in order to allow the establishment of a halfway house for persons discharged from mental institutions. The court ruled that the city government had determined that the use was not basically incompatible with other residential usage, and that since the board had been unable to support a finding of injury to nearby property, it would have to grant the exception.

At least one court, again in New York, has found a constitutional right on the part of deinstitutionalized patients to live where they wish. In *Stone* v. *Miller*,[61] the Federal District Court of the Eastern District of New York in 1974 declared that a local ordinance prohibiting people on medication from living in hotels or requiring the informing of the landlord of a prior history of mental illness, as a precondition to renting the apartment, was unconstitutional because it violated the rights of the mentally handicapped to travel and to be treated in the least restrictive setting. The latter right has been enunciated in numerous Federal Court decisions and most compellingly in *Lessard* v. *Schmidt.*[62]

If clients of the mental health system are denied the opportunity to locate in community residences because of exclusionary zoning laws, they are being denied their right to treatment (the doctrine that one may not be institutionalized without treatment)[63] and the right to rehabilitation in the least restrictive setting.

Since the early 1970's when the issue of community rejection of group homes arose, the courts have become far more receptive to arguments supporting the existence of a right to establish community residences. In one instance, *Rosen* v. *Birchwood Association,*[64] in an action brought pursuant to the New York Civil Rights Law, the plaintiffs sued a large real estate firm alleging that the defendant real estate firm violated the civil rights of the plaintiffs who wished to establish group homes in apartment houses. The court held that the real estate firm had, indeed, violated the plaintiffs' civil rights by refusing to rent to them for the stated purpose. Another New York court[65] has held that a large mansion on 29 acres of land could be used as a group home for mentally retarded persons even though the area was zoned for single family residential use. Similarly a Minnesota[66] trial court, deciding a case arising in a middle class suburb, refused to enjoin the use of a house for a small group home as violating the local "single family dwelling" covenant. An Ohio[67] court has sweepingly suggested that where such homes are operated by state agencies, the homes should be completely exempt from local covenants and zoning rules, based on the state's discharge of authorized governmental function and eminent domain.

The position taken by the Ohio court in *Brownfield* v. *Ohio*,[68] as well as that taken by some New York courts, reflects the principle that when a legislature has adopted a stated policy of deinstitutionalization, as embodied in statutes, local power to restrict the location of residential facilities is implicitly pre-empted and may not be used to thwart implementation of state policy.

Massachusetts courts have taken a different means of avoiding prohibitive zoning restrictions. The Court of Appeals in *Harbor Schools*

Inc. v. *Board of Appeals of Haverhill*[69] took the position that such residences fulfill a public educational function, and are thus exempt from local zoning regulations.

While the above discussion is not exhaustive, it illuminates the growing acceptance on the part of the judiciary, if not on the part of community neighbors, that chronic mental patients have the right to relatively normal community living.

B. Employment

Once the former mental patient has found a supportive community residence, foster home, group home or halfway house in which to live, the question of continued or new employment becomes important. In most states private discrimination in employment against those who were or are mentally disabled is not prohibited by law; moreover documentation of discrimination is difficult. However, given the continued public fear of the mentally ill, such discrimination undoubtedly exists.[70]

Since one must establish state or governmental action or involvement in order to challenge a practice or procedure on constitutional grounds,[71] discriminatory practices on the part of private agencies or businesses may continue unchecked unless remedial legislation is enacted. On the other hand, when the government discriminates in hiring, state action is involved and constitutional restraints of due process and equal protection of the law apply. A job applicant may bring suit under the equal protection clause of the Fourth and Fourteenth amendments to the constitution on the basis that the discrimination is not rationally related to a legitimate government interest.[72] Additionally, a job applicant may challenge the asking of questions about his/her mental health history as an impermissible invasion of personal privacy. However, courts are inclined to hold the government to a lesser standard when employment is concerned than when other rights such as freedom of speech or the right to liberty are concerned.[73]

There is a slowly emerging trend for state legislatures to enact legislation aimed at preventing employment discrimination of the mentally handicapped. One such statute was enacted in Illinois to implement the following 1970 provision of its constitution:

> All persons with a physical or mental handicap shall be free from discrimination in the sale or rental of property and shall be free from discrimination unrelated to ability in the hiring and promotion practices of any employer.[74]

The implementing legislation defines physical or mental handicap as a "handicap unrelated to one's ability to perform jobs or position available to him or promotions."[75] The statute explicitly excludes from evidence of inability to perform the fact that one "has been treated as a person in need of mental treatment as defined by the Mental Health Code of 1967 . . . or that the person has or is alleged to have undergone mental treatment or evaluation."[76] The statute further declares the refusing to hire, discharge or any other form of discrimination because of such mental handicap to be an unfair employment practice unless it can be shown that the particular handicap prevents the performance of the employment involved.[77] Similarly, labor organizations are prohibited from discriminating against mentally handicapped persons.[78]

An "antidiscrimination" statute like that of Illinois is limited by the difficulty and expense of proving discrimination. Massachusetts has attempted to overcome these limitations by enacting legislation which prohibits an employer from asking any questions of a job applicant or employee regarding past admissions to a mental hospital, provided that the applicant or employee has been discharged from the hospital or facility and can provide a physician's certificate to the effect that he/she is mentally competent to perform the job for which he/she is applying.[79] This confusing and contradictory statute also purports to permit the formerly hospitalized patient to refuse to reply to questions regarding hospitalization provided that he or she is no longer receiving treatment directly related to the hospital admission, and if he/she possesses a physician's certificate of competency.[80] Thus, the statutory language for all practical purposes denies the person the right to continue treatment and to concurrent employment. Although this statutory language has not yet been challenged in the courts, it probably would not withstand a constitutional challenge as being violative of the right to the least restrictive treatment.

A recent U.S. Supreme Court decision has thrown some light upon the vague requirement that the handicap be related to the position sought as it applies to handicapped persons. In *Southeastern Community College* v. *Davis*,[81] a hearing-impaired licensed practical nurse sought admission to the registered nursing program of the defendant college, a state institution receiving federal funds. Ms. Davis's application was rejected because the college felt that her hearing disability made it impossible for her to safely participate in the clinical portion of the program. That clinical portion included participation in operating-room procedures during which the participants would be wearing surgical masks. Suit was brought against the college pursuant to section 504 of the Rehabilitation Act of 1973[82] and the Fourth and Fourteenth amendments to the Constitution of the United States, which guarantee due process and equal protection of the laws. Section 504 of the Rehabilitation Act prohibits discrimination against otherwise qualified handicapped individuals in federally funded programs solely by reason of the handicap. Ms. Davis alleged that the action of the college in denying her admission not only violated her rights to due process and equal protection but also her rights under section 504. The court stated that an otherwise qualified person is one who meets all of the requirements of the program in spite of the handicap and that "mere possession of a handicap is not a permissible ground for assuming an inability to function in a particular context."[83] Addressing the question of "necessary physical qualification," the court found that the ability to understand without relying on lipreading is necessary for patient safety during the clinical phase of the program. Thus, without directly stating it, the court indicated that handicaps rationally related to job performance are those handicaps which should actually prevent performance.*

In an earlier case, *Glassman* v. *New York Medical College*,[84] a New York court found a former resident of a mental institution who had exhibited suicidal tendencies might be denied admission to a medical school on the basis that such tendencies, together with a record showing a pattern of interrupted studies, would render her unable to practice medicine and even to complete medical training. It should be noted that Ms. Glassman completed her undergraduate work while institutionalized. Since the *Glassman* case was decided in 1970 and on the basis of the New York Mental Hygiene law in force at that time, one might speculate that an action brought pursuant to the Rehabilitation Act of 1973 would be decided differently.

The chronic psychiatric patient faces employment issues even in community residences. The philosophy of the community residence movement is that the former patients should be provided a milieu which is both therapeutic and approximates a "normal" living situation or home environment. In such living arrangements certain maintenance tasks, perforce, are to be performed. It would be reasonable for the residents themselves to perform such tasks, thereby decreasing

**As discussed in Section A,* supra, *where no case precedent exists, attorneys look for analogous statutes and cases.*

the costs of the residential care. However, three questions arise regarding the residents' performing such tasks. First, should the residents be compensated for performing these tasks? Second, if the residents should be compensated for performing the tasks, should they be compensated for performing all tasks related to the care and upkeep of the premises, and what factors determine which activities are compensable? Third, what wages should the residents be paid for the compensable tasks?

In the 1973 case of *Souder* v. *Brennan*,[85] which involved institutionalized mentally ill patients, the District Court for the District of Columbia responded to the three questions in the following manner. The 1966 Amendments to the Fair Labor Standards Act of 1938 extended coverage under the maximum wage and overtime provisions of the Act to employees of public and private nonfederal hospitals and institutions for the residential care of the mentally ill. The court examined the statutory definition of "employ" (to suffer or permit to work) and applied the "economic reality" test of employment. The test revealed that "the reality is" that patient-workers perform work for which they are not handicapped (if handicapped, the patients might be paid a reduced wage), and the institution derived full economic benefit from the performance of such work. The work referred to by the court primarily involved washing dishes, helping in the kitchens and performing messenger services, which could be performed by nonhandicapped workers and did not include the maintenance of the patient's own quarters or tasks deemed to be "therapeutically beneficial." The *Souder* Court not only provided some guidelines as to the types of activities for which the institutionalized mentally infirm should be paid, it also held that patient-workers should receive the minimum wage.

However, in 1976, the United States Supreme Court in *National League of Cities* v. *Usery*[86] held that the minimum wage and hour provisions of the Fair Labor Standards Act cannot be constitutionally applied to state and local governments. Subsequent to the *National League of Cities* case, the National Labor Relations Board[87] assumed jurisdiction for collective bargaining purposes over a private nonprofit corporation which provided residential services to mentally disabled persons pursuant to a contract with the Commonwealth of Pennsylvania. If the community residence is funded by, but not operated by, a state mental health agency, it would appear that *National League of Cities* would not impact on the rights of the residents to be paid for performance of nonpersonal household tasks at the minimum wage. Moreover, some states by statute and/or regulation[88] have provided that "federal and state laws relating to wages, hours or work, workman's compensation and other labor standards" are applicable to residents who voluntarily perform labor; in this case, the residents would be paid the minimum wage.

While *Souder* set forth no specific standards for determining which tasks constitute labor, one test has been suggested: What would a tenant ordinarily do for himself? An activity which a tenant would ordinarily do for himself, such as vacuuming the rug, would not constitute labor. An activity which a landlord would ordinarily contract to have performed, such as painting the exterior of the building, would constitute compensable labor if performed by community residents. Certain activities such as lawn maintenance are not easily classified as labor or nonlabor and may become the subject of future litigation.

C. *The Vote*

Many states, generally by means of constitutional provisions, disenfranchise the "insane," "feebleminded," "mentally incompetent" and "idiots."[89] Most states have no criteria for determining who should be denied the right to vote because of mental disability, although adjudication of incompetency through guardianship proceedings, for example, would seem to be sufficient to disqualify one from voting.[90]

Practically, however, it would be extremely difficult to prevent a former resident of a mental hospital from exercising his/her voting right. Nor would there seem to be any reason for denying the right to vote to any person who is able to make a selection. Further, given the bases upon which the average American makes his/her choice, it is unlikely that mental patients, formerly or presently residents of state mental hospitals, will base their selections on any less rational criteria. Moreover, the mechanisms necessary to fairly evaluate competency to vote would be prohibitive in cost and would result in the disenfranchisement of vast numbers of citizenry. Thus, there have been no notable decisions in this area.[91]

D. *Election To Public Office*

While to date no appellate decisions have been reported regarding the denial of the right of a deinstitutionalized mental patient to seek public office, the case of Senator William Eagleton fairly illustrates public attitude towards potential office holders who have become involved with the mental health system. After his selection as presidential running mate in 1972, an investigation into his background revealed that Eagleton had undergone psychiatric treatment, namely, electric shock therapy. Upon the revelation of this fact, Eagleton "requested" that his name be withdrawn from consideration and apologized abjectly for any embarrassment caused his running mate.[92]

In general, the only qualification for seeking or holding public office is that the candidate be a qualified voter, that is, able to meet age and residential requirements. There are procedures available in virtually all jurisdictions by which office holders who do not perform their official functions may be removed. Thus, there would appear to be no need for 1) violating the privacy of a former mental patient who has provided no grounds for the assumption of incompetency by forcing the revelation of such intimate personal information or 2) disqualifying candidates who have sought psychiatric treatment either on an inpatient or outpatient basis. Procedures for removal of a public office holder on any ground, including inability to function because of a psychiatric disorder, should include a full hearing at which it would have to be proved that the official had not adequately performed his duties.

E. Right To Contract

Contracts for goods and services

A contract made by a person who has not been adjudicated as incompetent may be avoided by that person upon a showing that at the time of contracting he/she was in such a state of insanity as to "render him incapable of transacting the business."[93] When the fact is established, it is no defense to the voiding of the contract that the other party acted fairly and without knowledge of any circumstances which should have made him question the ability of the individual to form a contract. It is the inability of a person to understand the nature, quality and significance of a transaction which causes him to be incapable of forming a valid contract. Although the individual may avoid the contract, he/she would still be held liable for the fair market value of "necessaries" which are not returned. The term necessaries is a flexible term which generally includes food, clothing, medical attention, shelter and even education.

A few courts do not permit the avoidance of contracts where the other party acts in good faith and without knowledge of incompetency and cannot be returned to the status quo.[94] Where this doctrine prevails, the right to avoid is conditioned upon the return of the goods purchased.

The general rule is that a mentally ill person who has entered into a contract during a period of nonlucidity may ratify that contract when he/she becomes lucid or sane. If he/she chooses not to ratify the contract, he is not required to return any goods as a condition of avoiding the contract, although as noted above, he would be responsible for paying the fair market value of any necessaries. The rationale behind this principle is the protection by law of those who are unable to protect themselves. Thus, a person whose mental illness is controlled by medication would be required to fulfill any contractual obligation into which he entered. However, should that same person cease his medication, become irrational and enter into a contract to buy stocks, for example, he could later either, with impunity, refuse to honor the contract, or continue with the purchase of the stocks.[95]

F. Marriage Contracts

At common law, the marriage of an insane person was held to be void from the beginning. Some states still hold this position. Thus, the marriage would be as if it had never existed. Other states look at the marriage of a mentally incompetent individual as voidable as any other contract may be voidable. Both views are based upon the premise that for a contract to be valid, the parties must understand the nature of the contract and the duties and responsibilities which it creates. Interestingly, some courts have held that if a marriage is contracted during a "lucid interval" or is later ratified in a lucid interval, it is valid even though the party is mentally ill.[96]

Mental incompetence also is a ground for annulment of a marriage by the competent party, just as in many states it provides the grounds for divorce. The definitions of incompetence range widely, but most often reject rigid definitions and scrutinize the facts of each case in arriving at a determination of competency.[97] The public policy against marriage by incompetents is viewed against the common-law desire to safeguard the voluntary nature of the marriage contract; thus, the test of understanding the duties and responsibilities created by the contract. Some cases, however, have held that the only requirement is that a party entering into a marriage contract need understand the legal consequences of the contract. While this distinction may be more apparent than real, the courts which have adopted the latter view have held that "mere weakness of intellect or imbecility, eccentricity of partial dementia do not disqualify one for marriage."[98] It is unfortunate that the language by courts disregards such factors as the individual's ability to meet the demands of a stable and lasting relationship or to provide for any children of the marriage.

G. Wills

One's last will and testament may be deemed to be a form of contract, a contract between the testator and his or her beneficiaries. Thus, a will may be attacked by relatives who feel that they have been improperly omitted from a will on the grounds that the testator was not of sound mind when he/she signed the will. The persons who witness the signing of the will indicate that the testator signed the will in their presence, and that the testator was of sound mind at the time of the signing. However, the validity of the will may still be challenged on the basis of the incompetence of the testator.[99]

IV. THE AUTHORITY OF GUARDIANSHIP-CONSERVATORSHIPS

Virtually every state has laws providing for the appointment of guardians or conservators for those persons incapable of caring for themselves by reason of mental illness. Such appointments may provide the guardian or conservator with the power to commit the wards for the purpose of treatment for mental illness. Recent legislations and judicial decisions, however, have imposed constraints upon the authority of such guardians or conservators to commit their wards for treatment.

In Massachusetts, for example, such authority is denied a guardian unless . . . "The court specifically finds the same [treatment] to be in the best interest of such persons and specifically so authorizes such admission or commitment by its order or decree."[100] The court may not authorize commitment or admission unless a hearing has been held at which the ward is present and represented by an attorney. In *Fazio* v. *Fazio*[101] the Supreme Judicial Court of

Massachusetts held that in addition to a showing of mental illness there must be evidence that the proposed ward is unable to think or act for himself/herself in matters of personal health, safety and welfare. In a 1979 decision, *Doe* v. *Doe*,[102] the same court held that the "best interest" requirement can only be satisfied by a showing of a likelihood of the occurrence of serious harm to the ward or others. Further, the court found that a finding of serious harm must be supported by proof beyond a reasonable doubt—the standard applied in court-ordered (involuntary) civil commitments in Massachusetts.[103]

Similarly, the California Supreme Court in *Heap* v. *Roulet*[104] has ruled that before a proposed conservator can be appointed under California statute with power to involuntarily commit a proposed conservatee, a finding must be made that the proposed conservatee is gravely disabled as the result of a mental disorder. That finding must be proved beyond a reasonable doubt, and when a jury is requested, it must be decided by a unanimous verdict.

V. COMMITMENT REQUIREMENT—STANDARDS OF PROOF

Since the issuance of the Massachusetts and California opinions, the United States Supreme Court in *Addington* v. *Texas*[105] held that the standard of proof to be applied in civil commitment cases is that of "clear and convincing" evidence. The court rejected the argument that the deprivation of freedom in civil commitment cases is as extreme as the deprivation in criminal cases and therefore refused to require the criminal standard of beyond a reasonable doubt. The court based its opinion in part upon the fact that uncertainties of psychiatric diagnoses might render the standard's imposition of an unreasonable barrier to needed medical treatment.[106]

The function of the standard of proof is to "instruct the fact finder concerning the degree of confidence our society thinks he should have in the correctness of factual conclusions for a particular type of adjudication."[107] The standard allocates the risk of error of the decision between the litigants and shows the relative importance of the ultimate decision. There are generally three standards of proof imposed, reflecting differing degrees of certainty. The least restrictive standard is the preponderance of the evidence, the standard applied in the typical civil case involving monetary disputes. In criminal cases the interests of the defendant are so great that historically they have been protected by a standard of proof intended to eliminate so far as possible the likelihood of error in judgment. The intermediate standard of "clear," "cogent," "unequivocal" or "convincing" evidence is applied in civil cases involving allegations of fraud or other activities of a quasicriminal nature.[108]

The holding of the *Addington* court does not negate either the California or Massachusetts holdings or the statutes and decisions of the other eleven states requiring proof beyond a reasonable doubt of the need for commitment. As stated by Chief Justice Burger, "The essence of federalism is that states must be free to develop a variety of solutions to problems and not be forced into a common, uniform mold. As the substantive standards for civil commitment may vary from state to state, procedures must be allowed to vary so long as they meet the constitutional minimum."[109]

SUMMARY

As the decisions discussed in this chapter illustrate, this decade has been characterized by increasing attention by the judiciary to the rights of the mentally disabled. Those rights include the right to treatment, the right to treatment in the least restrictive setting and the right to refuse treatment. Because of judicial attention to these rights and the community mental health movement, the chronically mentally disabled are less isolated from society, have expanded opportunities to engage in gainful employment and are less often stigmatized by the fact of their illness or disability.

However, exercise of the right to refuse treatment conceivably could result in the curtailment of extended rights and opportunities. If, as suggested, patients who refuse treatment must be discharged from hospitalization, their ability to avail themselves of or to benefit from the expanded community opportunities is problematic. Mental health professionals are now confronted with a dilemma which by logic and training they should be equipped to resolve. Nevertheless, resolution of medical legal questions of this nature is the province of the courts whose action is imminent.

NOTES

1. Rule 23, Fed. R. Civ. Pro., 28 USCA.
2. *Saikewicz* v. *Superintendent of Belchertown State School*, 370 N.E. 2d 417 (Mass. 1977).
3. *In re Karen Ann Quinlan*, 355 A.2d 647 (N.J. 1976).

4. See, e.g., 21 USC s 360(g), Federal Food, Drug and Costmetic Act provides for judicial review of Food and Drug Administration orders by the United States Circuit Court of Appeals for the District of Columbia or for the circuit where the affected individual has his place of business.
5. U. S. Constitution, Article III s 1,2.
6. Id. Note 5.
7. e.g., Massachusetts, New Hampshire, Maine, Rhode Island, Florida, Colorado and South Dakota. See generally, Field, "The Advisory Opinion-An Analysis," 24 Ind.L.J. 203 (1949).
8. M'Naughten's Case, 8 Eng. Rep. 718 (House of Lords 1843). The M'Naughten Rules are stated, in part, as follows (the right and wrong test):

   > [T]hat to establish a defense of insanity, it must be clearly proved that at the time of the committing of the act the party accused was labouring under such a defect of reason, from disease of the mind as not to know the nature of the act he was doing: or if he did know it, that he did not know what he was doing wrong.

   This test was later supplemented by the "irresistible impulse test" or the diminished responsibility test. However, thirteen states and all the federal districts have adopted the American Law Institute test:

   > A person is not responsible for criminal conduct if at the time of such conduct as a result of mental disease or defect he lacks substantial capacity either to appreciate the criminality (wrongfulness) of his conduct or to conform his conduct to the requirements of law.

9. 373 F. 2d 451 (D.C. Cir. 1976).
10. 233 N.E.2d 908 (Mass. 1968).
11. Id.
12. *Lake* v. *Cameron*, 364 F.2d 657 (D.C.Cir. 1966).
    Wyatt v. *Stickney*, 325 F.Supp. 781 (1971), affirmed in part, reversed in part sub.nom. *Wyatt* v. *Anderholt*, 503 F.2d 1305 (5th Cir. 1974).
    Burnham v. *Department of Public Health of State of Ga*, 349 F. Supp. 1335 (1971).
    Suzaki v. *Quisenberry*, 411 F. Supp. 1113 (D.C. Hawaii 1976).
13. 325 F. Supp. 780, 784 (1971).
14. *Wyatt* v. *Stickney*, 344 F.Supp. 387, 390 (1971).
15. 493 F. 2d 507 (5th Cir. 1974).
16. *O'Connor* v. *Donaldson*, 95 S.Ct. 2486 (1976).
17. Supra, Note 15.
18. Supra, Note 16 at 2488.
19. Id.
20. *Lessard* v. *Schmidt*, 349 F.Supp. 1018, 1096.
21. Id.
22. Supra, Note 12.
23. 386 F. Supp. 378 (MD. Ala. 1974).
24. Supra, Note 12.
25. *Dixon* v. *Weinberger*, 405 F.Supp. 974, 976 (1975).
26. Id.

27. 42 USCA ss 2681-2687.
28. *New York* v. *State Association for Retarded Citizens* and *Parisi* v. *Carey*, 466 F. Supp. 487 (E.D.N.Y. 1979).
29. *Schloendorf* v. *Society of New York Hospital,* 211 N.Y. 125, 105 N.E.93, 93 (N.Y. 1914).
30. 464 F. 2d. 772 (D.C.Cor. 1972).
31. 8 Cal. 3d. 229, 104 Cal Report. 505 (1972).
32. Supra, Note 24.
33. Supra, Note 25.
34. Michigan Circuit Court for Wayne County, Civil No. 73-19434-AW, 2 Prison L. Reprt. (1973).
35. Supra, Note 3.
36. Supra, Note 2.
37. Supra, Note 28.
38. See, eg., Ore. Rev. Stat. ss 426.700 et seq. (1973);
Cal. Penal Code s 2670 et. seq. (West Supp. 1976);
Ohio Rev Code ss.512.271 (A) (7), (B).
39. *Rennie* v. *Klein,* in fra, note 37 and cases cited therein.
40. 446 F. 2d. 65, cert. denied, 404 U.S. 985.
41. See, *In re Boyd,* 403 F. 2d. 744 (D.C.Cir. 1979). When a legally incompetent patient asserts his First Amendment right not to receive psychotropic drugs and those drugs are not needed to save the patient's life, the court in deciding whether to order medication looked at must first decide: (1) whether prior to becoming incompetent the individual had rejected medication absolutely on religious grounds; (2) whether evidence exists which demonstrates on the part of the patient a strong adherence to the tenets of the faith;and (3) whether there is no countervailing evidence of vacillation.
42. The constitutional right to privacy was first enunciated in *Griswold* v. *Connecticut,* 381 U.S. 479 (1965) in which it was found to lie in the penumbra of the rights guaranteed by the First Amendment to the Constitution.
43. 462 F. Supp. 1131; No. 77-2624 (D.N.J. Sept. 14, 1979).
44. *In the Matter of the Hospitalization of B,* 383 A.2d 760 (N.J.Super. 1977).
45. 42 USCA 1983 provides for relief for persons whose constitutional rights are violated by persons "acting under color of" state or territorial law.
46. Supra, Note 43.
47. Supra, Note 43.
48. Supra, Note 43.
49. 478 F. Supp. 1342 (1979).
50. Id.
51. Id. at 1361.
52. Id.
53. Supra, Note 16.
54. Becker, A., Schulberg, H. Phasing out state hospitals, a psychiatric dilemma. *N. Eng. Jnl. Med* 294: 255.
55. 70 N.J. Super. 381, 175 A.2d.500 (1961).
56. 60 Wisc. 2d 182, 208 N.W. 2d 121 (1973), cert denied, 416 U.S. 936 (1974).
57. Id.
58. 416 U.S. 1 (1974).

59. Id. at 2.
60. 72 Misc. 2d 523, 339 N.Y.2d 511 (Sup.Ct. 1973).
61. 377 F. Supp. 177 (E.D. N.Y. 1974).
62. Supra, Note 12.
63. Supra, Note 16.
64. No. (S) H-D-60289-78 (N.Y. Div. of Human Rights, 1978).
65. See, *English* v. *Zoning Board of Appeals of Town of Evans*, N.Y. Sup. Ct., Ma7 8, 1978).
66. *Alexander* v. *Minnesota Jewish Group Homes*, No. 746834 (4th Jud. Dist. 1978).
67. *Brownfield* v. *Ohio*, No. 77-12-2995 (Ohio Summit Court, 1978).
68. Id.
69. Mass App, 366 NE.2d 764 (1977).
70. Eg. Recently a school official was reportedly fired because he was undergoing treatment for mental illness, Boston Globe, Dec. 14, 1979.
71. 28 USCA 1343.
72. PL 94-141.
73. See, e.g. *Arnette* v. *Kennedy*, 416 U.S. 134 (1974).
74. Ill. Const. Art. 1 s. 19.
75. Equal Opportunities for Handicapped Act, *Ill. Ann Stat.* ch. 38 ss 62-21 to 65-31.
76. Id. s 65.22.
77. Supra, Note 12.
78. Id.
79. M.G.L. ch. 151B s 4 (9A)
80. Id.
81. 98 S.Ct. 2361 (1979).
82. Id. at 2367.
83. Id. at 2366.
84. 64 Misc. 2d 466, 315 N.Y.2d 1 (1970).
85. 367 F.Supp. 808 (D.D.C. 1973).
86. 426 U.S. 833 (1976).
87. Mon Valley United Health Services, 99 LRRM 1332 (1978).
88. e.g. 104 CMR 14.03 (7), Mass.
89. See generally, *American Bar Foundation, The Mentally Disabled and the Law* (Brakel and Rock, eds., 1971).
90. Id.
91. Id.
92. Id.
93. 2 Williston Contracts s 251 (3d ed. 1959).
94. Simpson contracts s 112 (2ed. 1965).
95. Id.
96. Id.
97. Clark Domestic Relations s 13.2 (1st ed. 1968).
98. Id. s 2.15.

In determining whether to terminate the rights of a mentally disabled parent to the care and custody of his/her minor children, courts weigh the parents traditional interest in such care and custody against the interest of the child in a safe environment. In recent decisions the courts have looked at the parent's present ability, not at proof of a mental disorder, past or present.

See, e.g., *In re Mark "GG"*, 419 N.Y.S. 2d 275 (N.Y. Sup Ct. App. Divn. 1979); *In re Custody of a Minor*, 339 N.E. 2d 379 (Mass. 1979); *Price* v. *Price*, 255 S.E.2d 652 (N.C.1979); *In re Baby Suchy*, 281 N.W.2d 273 (Minn. 1979).

99. *Addington* v. *Texas*, 39 CCH S. Ct. Bull B2271.
100. M.G.L. ch. 201 s 6 as amended St. 1972 ch 567 s 1.
101. Mass Adv. Sh., 378 N.E.2d 951 (1978).
102. Mass Adv. Sh., 385 N.E.2d 995 (1979).
103. Id.
104. 50 P. 2d 1 (Cal. 1979).
105. Supra, Note 87.
106. Id.
107. Supra, Note 87 at B2275 citing *In re Winship*, 397 U.S. 358 (1970) (Harlan, J. Concurring).
108. McCormack Evidence s 320 (1954).
109. Supra, Note 87 at 2283;
Haw. Rev. Stat. s 334-60 (4) (I); Idaho Code s 66-329 (i); Kan. Stat. Ann. s 59-2917; Mont. Rev. Codes Ann s 38-1305(7); Okla. Stat. Tit. 43A s 54.1 (C); Ore. Rev. Stat. s 46.130; Utah Code Ann. s 64-7-36(6); Wis. Stat. s 51.20 (14) (c); *Superintendent of Worcester State Hospital* v. *Hagberg*, Mass., 372 N.E. 2d 242; *Proctor* v. *Butler*, 380 A. 2d 673 (N.H. 1977).

PART VI

OVERVIEW

CHAPTER 21

ESSENTIAL PRINCIPLES IN THE DELIVERY OF ADEQUATE CLINICAL CARE TO THE CHRONIC PSYCHIATRIC PATIENT IN THE COMMUNITY

RICHARD D. BUDSON, M.D.

Effective management of the chronic psychiatric patient in the community requires recognition of its complexity in a variety of ways. First, when one attempts to define the chronic patient, it is immediately apparent that a broad group of psychiatric patients could be so labelled. In particular, schizophrenic and paranoid disorders, the affective disorders and the personality disorders can all persist for years or typically run a course of remissions and exacerbations throughout a person's lifetime. Further, the degree of disorder, irrespective of diagnosis, can be extremely variable. Some patients are easily managed by a single clinician who is able to achieve a working alliance with the patient who is insightful and cooperative. Others are extremely vulnerable to totally disabling aberrations of thought and behavior, have no insight, and have little motivation to work with an entire team of rehabilitative mental health professionals, who find themselves exhausted at the effort.

In particular, the issue which is most pressing is that patients who are very difficult to manage for a variety of reasons, who in past decades would most assuredly have been managed in the completely closed setting of psychiatric hospital, must now be managed entirely in the community. In fact, the urgency of this book is in the concern that these patients, who at least in the past were safe within the confines of a medical institution in spite of its rehabilitative shortcomings, are now potentially inadvertent victims of neglect, for whatever reason—a condition which can lead to deterioration and misery. Within the mental hospital were performed a whole host of functions which, in fact, provided the patient with vital supports—housing, adequate diet, routine and emergency medical and dental care, clothing and, generally, protection from the pressures of outside living. The dangers of crime as experienced in the lowest socioeconomic sections of the urban environment, to which these patients are likely to drift once in the community, was not an issue; nor was there any necessity for the patient to negotiate his financial support with impersonal, often unresponsive, governmental agencies.

Thus, there is a concern for that patient, whatever diagnosis, who has a persistent or remittent mental disorder, and who in the past would likely have been hospitalized, but who now has to fend largely for himself in the community. Further, an inescapable moral issue facing all concerned parties is that for some patients without adequate treatment and rehabilitative measures, a likely outcome will be one which ought to be unacceptable to a civilized society. These occurring but heinous potentialities include the most objectionable—suicide, homicide, death through starvation, exposure or murder. No less acceptable is the slow deterioration of total social isolation, emptiness and gradually failing mental functioning, with the onset of hallucinations and delusions, resulting in a nonfunctioning, often terrified, subtly self-destructive, empty shell of a human being who is unable to care for himself in any effective manner; nor is yet another possibility any more acceptable—the persistent self-mutilation of limbs and torso in an escalating exercise in gradual self-destruction. And finally, equally unacceptable, is the episodic, wild, excited state of social provocation which repeatedly results in a person's being assaulted and dangerously injured.

These are the chronically mentally ill with whom we are especially concerned. There is no question but that a formidable goal is the acquisition of adequate financial resources to care for the thousands of patients so affected. But, putting that issue aside, we are at the same time in the infancy of learning how to best clinically manage these patients outside the confines of medical institutions. For these are the patients for whom adequate community treatment is most difficult to deliver. The length and comprehensiveness of this text is testimony to the difficulty of the task. Yet, indeed, it is not inclusive. Our medical libraries are filled with tomes of additional information and other valid points of view. But what is the single clinician to do? What is to guide the team of professionals? How can one possibly hope to approach a patient in all his complexity? What follows are some basic principles of care as they have evolved through the author's experience with such a population over a period of eleven years during which some 400 patients in the community were treated.

First, the chronically mentally ill are not a monolithic mass of troubled humanity as is so often implied in the literature. Rather, it is essential to clinically approach these patients, recognizing that they are represented by a number of different diagnostic groups. Two studies of "young" chronic patients in New York State Mental Health Centers portray this general reality. In the Rockland County Community Mental Health Center, of 900 patients between 18 and 30, 300 were categorized as chronic; and of these, 169 or 56% were schizophrenic, 12% had personality disorders and 7% had an effective disorder. Similar results were found in Hutchings Psychiatric Center in Onondaga County, New York, where 44% of the patients seen were between the ages of 18 and 34, and of those, 369 or 36% were judged to be chronic. Here again, of this 18 to 30 group, of 344 young adult, chronic patients, 171 were diagnosed as schizophrenic, 24 had major affective disorders, 32 personality disorders 25 neuroses, 8 substance abuse or dependency and 16 organic brain syndrome. Additionally, a major issue that comes up in all populations is suicide. In the Rockland County study, 42% of the 300 young chronics had suicide as a major issue (Pepper 1981).

Given this variability within the chronic population, a cardinal principle is that there is no substitute for a careful and accurate diagnosis. This is clearly because significant physiological, psychological, social and behavioral characteristics vary according to diagnosis and alter characteristic patterns of illness as manifested over time, which absolutely dictate the method of treatment. This is particularly so in regard to pharmacotherapy. At the same time, it is acknowledged that sometimes diagnosis is difficult to achieve. Even the most sophisticated clinicians and researchers are today debating whether schizoaffective illness exists or not—as opposed to either one or the other—schizophrenia or manic-depressive illness. But there is at the same time not one iota of debate that it is a tragic error to mistake a psychotic depression for schizophrenia and thereby to deprive the patient of antidepressant treatment which could dramatically obliterate the symptoms and restore him to health—the omission of which could lead to months of lack of treatment for symptoms of lethargy, inability to concentrate and withdrawal, which are sometimes mistaken for schizophrenic signs of social apathy instead of recognized as those of depression. Further, the impulsivity, unstable interpersonal relationships, affective instability, identity disturbances and chronic feelings of emptiness of the borderline personality disorder should not be mistaken for schizophrenia with the unfortunate, unnecessary utilization of phenothiazines and a subsequent gratuitous risk of tardive dyskinesia.

It is also important to note that there are significant diagnostic differences in the way patients respond to selected individual and group encounters. For instance, it has been found that the same active supervision and interaction of mental patients in foster homes, which results in improvement of nonschizophrenics, leads to deterioration in schizophrenics (Linn 1981). Such a research finding has important program planning ramifications which cannot be ignored. Similarly, an escalating hypomanic will need a structured, closely supervised milieu program, which is precisely what may be noxious to the schizophrenic. An additional important diagnostic consideration is the recognition that, in a patient with manic-depressive illness in remission, increased rage or a sudden ability to cause others to laugh may mean incipient psychosis. These affective states must not, then, be taken only at their face value without due caution and assessment in relation to diagnostic considerations.

The second vital consideration, after diagnosis, is the overall necessity for any significant person involved in the treatment of a patient to be truly knowledgeable about the patient and concerned for his well-being. A comprehensive assessment of the individual mental health worker's role with the chronic patient reveals a series of interrelated issues which must be addressed. First of all, there are a number of tasks which must be performed that are crucial to the welfare of the patient—helping to see to it that there are adequate housing, medical care, vocational training, family liaison meetings, financial aids, medication and so forth. These must be coordinated by a person who is most knowledgeable about the patient. Having *adequate, thorough knowledge* about the patient and all of his strengths and vulnerabilities, then, is the second requirement of the mental health professional. This, in particular, includes two very special kinds of knowledge. The first is knowing that particular situation which is characteristically experienced as stressful by the patient and which has been shown through experience to precipitate exacerbation of the illness and relapse. The second is the awareness of those specific patterns of behavior which typically are early premorbid signs of incipient relapse. This kind of in-depth knowledge, however, is best acquired through therapeutic closeness to the patient. In particular, when the clinician is able to be close to the patient, he learns firsthand about the patient's sensitivities and the reasons for them. In this way, he learns both through thoughtful observations and directly from the patient's own explanations and verbal expressions. At this point, the clinician encounters a dilemma—namely, that it is very difficult to be close to some of the chronically ill. Here there is a significant diagnostic difference. The manic-depressive patient in remission is often seemingly normal and easy to work with interpersonally. The borderline patient is easy to approach, and the problem is usually one of careful limit setting, done in such a manner so as to communicate firmness and reality limitations without communicating rejection to the patient. To achieve closeness with the schizophrenic patient requires the most skill. This is particularly so in two different stages: the initial phase of treatment and over the long haul. The initial phase has been described as the out-of-touch phase, and the long-haul phase is fraught with the vulnerability to staff burnout due to staff's high expectations for rapid movement of the patient.

Harold Searles has described an initial "out of contact" phase. The therapist feels that the patient does not perceive him as a person in the here and now since the patient is often lost "in a world of chaotically disturbed and distorted perceptions." In this potentially extended phase, the patient is out of touch with his feelings. Instead, his feeling-potentialities have long ago become condensed into bizarre symptomatology—hallucinations, delusional and neologistic utterances, and stereotyped and manneristic nonverbal behavior. The clinician consequently "experiences little in the way of his own feeling responses to the patient's behavior, except for a sense of strangeness and of allienness" (Searles 1965). Studies have shown that in response to this sense of strangeness and alienation, the mental health worker has often experienced intense personal anxiety and discomfort. The net result is often a pattern of avoidance of the patient by the professional and a defensive gravitation toward the safety of relating with other available professional colleagues. This kind of avoidance, in general, would be considered antitherapeutic. However, in schizophrenia, the problems of individual closeness, as considered here, and group relatedness, as considered below, are increasingly recognized as very difficult.

In schizophrenia, there is a dilemma in balancing the need for some social relationships on the one hand with the need to avoid a noxious level of emotional intensity on the other. Wing (1978) has adroitly addressed this problem in reviewing the work of Goldberg, Schooler and Hogarty (1977), Stevens (1973), and Stone and Eldred

(1959). These studies identify that patients living in a sheltered environment relapse very quickly when they are exposed to a program of rehabilitation that asks too much of them. Then again he describes the "clinical poverty syndrome" characterized by social understimulation. He concludes that patients who suffer from schizophrenia "remain vulnerable to social stresses of two rather different kinds. On the one hand, too much social stimulation, experienced by the patient as social intrusiveness, may lead to an acute relapse. On the other hand, too little stimulation will exacerbate any tendency already present toward social withdrawal. . . . Thus the patient has to walk a tightrope between two different types of danger and it is easy to become decompensated either way."

Contributing to this area of investigation is the concept of high and low "expressed emotion" (EE), identified by Brown, Birley and Wing (1972) and recently further developed by Vaughn and Leff (1981). These investigators have correlated high rehospitalization rates (58%) of patients returning to families with high EE which present attitudes of intrusiveness, disappointment and pressure on the patient to act normally; whereas patients returning to low EE families (nonintrusive, tolerant of symptom behaviors and understanding of the illness) had much lower relapse rates (16%).

Thus, the field of social supports and schizophrenia is a complicated one. As C. Christian Beels (1981) in an excellent review of the field observed, "There are patients who appear to survive crises with the help of friends, relatives and therapists. On the other hand . . . some patients are overwhelmed instead of supported by their social connections in ways that are not easy to define."

Recognizing these dilemmas, the clinician initially makes a carefully considered effort to be close to his patients, and is always sensitive to his degree of tolerance for social intimacy.

An additional reason to strive for such therapeutic closeness is the necessity to have an alliance with the patient. Again, diagnostically, there are different issues. Alliance means that with the borderline, the patient is increasingly able to tolerate limits, to have an observing ego so that he can tolerate increasingly painful affect, and autonomy gradually ensues which enables him to have a healthier life. In the case of the manic depressive, alliance is the trustworthy taking of lithium, and working with the therapist in order to tolerate the realities of a euphoria-free, normal, affective state—or even allowing oneself to experience sadness—as opposed to the patient who purposefully stops medication in order to achieve a psychotic state of mania to forestall any painful feelings. Alliance, in working with the depressive, is crucial for the preservation of life. In suicidal patients, the foremost focus of treatment is working through the recognition that in many cases the suicidal wish is a desire for relief of pain, which is transient and can be resolved in more constructive, life-sustaining ways. In the case of schizophrenics, as well as in all of the others, alliance is required in order to facilitate the increasing development of self-knowledge. The attainment of the patient's self-understanding ought to be a primary goal of both patient and therapist. The patient's recognition of his weaknesses as well as his strengths approaches the goal of a capacity to cope, and subsequently fosters increasing independence and inherent individual dignity. The attainment of self-knowledge allows *the patient* to increasingly learn of his vulnerabilities so that he can avoid noxious situations or, if unavoidable, take action to provide increased supports in times of predictable, emotional crises. The concept of preparation for stress is vital to the successful avoidance of breakdown under its pressures.

Finally, the attainment and working through of a successful alliance, through which self-knowledge is gained, is the matrix and basis upon which is developed the understanding of the importance in life of altruistic feelings and care about one's fellow man. This approaches the patient's sharing with the therapist the ethical concept of the responsibility of one human being for another in the family of mankind. In this context, the patient learns that not only can he benefit from the therapist's commitment to his well-being and his own knowledge about it, but he himself can gain and benefit from rendering care, understanding and concern for others. The capacity to care for others is then an attestation of yet another crucial principle: namely, that man lives naturally in the context of social networks and that interdependent social networks form extended psychosocial kinship systems that help to sustain the health of all concerned. The successful attainment of a caring, working alliance with a therapist, thus leading to the development of the ability to care for others, ultimately helps the patient to be part of an extended psychosocial kinship system that preserves and sustains health and well-being, and that also gives a feeling of being meaningfully engaged in society. From emptiness, isolation and withdrawal, treatment, under ideal conditions, can thus help the patient to attain the fullness of a meaningful life.

The third cardinal issue in treating the chronic psychiatric patient in the community is the recognition that all of the clinicians providing services to the patient in the different sectors—outpatient medication clinic, vocational training, social club, community residence, social services, family liaison—must work together collaboratively to provide the patient with a comprehensive, integrated, consistent treatment. This ideally comes about *not* through a single person who is denoted the "broker" of services, but rather through a process of the *entire* team meeting together as a whole periodically and sustaining additional communication as required. This is vital because the treatment team, in fact, becomes a crucial part of the patient's social network. Further, I would make the argument that when the staff works closely together it becomes, in Hammer's (1981) terms, a *supported* social network for the patient. By having linkages within its own ranks and not only to the patient, the network (in this instance, clinicians) is more likely to be effective in supporting the patient in a variety of crisis situations. This is because the participants are in a position to more naturally collaborate, first in recognizing impending stress, then in making it more likely preventable, as well as in managing an already manifest situation.

There are yet broader ramifications of the need for the staff to relate collaboratively as a supported social network. It is important to recognize that, irrespective of how the clinical team works together, the patient himself has to relate to, and is affected by, each of its component parts. Even if the team does not work at coordinating the treatment, the fact is that the patient is ultimately faced with this integrative task. If the clinicians don't work together, then the patient is put in a position of having to deal with a crucial reality which is ignored by the very people who are supposed to be helping. This can become an independent, iatrogenic stress introduced by the treatment system and significant in a variety of ways. First of all, the lack of intercommunication within the team can produce unclear and conflicting messages to the patient, which can replicate the adverse situation occurring in pathologic, conflicted and chaotic families (Lewis 1979). Such families have fragmented, unclear, disorganized communications and conflicting power structures that often lead to withdrawal, anxiety and confusion among family members, which contributes to patienthood. If, on the other hand, the patient can experience a consistent, coordinated, sustaining, thoughtful, caring group of clinicians, all of whom communicate well together and universally show the patient that his best interest is their first priority, then this very integration of the treatment can, in and of itself, be tantamount to a corrective, emotional, therapeutic experience.

The importance of this principle is demonstrable in several different ways which are characteristic of the different diagnostic groups. Typically, chronic, schizophrenic patients have been found to have very small social networks. It is not clear whether these patients started out with small networks or lost their networks due to their illness. There is evidence that there is a clustering among kin rather than nonkin. In such patients, there are suggestions that even when there are some nonkin persons in the network, they are often unsupported connections. In Hammer's (1981) terms, the network is not *clustered* because the individuals the patient relates to do not relate to each other. And finally, it has been observed that "for schizophrenic patients as well as for normal subjects, connections which are not structurally supported by common other connections have a relatively high likelihood of being severed." The point here is that the schizophrenic patient in treatment in the community ought not to find himself with a treatment team which is similarly unconnected. The patient himself may well tend to relate to the different spheres of his life in a very disconnected manner, which tends to enhance the different clinicians' isolation. The clinical team's response to this is paramount. For example, an impending visit of a patient's relative, which is known only to the family worker, may cause increasing agitation, delusions and sleeplessness, known to the pharmacotherapist; it will interfere with punctuality and concentration at the workshop, known only to the vocational counselor; and it will be disruptive to the community residence, known solely to its manager. If these four mental health professionals do not communicate, they may entirely miss the significance of the overall picture and respond in an inadequate, fragmented manner—no single clinician understanding either why there is a pathologic change or that there is a simultaneous deterioration in every sphere. Without communication, any one of these clinicians may sever the patient's connections to his unique program, ultimately resulting in the patient's total relapse and return to the hospital, disconnecting him from his entire community program. Communication, on the other hand, of all parties, could lead to a coordinated effort to support the patient in his efforts to deal with the family member, to provide a temporary increased level of medication, to offer a lightened workload at the workshop, as well as to mobilize group peer support at the residence.

It is not infrequent that borderline patients have had that family experience in which a parent will relate to them in a positive manner only upon the condition that the patient participates in a covert alliance against the other parent. These patients promote splitting amongst staff members with apparent ease, selecting certain staff members to be the positively held object who can do no wrong. Other staff members can be the objects of solely negative feelings. If the staff doesn't talk together, those related to positively may unwittingly begin to believe the patient's negative characterizations of the patient's pathological splitting. It can be, indeed, a unique therapeutic experience for such a patient to have a team of professionals who work together harmoniously in spite of all the patient's efforts to see them as either "bad or good guys." Such patients can also repudiate their own rage but can act in such a manner so as to cause the clinician to experience rage himself, which is then experienced vicariously by the patient, but which also causes guilt in the clinician. This phenomenon of "projective identification" used as a defense by the patient is most effectively identified and managed when the clinician can share with his colleagues the difficulty of handling such a situation.

Suicidal patients in particular are most effectively managed when the network of clinicians works closely together. There should be a prearranged agreement among all clinicians that when any one of them has an increased sense of suicide risk that it should be communicated to all of the others. This, experience has shown, often confirms that others have similarly had an increased sense that conditions were leading to an increased risk. Early intervention, often including a clinical team meeting, can prevent destructive action by the patient and can carefully delineate the precipitating circumstances leading to the deteriorating situation.

Finally, in dealing with all of the chronically ill in the community, it must be recognized that these are difficult patients for staff to treat over the long haul. Sometimes, patients who seem to be hardly improving at all create a feeling of uselessness within the staff. Other times, patients provoke anger and turmoil in the staff, who question whether it is all worth it. This is all the more true in the face of seeming ingratitude by a society which sees fit to consistently fund the public mental health programs inadequately. Such are the conditions which breed burnout. Through mutual support and communication, staff can enrich their therapeutic work through new insights and can comfort each other in their unique discomfort.

A fourth critical principle is the recognition that the structured use of a patient's time during the day, especially through work, at whatever level the patient can manage, can have an important therapeutic effect. While the critical components of the work personality are formed during the period of latency-childhood and adolescence, some children are so traumatized in their earlier years that their subsequent psychological development, including their capacity to work, is seriously harmed. This is often the case for hospitalized mental patients. When a mental patient is recovering and considering entering the world of work, a host of early psychological issues are extremely relevant. These act as a double-edged sword in that a potentially conflict-free work setting may be extremely helpful in stabilizing the patient's life whereas an unduly stressful work setting could lead to relapse. In particular, the author has over the years noted a variety of work issues which are intimately bound to psychological development in the first three stages of life. Attention paid to these issues can make all the difference in effective placement of patients in work settings. Specifically, for the rehabilitating mental patient, going to work can mean a great deal more than having an opportunity to "drain off unacceptable impulses" or having a defense against frightening fantasies. Rather, the work setting itself can be experienced by the vulnerable person with a recent mental illness as providing a significant holding environment—a structured, daily setting to which the patient goes and which gives him a sense of security and identity, regularity and sameness.

A regressed hospitalized patient with an acute paranoid psychosis often experiences problems relating to early oral deprivation. He typically has a sense of distrust if not frank paranoia regarding his environment—feeling his world to be often chaotic, unpredictable, frightening and menacing. He feels alienated and hostile, isolated and abandoned, helpless and weak—having no recognized role, place or identity. Surely, with hospitalization, tranquilizing antipsychotic drugs, milieu management and individual psychological counseling, this patient may have recovered from many of these fearful experiences. However, at a time of stress, such as reentering the outside community, such a patient typically has a very real vulnerability to reexperiencing similar symptomatology. This is particularly so when the person, rehabilitated to this critical point, has no other identity except that of patient. Community placement in such facilities as halfway houses, cooperative apartments or single occupancy hotels with no meaningful daily program resulting in idleness will often lead to such psychological deterioration. It has been observed, however, that engagement in a suitable job may forestall and often prevent such deterioration. To what do we attribute this ameliorating effect of work?

The work experience can provide a profound sense of order replacing chaos. The work day provides a temporal structure and a routine schedule: a time to arise, to bathe, to groom, to eat, to leave the residence for work and to arrive on time; a time to leave work for home, to rest, to socialize, to eat and to retire. The same routine again and again, day after day, in a rhythm of regularity and predictability, yields order and contributes to a sense that the world is safe in its predictability rather than forboding, chaotic and disordered. The constancy of the work setting replaces peripatetic idleness. There is something comforting about returning to the same workbench, in the same spot, with the same coworkers on either side and the familiar supervisor and time clerk. The worker is required to concentrate attention upon a given, worthwhile, predictable task instead of being idle, left to drift into autistic, tormented fantasies. The task accomplished draws warm, comforting praise from a sympathetic, supportive supervisor, filling the person with a sense of pride, warmth and value and contradicting inner feelings of worthlessness and uselessness. The task accomplished, the praise received, yields a sense of identity—"I am a maker of this; I am a finisher of that"; instead of "I have no use; I am nobody; I am a defective, social reject." The experience of sharing this identity sense with a coworker—"We are workers here together," sharing in this experience, aware of each other, helping each other, eating lunch together, taking public transportation together—replaces isolated anomie. The entire feeling tone in which we have thus immersed our hypothetical ex-mental patient is the rhythmic constancy and warmth of early oral life which significantly contributes to an inner sense of basic trust—the world is a safe place. Optimism develops in such a setting, and the developing person is thus readied for new growth. The schedule fulfilled, the familiar place taken, the task accomplished, the praise received and the fellowship experienced make the world seem a rhythmic, predictable, loving, safe place.

Admittedly, we have portrayed the ideal, emphasizing the potential benefits of the addition of work to the life of a rehabilitating patient. If, on the other hand, the work experience is chaotic, with changing schedules, supervisors and coworkers—where tension and criticism and animosity are prevailing—it can precipitate regression into the previous paranoid state. What is more usually a favorable work environment, from time to time is normally subject to change and stress. Through misunderstanding and happenstance, a worker can feel unappreciated, criticized, extruded or treated unfairly. It is at such times that crisis intervention is indicated in order to clarify the issues, to help the worker to avoid generalizing the experienced insult, to help recover his sense of well-being so that he can continue in his position.

Certain aspects of the work situation call upon personality traits which are developed in the second or anal stage of life. Once secure in the job setting, other issues may be addressed and mastered. The new worker can develop the attributes of punctuality and neatness—requisites in the work arena, while in the hospital or community residence they may have been only matters for struggle with the staff. A sense of competence and mastery accompany task achievement, and the ultimate receipt of monetary compensation enhances the recognition that the work experience contributes to true autonomy. A sense of humiliation and shame is replaced with self-respect. Here again, the sensitive handling of the worker by supervisors in the work setting contributes to the attainment of a sense of autonomy instead of shame. This is particularly so in the initial phases of the worker learning a new work skill.

Finally, for the healthier worker, the job experience is an outlet for competition and initiative instead of intimidation and compliance. Initiative in this setting should be rewarded—such as the common practice of an award for the best suggestion of the month in a "suggestion box." This is in marked contrast to the outright subjugation to which the former patient often has been subjected in the rigid life of the state mental institution, where patient initiative involving life situations was almost entirely squelched.

I have just explored four critical principles in the delivery of clinical care to the chronic psychiatric patient in the community. These have included the importance of accurate diagnosis, the requisite of the clinician being meaningfully close to the patient, the relevance of the entire clinical team collaborating in the delivery of a comprehensive care system, and the significance of the way in which a patient uses his daily time. It should be observed that each of these four principles represent, in part at least, an expression of four basic components of the patient's mental life—namely, the psychophysiological, the psychological, the psychosocial and the behavioral.

The reader cannot but be impressed with the complexity of the task when he contemplates all that has been involved in the consideration of only four principles. It is clear that there are many more issues to be considered in a thorough review of this topic. Nevertheless, these several issues have been enunciated because it is essential that those issues which are the *sine qua non* of adequate care not be ignored or forgotten. It is this author's experience that by carefully practicing the principles as herein described, the clinician will, at a minimum, be engaging the patient in a treatment program which has basic quality.

Ultimately, considering the patient in a comprehensive fashion, such as suggested here, has a meaning which cuts to the core of what quality medical care is all about. This is the devotion of the clinician to acquiring as authentic a picture of the patient as he is able. Not only is this practicing medicine in the best scientific tradition; it is also an expression of the highest medical ethic. This is the ethic of man's altruistic care for his fellow man.

REFERENCES

Beels, C. C. Social support and schizophrenia. *Schizophrenia Bulletin* 7(1): 58-71 (1981).

Brown, G. W., Birley, J. L. T., and Wing, J. K. Influence of family life on the course of schizophrenic disorders: A replication. *Br. J. Psychiatry* 121: 241-258 (1972).

Goldberg, S. C., Schooler, N. R., Hogarty, G. E., et al. Prediction of relapse in schizophrenic outpatients treated by drug and sociotherapy. *Arch. Gen. Psychiatry* 34: 171-184 (1977).

Hammer, M. Social supports, social networks, and schizophrenia. *Schizophrenia Bulletin* 7(1): 45-57 (1981).

Lewis, J. M. *How's Your Family?* Brunner/Mazel, 1979.

Linn, M. W. Can foster care survive? in *Issues in Community Residential Care,* A New Directions in Mental Health Services Quarterly Sourcebook. Edited by R. D. Budson, ed. San Francisco, CA: Jossey-Bass Publications, 1981.

Pepper, B., Kirschner, M. C., and Ryglewicz, H. The young adult chronic patient: overview of a population. *Hospital and Community Psychiatry* 32(7): 463-469 (1981).

Searles, H. F. Phases of patient-therapist interaction in the psychotherapy of chronic schizophrenia, in *Collected Papers on Schizophrenia and Related Subjects.* New York: Int. Univ. Press, 1965, 525-531.

Stevens, B. Evaluation of rehabilitation for psychotic patients in the community. *Acta Psychiatr. Scand.* 49: 169-180 (1973).

Stone, A. A., and Eldred, S. H. Delusion formation during the activation of chronic schizophrenic patients. *Arch. Gen. Psychiatry* 1: 177-179 (1959).

Vaughn, C. E., and Leff, J. P. Patterns of emotional response in relatives of schizophrenic patients. *Schizophrenia Bulletin* 7(1): 43-44 (1981).

Wing, J. K. The social context of schizophrenia. *American Journal of Psychiatry* 135(11): 1333-1339 (November 1978).

ACKNOWLEDGMENT

The author gratefully acknowledges the thoughtful discussions of the content of this chapter by Rona E. Klein, M.D.

CHAPTER 22

COMMUNITY SURVIVAL OF THE CHRONIC PSYCHIATRIC PATIENT: RESEARCH PRIORITIES

IVAN BAROFSKY

INTRODUCTION

As indicated by the content of this text, the care of the chronic psychiatric patient in the community consists of two major elements—the psychosocial therapies and the pharmacotherapies, as set in different care sites. The delivery of these therapies occurs within a complex administrative and legal structure, a structure that is designed to insure that patients have *access* to such care and that the care provided is of *optimal* quality. The major events that have led to what is now considered standard care for the chronic patient include the development of the major tranquilizers starting in the mid 1950s, deinstitutionalization, which started in the 1960s, changes in the legal status of the chronic patient in the 1970s and the slow development during this period of community care programs which are now becoming mature in form, quality and numbers.

What has been learned during this period is that no one *element of care*, in and of itself, is sufficient to manage the symptomatology of—much less "cure"—a majority of patients. What has become necessary, as has been found for many other chronic diseases, is the development of multimodality therapies. The underlying assumption of a multimodality therapy is that by combining therapies with different "sites of action," a combination can be found which would be more effective than individual therapies alone. The "sites of action" for therapies might be the psychopathology of the patient's family, the patient's response to stress, the patient's symptomatology, the

Table 1 Alternative Care Sites for the Chronic Psychiatric Patient

Hospital Care:	Acute Treatment Ward
	Locked Continued-Treatment Ward
	Open Continued-Treatment Ward
Community Care:	Day Hospital
	Nursing Homes
	Long-term Group Residents
	Transitional Halfway Houses
	Cooperative Apartments
	Foster Care
	Board and Care Homes
	Hotels
	Lodge Programs
	Work Camps
	Crisis Centers

presence of medication noncompliance, the work status of the patient, the patient's interpersonal relationships, etc. The construction of a multimodality therapy is based on a provider's assessment of the needs and potential of a patient, as modified by experience with the patient. A very obvious research task is to make this process as rational as possible.

The event that precipitates care is, of course, an initial or recurrent psychotic episode. If the psychotic episode alerts the person's family or a provider to the need for care, then the patient may be prescribed treatment in a hospital (e.g., an acute treatment ward) or in the community. The care provided at these facilities is usually arranged so that an individual's opportunities for independent functioning are matched to his clinical status. Sometimes an individual will move from facility to facility as his clinical status changes. Most often, however, the chronic patient remains at a facility for an extended period so that a more realistic concern becomes sustaining the rehabilitative program that had been initiated for the patient. Table 1 summarizes these facilities, or care sites.

Where the patient's received care, however, represents more than a physical place, it is also a social, cultural, financial, political and therapeutic environment. The successful organization of elements of care, as modified by characteristics of the care site, into a *program of care* is a major determinant of the outcome of care. Evaluation of the implementation of such programs of care also constitutes an obvious research task.

Given a number of effective therapies delivered in an appropriate manner, there still remains the issue of whether the care provided is an integrated and individualized program of care. *Integration*, at any one time or over time, represents the adjustment of a care program to an individual patient's needs, an adjustment which is also essential to ensure the quality and outcome of care. The implementation of such a program was discussed by Budson in the previous chapter.

The present discussion has highlighted three interrelated issues, each of which represent a different type of analysis of the care the chronic patient receives. These issues are:

- What components of care are effective, and which will lead to an optimal outcome?
- Will the outcome of care vary with the program designed to implement care?
- What role does integrating and individualizing the components of care play in determining the outcome of care?

The following discussion will attempt to summarize what is known about each of these questions.[1] This will help us evaluate the empirical rationale for providing care for the chronic psychiatric patient in the community, and in so doing will help identify the research priorities required for providing more effective care.

EVALUATION OF TREATMENTS FOR THE CHRONIC PSYCHIATRIC PATIENT IN THE COMMUNITY

The chronic psychiatric patient who typically receives one or two types of drugs (antipsychotic, antiparkinsonian) and various types of psychosocial therapy (individual or group psychotherapy, vocational training, recreational therapy, etc.) is, in fact, receiving a complex therapeutic regimen. The effectiveness of such a regimen is not only dependent on the specific site of action of each component of the regimen but also on the interaction that may occur among the therapies themselves or among the consequences of the therapy. For example, the combination of individual and group therapy has been found to be more effective than each separately (e.g., Mosher and Keith 1981), whereas the consequence of one form of a drug facilitates social learning more than another (e.g., Gillis and Parkinson 1981). This section will review what is known about the interaction

Table 2 Types of Studies Evaluating the Care Provided the Chronic Psychiatric Patient in the Community

Treatment Evaluation
Drugs vs. Placebo/Drug
Drug vs. PST*
PST vs. No PST/PST
Program Evaluation
Aftercare vs. No Aftercare/Aftercare
Hospital (Inpatient) vs. Day Hospital Care
Hospital (Inpatient) vs. Community Care
Early Discharge Studies

*PST—Psychosocial Therapy

of elements that make up a therapeutic regimen. Table 2 summarizes the various types of studies that have been reported.[2] The studies to be discussed were limited, to the extent possible, to schizophrenic patients in the community.[3]

a. *Drug Studies*

The available data indicate that the symptoms of most acutely ill psychotic patients will be reduced in response to the major tranquilizers, but that when administered chronically, a measurable proportion of the patients will experience relapse in the presence of drug. In addition, there appears to be a subgroup of patients who remain symptom free in the absence of drug, and a subgroup who essentially never respond to drug (May and Goldberg 1978). The Barofsky and Connelly paper (see this text) revealed that while noncompliance rate varied as a function of method of administering the phenothiazine, the rate of relapse did not (i.e., a comparison of oral and long-acting phenothiazines). They also found that a host of patient-related factors determined whether or not the patient was noncompliant, only one of which was the patient's psychiatric background. Finally, a large percentage of the patients on the neuroleptics will develop basal ganglion side effects, which will require the administration of antiparkinsonian drugs (e.g., Jeste and Wyatt 1981). This brief summary of the state of pharmacotherapy for schizophrenics reveals that the available drugs are not as *effective* as required, that the failure of drugs to be effective cannot be *blamed* simply on the patient's noncompliance or psychiatric status and that the *choice* between methods of administering drugs (oral, or as long-acting phenothiazines) is one of convenience, not differential effectiveness. With this background the following research is proposed:

- New biological approaches are required to develop drugs which have fewer nonspecific effects (Baldessarini, this text; Davis et al. 1981).

- Currently available drugs have to be used with greater precision. This can be done by identifying premorbid factors (e.g., Goldstein et al. 1978), by developing test-dose procedures (May 1974) or by using subjective responses to initial drug administrations (Van Putten et al. 1981) to predict the patient's response to prolonged drug administration. In addition, diagnostic procedures have to be improved so that the relationship between response to drug and psychiatric status can be improved. The precision with which a physician makes clinical decisions (e.g., modifying a drug dose) can also be improved by the development of rapid inexpensive clinical procedures which detect (in blood or urine) the level of drug consumed (this is relevant for both antipsychotic and antiparkinsonian drugs).

- Factors which predict drug noncompliance have to be established. This knowledge could then be used to develop interventions that reduce medication noncompliance (particularly for oral medications). If it can be shown that the patient is compliant and the therapy ineffective, then drug doses can be reduced or eliminated, or a different drug used. In this way, the patient's right to refuse treatment will have both legal and medical support.

- Studies of antiparkinsonian drug compliance have to be done. These studies, combined with compliance studies of antipsychotic medication, provide a unique research opportunity since they permit an investigator to study compliance with two or more drugs in the same patient.

- Cost-benefit studies have to be done comparing patients on chronic medications with those who are provided drug holidays, intermittent drug administration, etc.

b. Drugs and Psychosocial Therapy Studies

There are three major studies that evaluate drugs with or without psychosocial therapies.[4] One study deals with acutely ill, mostly first-admission schizophrenics (Goldstein et al. 1978). This study was limited to a 6-month followup of patients who received low or high doses of long-acting phenothiazines with or without crisis-oriented family therapy (therapy which was provided within the first 6 weeks of returning to the community). In a second study chronic schizophrenics were studied over a 2-year period (Goldberg et al. 1977; Hogarty et al. 1973, 1974, 1976). They received either placebo or oral phenothiazine, with or without major supportive role therapy. In a third study chronic schizophrenics (Hogarty et al. 1979) were given either an oral or long-acting phenothiazine, with or without "social therapy." This study also followed patients for 2 years.

These studies established that drug therapy was a necessary but not sufficient condition for community survival and that psychosocial therapies could be either beneficial or "toxic" depending on the clinical status of the patient. The combination of drug therapy and psychosocial therapy consistently resulted in the largest proportion of community survival per study. Various measures of premorbid adjustment were found to be complex predictors of response to therapy. In all three studies the sex of the patient was an important predictor or covariate of community survival, with women, in general, responding better to therapy. In both long-term studies, the contribution of the psychosocial therapies to community survival became obvious only during the second year of the study. This suggests that drugs and the psychosocial therapies differ in terms of the time it takes for them to have their optimal therapeutic benefit. In both long-term studies there were groups of patients who did not respond to therapy and groups of patients whose continued response to therapy appeared dependent on the absence of environmental or family stress. These studies suggest that characteristics of the patient, particularly his psychophysiological state and his environment, were major contributors to the probability of relapse. The research to date suggests the following studies:

- If, as appears to be, the schizophrenic cannot tolerate the stress that other persons can, then it is necessary to identify what these stresses are and how they override the benefit provided by the available therapies. With this knowledge it should be possible to design studies that include more specifically directed therapies. For example, if the patient's family is a major source of stress, then which therapy would lead to better survival in the community: crisis-oriented family therapy, regular (once-a-month) family therapy (all members of the family participate), or removal of the patient from the family?

- If the therapeutic benefit that the psychosocial therapies provide takes time to develop, then more has to be learned about the specifics of what it is that is developing with time. These descriptive studies should provide the basis for designing new interventions that would hasten the development of the benefit of the psychosocial therapies.
- Studies of the relationship between drug noncompliance and psychosocial therapy compliance (e.g., appointment keeping) have to be done, although the little that is known does not suggest a simple relationship (e.g., Hogarty et al. 1976). It would also be of interest to determine if interventions designed to deal with one type of noncompliance would impact upon another type of noncompliance.
- Studies have to be done to determine if, as has been stated, drugs "set the stage" for implementing psychosocial therapy, or if drugs disrupt the rehabilitation process (e.g., Anthony et al. 1978; Gillis and Parkison 1981).

c. *Psychosocial Therapy*

Do schizophrenics survive longer in the community if the care they receive includes one type of psychosocial therapy but not another? Table 3 summarizes the major psychosocial therapies. The available literature (see Mosher and Keith 1981) indicates the following:

Table 3 Types of Psychosocial Therapy

Individual Psychotherapy
Group Psychotherapy
Family Therapy
Role Therapy
Recreational Therapy
Vocational Rehabilitation

- Only one (Purvis and Miskimins 1970) of four controlled studies (Herz et al. 1974; Levene et al. 1970; O'Brien et al. 1972) found that *group therapy* significantly delayed rehospitalization when compared with *individual therapy*. There was little evidence that social and vocational adjustment were differentially affected by the two therapies, although patients and providers expressed more satisfaction with group therapy.

- Comparison of *group therapy* to a nongroup therapy control revealed that in two of three studies (Barowski and Tolwinski 1969; Claghorn et al. 1974; Shatten et al. 1966) symptomatology was reduced with group therapy. There was also evidence for fewer readmissions in one study (Shatten et al. 1966) and improvement in psychiatric status in another (Claghorn et al. 1974).

- Controlled studies have also been reported comparing *family therapy* with no therapy (Goldstein et al. 1978), inpatient therapy (Langsley, Machotka et al. 1968) or individual therapy (Ro-Trock et al. 1977). Relapse/rehospitalization rates were lower for family therapy for each study, although the data suggested (e.g., Goldstein et al. 1978) that drugs were required for this observation.

- The importance of social *role therapy* in maintaining social functioning of the patient in the community has been studied by comparing drug with no-drug conditions (Hogarty et al. 1973, 1974, 1976) or with oral or long-acting phenothiazines (Hogarty et al. 1979). Both sets of studies indicate that maximum community survival comes from a combination of role therapy and drug.

Vocational and recreational therapy have usually been studied as specific parts of service systems, so no effort will be made here to present them separately (Anthony et al. 1978).

A psychosocial therapy, as defined here,[4] is a set of activities or procedures which a provider and patient do together and which can be applied at one care site or another. It is the transposibility of the procedures from site to site which identifies this therapy as a treatment separate from a community-based program of care. However, the success of a psychosocial treatment is also dependent on the match among patient, therapist and setting characteristics. In addition, there is much yet to learn about which psychosocial therapy is best for which group of schizophrenics, how a particular therapy can be optimally administered and how success or failure with a treatment can be determined. With this background the following research can be proposed:

- Studies should be done comparing the *outcome* of different psychosocial therapies, individually or in combination. Thus, would occasional crisis-oriented family therapy, as a supplement to regular group therapy lead to better community survival than either therapy alone? Is the maintenance of social functionings, as mediated by social role therapy, as adequate an approach to community survival as the insight therapy provided by individual psychotherapy? Does each type of therapy have a specific, but limited objective in the total care of the patient, or is one type of therapy "better" than another? What empirical evidence can be provided to support the process of selecting one psychosocial therapy instead of another or combination of therapies?

- In addition to the need to know the relative efficacy of individual therapies and combinations of therapies, it is also necessary to know that each is administered under optimal conditions (*the process*). To establish this will require studies which systematically vary the frequency with which a person participates in therapy, the intensity of the therapeutic intervention (e.g., Lamb and Goertzel, 1977) and the nature of the therapy. Many aspects of this task are the objects of current clinical concern and evaluation—these are not new issues. What would be new, however, is the systematic evaluation of alternative administrative procedures as part of controlled studies of the chronic patient in the community. The current practice of allowing the provider to individualize the administration of a psychosocial therapy in a study may be clinically and ethically necessary, but it has the consequence of leaving open the question of whether the therapy has been optimally administered.

- A final set of studies would deal with the interaction between psychosocial therapies and antipsychotic drugs. Studies addressing this issue have been discussed earlier.

EVALUATION OF PROGRAMS OF CARE FOR THE CHRONIC PSYCHIATRIC PATIENT IN THE COMMUNITY

The success of efforts to provide care for the chronic patient in the community are dependent on having available effective therapies —therapies which are optimally implemented and delivered, yet individualized for the patient. In the previous section we reviewed what was known about the efficacy of individual treatments, and on the basis of this identified a set of research tasks. In this section we will evaluate various efforts at implementing care programs and suggest additional research activities. The final section will deal with the individualization of treatment.

The implementation of a care program is critically dependent on a wide range of organizational issues—issues that evolve out of efforts to provide care in different care settings. Factors which determine the success of such efforts include the physical characteristics of the care site, the cultural and financial resources of the community, legal restrictions on a community residence (e.g., zoning regulations), the presence of advocates and other persons interested in the welfare of the chronic patient, the acceptance by the community of the chronic patient, the availability of third-party payments, the social network of the patient, the number and skill of available providers and many other related issues. These variables are important determinants of a patient's access to and utilization of services.

A wide range of model programs have been developed, each of which represents a particular "solution" to the problem of how to provide care for the chronic patient in the community. Sometimes these demonstration projects reflect a conceptual orientation, but always they are organized with careful attention to the realities of community living for the chronic patient. Since such model programs represent the point of care, they will inevitably be the building blocks of a community-wide system of care. As Bachrach (1980) has indicated, however, a collection of such programs should not be considered to add up to a mental health system. To make a mental health system requires that the relationship between the different care programs and the community as a whole be specified, an issue that can not be addressed here. Rather, what we are concerned about is what has been learned and what remains to be discovered about the various programs of care. We will review only those programs which have been evaluated by some systematic procedure (e.g., random assignment of patients between treatment). What has been learned is the following:

- *Aftercare*, independent of its specific nature, leads to longer community survival than no aftercare, although some aftercare programs are more effective in maintaining the patient in the community than others (e.g., Beard et al. 1963; Caffey et al. 1971; Claghorn and Kinross-Wright 1971). Aftercare may involve recruiting volunteer therapists to monitor the chronic patient (Katkin et al. 1971); using alternative care sites such as a day hospital, an outpatient department, or a general practitioner; (Sheldon 1964); or varying the intensity of the aftercare (Lamb and Goertzel 1972).

- More specifically, it has been shown that *day hospital* care is an effective alternative to inpatient care, although this advantage disappears by the second year of followup (relevant studies summarized in Linn et al. 1979). In addition, day hospital care was also found to be more effective than outpatient care (Gut et al. 1969; Meltzoff and Blumenthal 1966).

- In terms of preparing a patient to remain in the community, *community-based* treatments were found to be as effective as, or better than hospital treatment with aftercare. A wide range of community care programs has been evaluated, including *home care* (Langsley et al. 1968; Pasamanick et al. 1967; Rittenhouse 1970), *nonfamilial residences* (Mosher et al. 1975; Polak and Kirby 1976), *foster care* (Linn et al. 1977, 1980), *lodge programs* (Fairweather 1964, 1969, 1980) and *training in community living programs* (Stein et al., this text, 1975, 1980; Marx et al. 1973). Removing patients from these programs inevitably removes the advantage that the community-based treatment programs had over hospital care. Several other types of community care are in use (Table 1) but have not been evaluated in controlled studies.

- *Early hospital discharge* with systematic community support leads to as effective a community adjustment as "optimal" hospitalization (Caffey et al. 1971; Glick et al. 1976; Herz et al. 1977; Hirsch et al. 1979; Weisman et al. 1969). Moreover, efforts at designing an inpatient treatment program effective in sustaining community survival have, in general, not succeeded (Anthony et al. 1972; Ellsworth et al. 1979), although the recent report of Paul and Lentz (1977) suggests otherwise.

In summary, these studies demonstrate that community care represents an effective alternative to hospital care, and that maintenance of the patient in the community is dependent on the continued presence of these care programs. Programs which succeed are designed around the specific characteristics and needs of the patient (e.g., sensitivity to stress, family psychopathology, skills required for community participation, etc.), and make the transfer from the training situation to real life as simple and direct as possible.

The work of Stein and his colleagues (Marx et al. 1973, 1975, 1980) probably represents the leading edge of current efforts to develop community-based treatment programs. The reason for this is largely that their model represents a sophisticated approach to individualized care yet also appears generalizable across care sites (urban, suburban and rural). In addition, by training patients in the community, potential problems in transferring what the patient has learned to the site of use can be minimized. The cost of this program also seems competitive (Weisbrod and Stein 1980). We will use Stein's work as the backdrop to generate a research agenda with the proviso that issues that cut across any other program of care can also be raised.

- Although evidence exists that model programs such as Stein's succeed, there is still the opportunity to study whether the procedures used will lead to an optimal outcome. For example, training patients to cope with real life situations is an essential element of Stein's intervention, yet there are many ways to teach a person to cope. Very few studies have been reported which experimentally manipulate and evaluate the procedures within a model program (e.g., Austin et al. 1976).

- Stein et al. (1980) have found, as had Langsley et al. (1971) and Davis et al. (1974) before them, that once a patient is transferred from the special training program to traditional community care, many of the improvements in social functioning are lost and use of the hospital is increased. Maintaining the impact of a program, however, is not unique to the chronic psychiatric patient in the community. It is a problem that is found with virtually all behavioral interventions (e.g., weight loss programs, life-style changes, etc.). The existence of the problem actually demonstrates the power of the program of care, and the practical solution of the problem involves diminishing the difference between the training setting and the application site. This can be done in two ways; by making the application site more like the training site, or vice versa. Irrespective of the particular approach taken, the solution to the problem requires a concerted research effort.

- The training program used by Stein et al. (1978) is actually a complex collection of treatments presented in a particular sequence designed for the individual involved, starting from the time of the psychotic episode or referral. What is done, when it is done and how it is done are all questions which require specific answers if the program is to be readily reproduced at another location. To date, Stein has not provided this level of detail. The experience of Fairweather (1964, 1969, 1980) in transferring his program to different care sites is an example of the effort that has to be provided. It is only with such procedural detail that the rhetorical question asked by Greenblatt and Budson (1976), "Once demonstration of an effective modality has been made, how do we export it?", can be answered. What seems clear is that reproduction of Stein's program is a technical task and not something that can be judged *a priori* to have characteristics that would prevent the procedure from being used elsewhere (Bachrach 1980).

If it can be shown that a model program can be developed which maintains improvement of the behavior and social functioning of the chronic patient, and that such a program can be constituted in a new setting, then the key tasks for developing a program of care for the chronic patient in the community have been satisfied. This does not mean that other tasks do not remain, including determining whether the community has the political will and economic resources to implement such a program; rather, it would mean that the *necessary* conditions for developing a mental health system for the chronic patient have been established. Since this is not yet the case, the primary task of research efforts in this area should be the development of more effective model programs.

THE INTEGRATION OF CARE FOR THE CHRONIC PATIENT IN THE COMMUNITY

Individualizing and integrating the various treatment elements into a total care program is the essence of what is meant by the term "clinical care"—it is what a provider is taught to do and is expected to do (see Chapter 21 by Budson). However, the nature of providing care for the chronic patient in the community significantly frustrates this process. Factors such as the ease with which a patient can be lost to followup, difficulties in measuring drug compliance in the community, problems of providing rehabilitative services in the community, etc., makes monitoring the status of the chronic patient a difficult task. One of the important accomplishments of the model programs has been that they have created a structure which not only provides a context for a treatment intervention, but also makes the patient accessible and available. Such structure would appear to be a necessary precondition for any effort at providing an individualized and integrated care program.

There does not seem to be a substantive research literature that has evaluated different methods of providing an individualized and integrated program of care for the chronic patient. What literature is available addresses limited issues over relatively brief periods of time. The kind of sustained commitment, in terms of time and effort, that is characteristic of clinical care for the chronic patient has not been viewed by clinicians as an opportunity to systematically evaluate alternative methods of treating the patient. Part of the reason for this may be that clinicians do not realize that statistical methods are available which permit valid conclusions to be drawn from single-subject studies (Barlow and Hensen 1973; Hensen and Barlow 1976). Another reason may be that clinicians resist manipulating procedures and techniques which they consider to require great precision and experience to apply (e.g., psychotherapy). In addition, they may want to avoid giving a patient less than what they consider optimal care for legal and ethical, as well as therapeutic reasons.

For a clinician to be convinced that it is appropriate for him to "experiment" with his patients, he has to be shown that the available treatments or procedures either do not work or are only partially effective and that viable options exist. To be convinced, for example, that a rehabilitative effort has reached the limits of its impact on a patient implies that the provider (or patient for that matter) has some sense of the potential of the patient and the power of the treatment. Clinical experience gives the provider an understanding of what can be accomplished with individual patients within practical time spans, and what is considered a successful effort is defined within this experience. To decide, however, that a treatment has been applied in an optimal manner and that the outcome reflects what can be expected to be accomplished implies that the provider has had extensive experience with the procedure. For a provider to gain such experience, however, also implies that he has had a prior commitment to the efficacy of the procedure; to feel otherwise would not be considered ethical. Such a commitment, however, could then become a barrier to change. What also happens is that the expertise required for different treatments seems to reside in different professionals; thus role conflicts can also confound the therapeutic evaluation and change process. Accordingly, much of the resistance to the systematic evaluation of treatments in an individual patient may be due to the psychology of providing care rather than to efficacy of the treatment.

There is another approach to the study of integrated care, and that is at systems level—how can the various services needed by the chronic patient be delivered in a reliable and timely manner? Other authors in this text have addressed this issue, and by not discussing it we do not mean to underestimate its relevance or importance. Rather, we are convinced that highest priority should be given to research efforts which focus on the most critical events in the care process, and these events occur within programs of care, not with the system of care.

SUMMARY

The research agenda outlined above reflects the view that events critical to the care of the chronic psychiatric patient in the community occur at several levels of analysis. These levels of analysis include individual treatments, programs of care, and community-wide systems of care. When evaluating individual treatments, programmatic and systems issues are allowed to vary between patients and settings. When dealing with programs of care, treatments are specified, but their combination and implementation are systematically varied and evaluated. When dealing with systems of care, how best to maintain and service individuals and programs on a community-wide basis is considered. Organizational issues are present at each level of analysis; thus, whereas studies can be performed relatively independently at each level of analysis, it is also clear that a relationship exists among these levels as well. This approach explicitly rejects the view that one level of analysis, or type of study, is more important than another; but we would argue that priorities exist in the types of studies that should be done. What is being specifically promoted is an expanded research effort in developing effective treatments and their more efficient combination and implementation into programs of care. In addition, since any therapeutic regimen is going to consist of multiple components, the individualization and integration of such regimens is required. This too, however, is considered a researchable task.

Once research progress in these areas has been made, then mental health service systems can be efficiently and effectively organized. There would be nothing worse for the deinstitutionalization movement than to create an expensive and complex service system that would not be able to achieve its objective of optimizing the social functioning and community survival of the chronic patient because partially effective therapies or programs were utilized. Having said this, it is also important to say that having effective therapies would also not prevent the failure of deinstitutionalization if the patient did not have access to such services. Clearly, a therapeutic failure can result from having full exposure to an ineffective therapy (representing a program failure) or partial exposure to an effective therapy (representing a systems failure).

In establishing a research agenda, it is almost inevitable that certain specific research issues are not directly addressed. For example, what should be the measure of the success of a treatment or program of care? We have emphasized community survival, but would also agree that social functioning, employment, quality of life, etc., are viable alternatives. How to measure these outcome variables, what instruments to use, etc., are all questions that could be the focus of meaningful research activities. We have also avoided dealing with diagnostic issues by trying to confine ourselves to schizophrenics, but clearly this is not the reality of clinical practice. How the diagnostic heterogenity of clinical populations limits the applicability of individual treatment or the generalizability of programs of care can also be a meaningful research task. However, to be concerned about this issue before the characteristics of an effective treatment or program of care are known would appear to be inefficient usage of research time. Utilization data and patient satisfaction data would also be important research activities, but again, these would be dependent on the efficacy of available treatments for specific groups of patients.

The primary objective of research in this area must be the development of effective alternative therapies and/or programs of care. All other activities are important means of accommodating the relative efficacy of known treatments to clinical reality but should not be considered as ends in themselves.

NOTES

1. It will not be possible to provide the reader with a detailed review of the literature supporting many of the recommendations listed for future research efforts. It will sometimes not even be possible to spell out the specific direction this research should take. The reader, however, will be referred, where possible, to sources that will provide the appropriate level of detail.
2. There is a substantial literature which uses relapse/rehospitalization rates (community survival) as an outcome measure for studies of alternative within the hospital procedures (e.g., alternative drug treatments, individual psychotherapy, milieu therapy, token economies, etc.). These studies will not be reviewed here since they do not ordinarily experimentally manipulate the treatment the chronic patient receives *in* the community.
3. This was done so that recommendations that generated from this review would be consistent with thc Barofsky and Connelly paper (this text) which limited itself to studies dealing with schizophrenic patients.
4. A psychosocial therapy was defined in two ways. First, it could consist of a specific set of procedures that defined the relationship between the patient and the provider (e.g., individual or group psychotherapy). Second, it could describe a task that the patient and provider have to work together to solve (e.g., a family crisis, preparation for employment, an education objective, etc.) without necessarily specifying a specific procedure to achieve this objective. Psychosocial therapy is different from patient monitoring, where usually only medication taking and compliance behavior of the patient are investigated.

REFERENCES

Anthony, W. A., Buell, G. J., Sharratt, S., and Althoff, M. E. The efficacy of psychiatric rehabilitation. *Psychological Bulletin* 78: 447-456 (1976).

Anthony, W. A., Cohen, M. R., and Vitalo, R. The measurement of rehabilitation outcome. *Schizophrenia Bulletin* 4: 365-398 (1978).

Austin, N. K., Liberman, R. P., King, L. W., and DeRisi, W. J. A comparative evaluation of two day hospitals. *The Journal of Nervous and Mental Diseases* 163: 253-262 (1976).

Bachrach, L. L. Overview: Model programs for chronic mental patients. *American Journal of Psychiatry* 137: 1023-1031 (1980).

Baldessarini, R. Clinical pharmacology and side effects of anti-psychotic and mood-stabilizing drugs with chronic or recurrent disorders, in *The Chronic Psychiatric Patient in the Community: Principles of Treatment* I. Barofsky and R. D. Budson, eds. New York: Spectrum, 1982.

Barlow, D. H. and Hersen, M. Single-case experimental designs: Use in applied clinical research. *Archives of General Psychiatry* 29: 319-325 (1973).

Barofsky, I. and Connelly, C. A. E. Problems in providing effective care for the chronic psychiatric patient, in *The Chronic Psychiatric Patient in the Community: Principles of Treatment* I. Barofsky and R. D. Budson, eds. New York: Spectrum, 1982.

Beard, J. H., Pitt, R. B., Fisher, S. H., and Goertzel, V. Evaluating the effectiveness of a psychiatric rehabilitation program. *American Journal of Orthopsychiatry* 33: 701-712 (1963).
Borowski, T., and Tolwinski, T. Treatment of paranoid schizophrenics with chlorpromazine and group therapy. *Diseases of the Nervous System* 30: 201-202 (1969).
Caffey, E. M., Galbrecht, C. R., and Klett, C. J. Brief hospitalization and aftercare in the treatment of schizophrenia. *Archives of General Psychiatry* 24: 81-86 (1971).
Claghorn, J. L., and Kinross-Wright, J. Reduction in hospitalization of schizophrenics. *American Journal of Psychiatry* 128: 344-347 (1971).
Claghorn, J. L., Johnston, E. E., Cook, T. H., and Itschner, L. Group therapy and maintenance treatment of schizophrenics. *Archives of General Psychiatry* 31: 361-365 (1974).
Davis, A. E., Dinitz, S., and Pasamanick, B. *Schizophrenia in the New Custodial Community.* Ohio: Ohio State University Press, 1974.
Davis, I. M., Schaffer, C. B., Killian, G. A., Kinard, C., and Chan, C. Important issues in the drug treatment of schizophrenia. *Special Report: Schizophrenia 1980.* DHHS No. (ADM) 81-1064, 1981, pp. 109-126.
Ellsworth, R. B., Collins, J. F., Casey, N. A., Schoonover, R. A., Hickey, R. H., Hyer, L., Twemlow, S. W., and Nesselroade, J. R. Some characteristics of effective psychiatric treatment programs. *Journal of Consulting and Clinical Psychology* 47: 799-817 (1979).
Fairweather, G. W., ed. *Social Psychology in Treatment of Mental Illness: An Experimental Approach.* New York: Wiley, 1964.
Fairweather, G. W., ed. *The Fairweather Lodge: A Twenty-Five Year Retrospective.* San Francisco: Jossey-Bass, 1980.
Fairweather, G., Sanders, D., Cressler, D., and Maynard, H. *Community Life for the Mentally Ill: An Alternative to Institutional Care.* Chicago: Aldine Publishing Company, 1969.
Gillis, J. S. and Parkison, S. The effects of fluphenazine decanoate injection and chlorpromazine on symptom severity and learning in outpatient schizophrenics. *Current Therapeutic Research* 29: 551-566 (1981).
Glick, I. D., Hargreaves, W. A., Drues, J., and Showstack, J. A. Short versus long hospitalization: A prospective controlled study IV. One-year followup results for schizophrenic patients. *American Journal of Psychiatry* 133: 509-514 (1976).
Goldberg, S. C., Schooler, N. R., Hogarty, G. E., and Roper, M. Prediction of relapse in schizophrenic outpatients treated by drug and sociotherapy. *Archives of General Psychiatry* 34: 171-184 (1977).
Goldstein, M. J., Rodnick, E. H., Evans, J. R., May, P. R. A., and Steinberg, M. R. Drug and family therapy in the aftercare of acute schizophrenics. *Archives of General Psychiatry* 35: 1169-1177 (1978).
Greenblatt, M., and Budson, R. D. eds. A symposium: Follow-up studies of community care. *American Journal of Psychiatry* 133: 916-921 (1976).
Guy, W., Gross, M., Hogarty, G. E., and Dennis, H. A controlled evaluation of day hospital effectiveness. *Archives of General Psychiatry* 20: 329-338 (1969).
Hersen, M., and Barlow, D. H. *Single Case Experimental Designs: Strategies for Studying Behavior Change.* New York: Pergamon Press, 1976.

Herz, M., Endicott, J., and Spitzer, R. L. Brief hospitalization: A two-year follow-up. *American Journal of Psychiatry* 134: 502–507 (1977).

Herz, M. I., Spitzer, R. L., Gibbon, M., Greenspan, K., and Reibel, S. Individual versus group aftercare treatment. *American Journal of Psychiatry* 131: 808-812 (1974).

Hirsch, S. R., Platt, S., Knights, A., and Weyman, A. Shortening hospital stay for psychiatric care: Effect on patients and their families. *British Medical Journal* 1: 442–446 (1979).

Hogarty, G. E., Goldberg, S. C., and the Collaborative Study Group. Drug and sociotherapy in the aftercare of schizophrenic patients: One-year relapse rates. *Archives of General Psychiatry* 28: 54–64 (1973).

Hogarty, G. E., Goldberg, S. C., Schooler, N. R., Ulrich, R. F., and the Collaborative Study Group. Drug and sociotherapy in the aftercare of schizophrenic patients: III. Adjustment of non-relapsed patients. *Archives of General Psychiatry* 31: 609–618 (1974).

Hogarty, G. E., Ulrich, R. F., Goldberg, S. C., and Schooler, N. R. Sociotherapy and the prevention of relapse among schizophrenic patients: An artifact of drug?, in *Evaluation of Psychological Therapies: Psychotherapies, Behavior Therapies, and Their Interactions* R. L. Spitzer and D. F. Klein, eds. Baltimore: Johns Hopkins University Press, 1976, pp. 285–293.

Hogarty, G. E., Schooler, N. R., Ulrich, R. F., Mussare, F., Ferro, P., and Herron, E. Fluphenazine and social therapy in the aftercare of schizophrenic patients. Relapse analyses of a two-year controlled study of fluphenazine decanoate and fluphenazine hydrochloride. *Archives of General Psychiatry* 36: 1283-1294 (1979).

Jeste, D. V. and Wyatt, R. J. Changing epidemiology of tardive dyskinesia: An overview. *American Journal of Psychiatry* 138: 297–309 (1981).

Katkin, S., Ginsburg, M., Rifkin, M. H., and Scott, J. T. Effectiveness of female volunteers with treatment of outpatients. *Journal of Counseling Psychology* 18: 97-100 (1971).

Lamb, H. R., and Goertzel, V. High expectations of long-term ex-state hospital patients. *American Journal of Psychiatry* 129: 471-475 (1972).

Langsley, D. G., Kaplan, D. M., Pittman, F. S., Machotka, P., Flomenhaft, K., and DeYoung, C. D. *The Treatment of Families in Crisis.* New York: Grune and Stratton, 1968.

Langsley, D. G., Machotka, P., and Flomenhaft, K. Family crisis therapy: Results and implications. *Family Process* 7: 145-158 (1968).

Langsley, D. G., Machotka, P., and Flomenhaft, K. Avoiding mental hospital admission: A follow-up study. *American Journal of Psychiatry* 127: 1391–1394 (1971).

Levene, H. I., Patterson, V., Murphey, B. G., Overbeck, A. L., and Veach, T. L. The aftercare of schizophrenics: An evaluation of group and individual approaches. *Psychiatric Quarterly* 44: 296–304 (1970).

Linn, M. W., Caffey, E. M., Klett, J., and Hogarty, G. Hospital vs. community (foster) care for psychiatric patients. *Archives of General Psychiatry* 34: 78-83 (1977).

Linn, M. W., Caffey, E. M., Klett, C. J., Hogarty, G. E., and Lamb, H. R. Day treatment and psychotropic drugs in the aftercare of schizophrenic patients. *Archives of General Psychiatry* 36: 1055-1072 (1979).

Linn, M. W., Klett, J., and Caffey, E. M. Foster home characteristics and psychiatric patient outcome. *Archives of General Psychiatry* 37: 129-132 (1980).

Marx, A. J., Test, M. A., and Stein, L. I. Extrahospital management of severe mental illness: Feasibility and effects of social functioning. *Archives of General Psychiatry* 29: 505-511 (1973).

May, P. R. A., and Goldberg, S. C. Predictions of schizophrenic patients' response to pharmacotherapy, in *Psychopharmacology: A Generation of Progress.* M. A. Lipton, A. DiMascio, and K. F. Killam, eds. New York: Raven Press, 1978.

May, P. R. A., Van Putten, T., Yale, C., Potepan, P., Jenden, D. J., Fairchild, M. D., Goldstein, M. J., and Dixon, W. J. Predicting individual responses to drug treatment in schizophrenia. *Journal of Nervous and Mental Diseases* 162: 177-183 (1976).

Meltzoff, J., and Blumenthal, R. L. *The Day Treatment Center: Principles Application and Evaluation.* Springfield, Ill.: C. C. Thomas, 1966.

Mosher, L. R., and Keith, S. J. Psychosocial treatment: Individual, group, family, and community support approaches. *Special Report: Schizophrenia 1980.* DHHS No. (ADM) 81-1064, 1981, pp. 127-158.

Mosher, L. R., Menn, A. Z., and Mathews, S. Sotenia: Evaluation of a home-based treatment for schizophrenia. *American Journal of Orthopsychiatry* 45: 455-469, 1975.

O'Brien, C. P., Hamm, K. B., Ray, B. A., Pierce, J. F., Luborsky, L., and Mintz, J. Group vs. individual psychotherapy with schizophrenics: A controlled outcome study. *Archives of General Psychiatry* 27: 474-478 (1972).

Pasamanick, B., Scarpitti, F. D., and Dinitz, S. *Schizophrenics in the Community: An Experimental Study in the Prevention of Hospitalization.* New York: Appleton-Century-Crofts, 1967.

Paul, G. L., and Lentz, R. J. *Psychosocial treatment of chronic mental patients: Milieu versus social-learning programs.* Cambridge, MA: Harvard University, 1977.

Polak, P. R., and Kirby, M. W. A model to replace psychiatric hospitals. *Journal of Nervous and Mental Disease* 162: 13-22 (1976).

Purvis, S. A., and Miskimins, R. W. Effects of community followup on posthospital adjustments of psychiatric patients. *Community Mental Health Journal* 6: 374-382 (1970).

Rittenhouse, J. D. Endurance of effect: Family-unit treatment compared to identified patient treatment, in *Proceedings of the Annual Convention of the American Psychological Association.* Washington, D.C.: American Psychological Association, 1970, Vol. 2, 535-536.

Ro-Trock, G. K., Wellisch, D. K., and Schoolar, J. C. A family therapy outcome study in an inpatient setting. *American Journal of Orthopsychiatry* 47: 514-522 (1977).

Shartan, S. P., Dcamp, L., Fujii, E., Fross, G. G., and Wolff, R. J. Group treatments of conditionally discharged patients in a mental health clinic. *American Journal of Psychiatry* 122: 798-805 (1966).

Sheldon, A. An evaluation of psychiatric after-care. *British Journal of Psychiatry* 110: 662-667 (1964).

Stein, L. I., and Test, M. A. An alternative to mental-hospital treatment, in *An Alternative to Mental Hospital Treatment,* L. I. Stein and M. A. Test, eds. New York: Plenum, 1978, pp. 43-55.

Stein, L. I., and Test, M. A. Alternative to mental hospital treatment: I. Conceptual model, treatment program and clinical evaluation. *Archives of General Psychiatry* 37: 392-397 (1980).

Stein, L. I., Test, M. A., and Marx, A. J. Alternative to the hospital: A controlled study. *American Journal of Psychiatry* 132: 517-522 (1975).

Van Putten, T., May, P. R. A., Marder, S. R., and Wittmann, L. A. Subjective response to antipsychotic drugs. *Archives of General Psychiatry* 38: 187-190, 1981.

Weisbrod, B. A., Test, M. A., and Stein, L. I. Alternative to mental hospital treatment. II. Economic benefit-cost analysis. *Archives of General Psychiatry* 37: 400-405 (1980).

Weisman, G., Feirstein, A., and Thomas, C. Three-day hospitalization: A model for intensive intervention. *Archives of General Psychiatry* 21: 620-629, 1969.

INDEX

I

J

K

L

M